Women's Health in Primary Care

Women's Health in Primary Care

Second Edition

Edited by

Toni Hazell

Somerset Gardens Family Healthcare Centre

Florence Britton

Royal College of Obstetricians and Gynaecologists

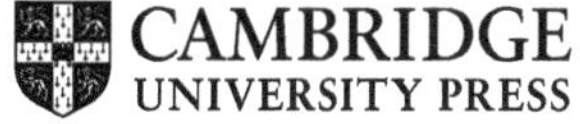

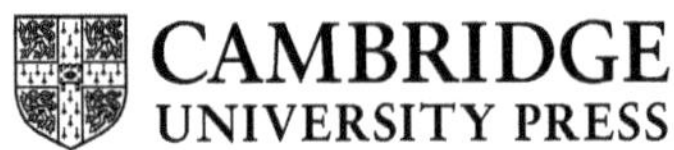

Shaftesbury Road, Cambridge CB2 8EA, United Kingdom

One Liberty Plaza, 20th Floor, New York, NY 10006, USA

477 Williamstown Road, Port Melbourne, VIC 3207, Australia

314–321, 3rd Floor, Plot 3, Splendor Forum, Jasola District Centre, New Delhi – 110025, India

Cambridge University Press is part of Cambridge University Press & Assessment, a department of the University of Cambridge.

We share the University's mission to contribute to society through the pursuit of education, learning and research at the highest international levels of excellence.

www.cambridge.org
Information on this title: www.cambridge.org/9781009492744

DOI: 10.1017/9781009492720

When citing this work, please include a reference to the DOI 10.1017/9781009492720

First published 2026

A catalogue record for this publication is available from the British Library

A Cataloging-in-Publication data record for this book is available from the Library of Congress

ISBN 978-1-009-49274-4 Paperback

Contents

Acknowledgements

We would like to acknowledge Naijia Aziz, Helen Barnes, Paula Briggs, Pam Brown, Victoria Corkhill, Christine Corrin, Sally Kidsley, Sally Louden, Robert A. Reichert, Carolyn Sadler, Tim Sayer, Judy Shakespeare, Clare Spencer and Jackie Tay for their work in authoring chapters in the previous edition.

Abbreviations

ALO	actinomyces-like organisms
ALP	alkaline phosphatase
AMH	anti-Müllerian hormone
APLS	anti-phospholipid syndrome
ARTs	anti-retroviral therapies
AUB	abnormal uterine bleeding
BASHH	British Association for Sexual Health and HIV
BCG vaccine	Bacillus Calmette–Guérin vaccine
BMD	bone mineral density
BMI	body mass index
BMS	British Menopause Society
BPS	bladder pain syndrome
BSCCP	British Society for Colposcopy and Cervical Cytology
BV	bacterial vaginosis
CAIS	complete androgen insensitivity syndrome
CBT	cognitive behavioural therapy
CFTR	cystic fibrosis transmembrane conductance regulator
CGIN	cervical glandular intraepithelial neoplasia
CHC	combined hormonal contraceptive
CIN	cervical intraepithelial neoplasia
CKD	chronic kidney disease
CNS	central nervous system
COC	combined oral contraceptive
COCP	combined oral contraceptive pill
COPD	chronic obstructive pulmonary disease
CoSRH	College of Sexual and Reproductive Healthcare
CSF	cerebrospinal fluid
Cu-IUD	copper-intrauterine device
DIC	disseminated intravascular coagulation
DMPA	depot medroxyprogesterone acetate
DPP	diabetes prevention programme
DRSP	drospirenone
DSG	desogestrel
DSM	Diagnostic and Statistical Manual of Mental Disorders
DVT	deep vein thrombosis
EC	emergency contraception
eGFR	estimated glomerular filtration rate
EOC	epithelial ovarian cancer
EPAU	early pregnancy assessment unit
ET	endometrial thickness
FAI	free androgen index
FBC	full blood count
FGM	female genital mutilation
FHA	functional hypothalamic amenorrhoea
FIGO	Federation of Gynaecology and Obstetrics
FSH	follicle-stimulating hormone
GDM	gestational diabetes mellitus
GMC	General Medical Council
GnRH	gonadotrophin-releasing hormone
GSM	genitourinary syndrome of menopause
hCG	human chorionic gonadotrophin
HCP	healthcare professional
HFI	hormone-free interval
HMB	heavy menstrual bleeding
HNPCC	hereditary non-polyposis colorectal cancer
HPO axis	hypothalamic-pituitary-ovarian axis
HPV	human papilloma virus
HRT	hormone replacement therapy
HSDD	hypoactive sexual desire disorder
IBD	inflammatory bowel disease
IC	interstitial cystitis
ICD	International Classification of Diseases
ICP	intrahepatic cholestasis of pregnancy
IBS	irritable bowel syndrome

IM	intramuscularly
IMB	intermenstrual bleeding
IUD	intrauterine device
IVF	in vitro fertilisation
LAM	lactational amenorrhoeic method
LARC	long-acting reversible method of contraception
LBC	liquid-based cytology
LH	luteinising hormone
LLETZ	loop excision of the transformation zone
LMBBS	Laurence–Moon–Bardet–Biedl syndrome
LMP	last menstrual period
LNG	levonorgestrel
LNG-IUD	levonorgestrel intrauterine device
MBL	menstrual blood loss
MDT	multi-disciplinary team
MMR	measles, mumps and rubella
MRKH	Mayer–Rokitansky–Küster–Hauser syndrome
MSU	mid-stream urine
MUI	mixed urinary incontinence
MVA	manual vacuum aspiration
NAAT	nucleic acid amplification technique
NDH	non-diabetic hyperglycaemia
NET	norethisterone
NGU	non-gonococcal urethritis
NHS	National Health Service
NHSCSP	National Cervical Screening Programme
NICE	National Institute for Health and Care Excellence
NSAID	non-steroidal anti-inflammatory drug
OAB	overactive bladder
OCD	obsessive-compulsive disorder
OCP	oral contraceptive pill
PCB	postcoital bleeding
PCOS	polycystic ovarian syndrome
PE	pulmonary embolism
PET	positron emission tomography
PFMT	pelvic floor muscle training
PGAD	persistent genital arousal disorder
PID	pelvic inflammatory disease
PMB	postmenopausal bleeding
PMD	premenstrual disorder
PMDD	premenstrual dysphoric disorder
PMI	postnatal mental illness
POI	premature ovarian insufficiency
POP	pelvic organ prolapse
POP	progestogen-only pill
PP	postnatal psychosis
PPH	postpartum haemorrhage
PPV	positive predictive value
PCR	postvoid residual
QALYs	quality-of-life years
RA	rheumatoid arthritis
RCGP	Royal College of General Practitioners
RCOG	Royal College of Obstetricians and Gynaecologists
RCT	randomised controlled trial
RMI	risk of malignancy index
ROCA	risk of ovarian cancer algorithm
SARA	sexually acquired reactive arthritis
SCJ	squamocolumnar junction
SHBG	sex hormone-binding globulin
SLE	systemic lupus erythematosus
SMM	surgical management of miscarriage
SNRIs	serotonin and norepinephrine reuptake inhibitors
SSRIs	selective serotonin reuptake inhibitors
STI	sexually transmitted infection
SUDEP	sudden unexpected death in epilepsy
SUI	stress urinary incontinence
TFT	thyroid function test
TPO	thyroid peroxidase
TSH	thyroid-stimulating hormone
TV	transvaginal
TV	*Trichomonas vaginalis*
TVUS	transvaginal ultrasound scan
TZ	transformation zone
UB	unscheduled bleeding
UI	urinary incontinence
UKHSA	UK Health Security Agency
UKMEC	UK medical eligibility criteria
UPA	ulipristal acetate
UPT	urinary pregnancy test
USI	urodynamic stress incontinence
UTI	urinary tract infection
UUI	urgency urinary incontinence
VIN	vulval intraepithelial neoplasia
VTE	venous thromboembolism risk
VVC	vulvovaginal candidiasis
VZIG	varicella immunoglobulin
WHO	World Health Organization

Chapter 1

The Physiology of the Menstrual Cycle and Its Impact on Menstrual Cycle Disorders

Practical Implications for Primary Care

Zoe Schaedel

Key Points

- The menstrual cycle is regulated by the hypothalamic-pituitary-ovarian (HPO) axis [1]; awareness of its physiology is the basis of understanding normal and abnormal menstrual bleeding.
- The International Federation of Gynaecology and Obstetrics' (FIGO's) PALM-COIEN classification system classifies nine causes of abnormal uterine bleeding (AUB) (PALM: polyp, adenomyosis, leiomyoma (uterine fibroids), malignancy and hyperplasia) and non-structural causes (COEIN: coagulopathy, ovulatory dysfunction, endometrial, iatrogenic and not otherwise classified) [2].
- In ovulatory disorders, the physiology of the normal menstrual cycle is disrupted; these are common causes of amenorrhoea, AUB and infertility [3].
- Ovulatory disorders include endocrinopathies such as polycystic ovarian syndrome (PCOS) and the anovulatory cycles that may be seen in adolescence and perimenopause [4].
- Anovulation is associated with infrequent menstruation, but bleeding when it does occur can be heavy.
- For women with uterine cavity abnormality, histological abnormality, adenomyosis or risk factors for fibroids, investigations should seek the cause of AUB prior to any treatment [5]. These may include transvaginal ultrasound, hysteroscopy and endometrial sampling.
- Progestogens are the mainstay of treatment for AUB and endometrial protection as part of hormone replacement therapy.

Case Scenario 1.1

Esme is a 47-year-old social worker with two adopted children, aged 20 and 18. She has been married for 24 years and has never used contraception, as her husband has azoospermia. She has always had irregular, infrequent periods, but over the last few years they have become heavier, with clots and flooding which keep her off work. Her last menstrual period (LMP) was six weeks ago. She has also gained weight; her body mass index (BMI) is now 41 kg/m^2. On examination, no clinical abnormality is detected.

Her haemoglobin is 90 g/L. A transvaginal ultrasound shows multiple small peripheral follicles on both ovaries, which have a polycystic pattern. It also shows an anteverted uterus with a thickened endometrium, suspicious of hyperplasia.

During the consultation Esme mentions her adopted daughter Jessica who, at age 18, is undergoing treatment for anorexia nervosa. She was having unpredictable and irregular periods since the age of 14 but has not had any menstrual bleeding for at least six months.

Hormonal Control of the Menstrual Cycle

The menstrual cycle is controlled by the HPO axis after puberty in females (Figure 1.1). It begins and ends with menstruation. The principal function of the cycle is to produce an ovum, enable its fertilisation and implantation, and allow growth and safe expulsion of the fetus. The menstrual cycle is divided by ovulation into two distinct phases: follicular and luteal. A woman's median cycle length is 28 days with most falling between 25 and 30 days; the luteal phase is around 14 days long. Real-world data from cycle tracking apps suggests there is significant variability in cycle and follicular phase length; even the luteal phase may deviate significantly from 14 days [6].

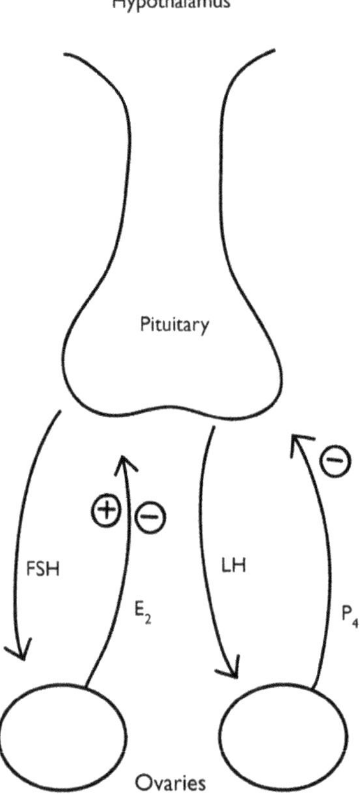

Figure 1.1 The hypothalamic-pituitary-ovarian axis. Source: Reproduced with permission from reference [1].

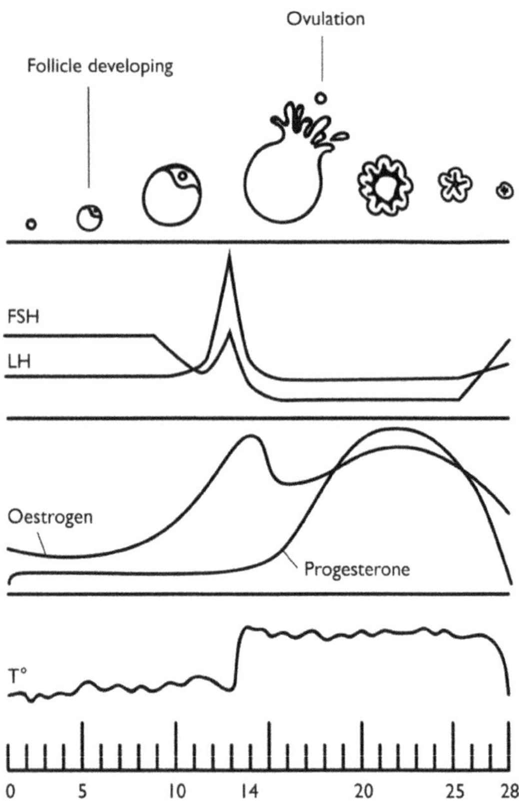

Figure 1.2 The menstrual cycle. Source: Reproduced with permission from reference [1].

The menstrual cycle may be affected by hormonal factors, ethnicity, BMI, stress and lifestyle factors. Normal functioning of the HPO axis is essential for reproductive health; the cyclical production of the hormones oestrogen and progesterone have widespread physiological effects including impacts on psychological, cardiovascular, metabolic and bone health.

Follicular Phase

Gonadotrophin-releasing hormone (GnRH) is secreted in a pulsatile manner from the hypothalamus via venous channels; it stimulates the anterior pituitary. The anterior pituitary releases two gonadotrophins, follicle-stimulating hormone (FSH) and luteinising hormone (LH), in a dose which is dependent upon the pulsatile pattern of GnRH release.

The release of FSH stimulates growth and development of the Graafian follicles in the ovary; LH is at basal levels throughout the cycle, except for the very important pre-ovulatory LH peak. At the beginning of every menstrual cycle (Figure 1.2), under the influence of rising FSH levels, a number of primordial follicles start maturing. As these follicles grow, the granulosa cells surrounding the oocyte secrete oestrogen. Oestrogen circulates throughout the body and affects many organs. It also acts on the HPO axis, suppressing FSH production via negative feedback. Only one of the developing follicles will generally continue to mature and will become the dominant follicle for ovulation.

Oestrogen secreted by the developing follicles causes the glands and stroma in the endometrium to proliferate prior to ovulation. This is also called the proliferative phase.

Ovulation

When the follicle is mature, as indicated by a critical level of oestrogen secretion, the LH peak, and a small FSH peak, are triggered from the HPO axis 24 hours before ovulation. This gives positive feedback to the ripe Graafian follicle (16–22 mm in diameter) situated on the surface of the ovary, which ruptures. The ovum is released, surrounded by cumulus cells, to be swept up by the fimbriae of the fallopian tube. The oocyte-cumulus mass travels down the fallopian tube, where it may be fertilised by spermatozoa.

Luteal Phase

Following ovulation, the remains of the follicle on the surface of the ovary forms the corpus luteum (yellow body). The colour is due to deposition of carotene in the theca cells. The corpus luteum secretes progesterone in addition to oestrogen. These two hormones in combination are responsible for the development of many tortuous endometrial glands, with cells rich in glycogen (secretory endometrium). This is also referred to as the secretory phase of the menstrual cycle. Physiologists divide the menstrual cycle into *follicular and luteal phases* and histologists refer to *proliferative and secretory phases*. The terms are interchangeable.

If conception does not occur, the corpus luteum disintegrates, oestrogen and progesterone levels fall, and the endometrium sloughs off (menstruation).

The menstrual cycle can be used to indicate whether ovulation is occurring. Regular menstrual cycles suggest ovulation; an absence of menstruation suggests the absence of ovulation or follicular development. Bleeding can, however, occur without ovulation, as follicles can develop independently. During follicular growth, oestrogen is secreted, which results in endometrial proliferation. When the follicle fails to ovulate and ceases to develop, oestrogen levels fall, resulting in endometrial shedding which is distinct from the menstrual cycle as described above.

In the absence of pregnancy, the corpus luteum has an inherent lifespan of 12–14 days.

If the oocyte is fertilised in the fallopian tube, the early embryo secretes beta human chorionic gonadotrophin (beta HCG) within days, maintaining the corpus luteum, which continues to secrete progesterone and oestrogen until the placenta takes over at seven to nine weeks gestation.

Bioassays of the Menstrual Cycle: Mucus and Temperature Changes

Mucus Changes

The quantity and quality of cervical mucus are dependent upon its salt and water content, which is regulated by the relative systemic levels of oestrogen and progesterone.

Oestrogen has the effect of stimulating copious amounts of watery/slippery mucus, which is described as being similar to egg white. The effect of progesterone, after ovulation, is to rapidly change the mucus into a 'gluey' consistency. In the days after menstruation, a woman will have low levels of oestrogen and little mucus is secreted. In the mid-follicular phase, as oestrogen rises, there is a corresponding increase in watery/slippery mucus. Just prior to ovulation there is a maximal level of unopposed oestrogen, with a corresponding increase in slippery mucus. This enhances the passage of sperm if sexual intercourse takes place in this fertile phase [7]. As soon as ovulation occurs and progesterone is secreted, the mucus changes to a 'gluey' consistency, impermeable to sperm. These physiological changes act as a bioassay to pinpoint various stages of the menstrual cycle and are the basis for natural family planning using the Billings method [8].

Basal Body Temperature

The effect of progesterone secreted in the luteal phase is to elevate body temperature. If a woman's temperature is measured on waking each morning (basal body temperature), and in the presence of ovulation, it will increase by approximately 0.5°C during the luteal phase. This can also be used retrospectively as a bioassay to determine the timing of ovulation and the efficiency of the luteal phase.

Esme's case history illustrates two common pathologies relating to a disturbance of normal menstrual physiology: PCOS and perimenopausal AUB.

Polycystic Ovaries/Polycystic Ovary Syndrome

This is the commonest endocrine condition to affect women and is complex, with multisystem repercussions. The diagnostic criteria are discussed in Chapter 14 of this book – they include hyperandrogenism. Weight gain increases the risk of PCOS due to decreased sex hormone-binding globulin (SHBG) levels, resulting in increased circulating free androgens, causing hirsutism and acne. Obesity also causes insulin resistance, which augments hyperandrogenism. Many women with irregular menstruation are likely to have PCOS [9,10].

Esme has typical symptoms of PCOS, with irregular cycles due to irregular and sporadic ovulation. Fertility interventions such as clomifene citrate or FSH injections could have been considered should she have wished for a pregnancy with donor sperm.

In women with PCOS and infrequent ovulation, there are long periods of unopposed oestrogen secretion due to the small follicles which produce oestrogen. In the absence of ovulation and without a corpus luteum forming, there is no progesterone produced to induce the secretory change in the endometrium, nor is there regular endometrial shedding. Consequently, the endometrium becomes hyperplastic, sometimes developing atypical changes, a precursor to endometrial cancer.

Obesity is associated with an increase in conversion of cholesterol to oestrogen and, in addition to the changes to the menstrual cycle, is an additional risk factor for endometrial cancer. Esme's BMI amplifies other risks, including potential insulin resistance predisposing to type 2 diabetes mellitus.

Esme has a number of risk factors for endometrial cancer, including obesity, nulliparity and having PCOS with infrequent ovulation and menstruation. As well as management of her PCOS (discussed in Chapter 14), she should be offered endometrial sampling to exclude cancer. Treatment options include progestogen to reduce endometrial hyperplasia, which will have the added benefit of reducing heavy menstrual bleeding (HMB). The most effective route of administration is a levonorgestrel intrauterine device, as this delivers the progestogen directly to the endometrium. Alternative options include oral progestogens.

Perimenopausal Heavy Menstrual Bleeding

Esme's HMB is likely to be exacerbated by the perimenopause. As women approach the menopause, anovulatory cycles become more common and, in the absence of progesterone secretion, the endometrium proliferates without secretory change or regular shedding. Unopposed oestrogen therefore has a similar effect to that seen in women with PCOS.

Progesterone, Progestogens and Progestins

There is sometimes confusion in the terminology used to describe progestogens. A progestogen is any hormone with progesterone-like activity on the endometrium, meaning that it induces secretory change. Following ovulation, the ovary secretes natural progesterone, which has unique pharmacodynamic activity and a unique safety profile compared to synthetically produced progesterone-like hormones, such as those found in oral contraceptives, which are called progestins. The function of progestins depends on their binding to a variety of nuclear receptors, and they may have different or even opposite effects to each other.

Esme's daughter Jessica is experiencing amenorrhoea which may be due to abnormal signalling between the hypothalamus and pituitary gland, resulting from her anorexia nervosa, leading to anovulation.

Hypothalamic Amenorrhoea

Deficient secretion of GnRH leads to insufficient LH and FSH levels to maintain full folliculogenesis and normal ovulatory ovarian function, with consequent oestrogen deficiency. This accounts for 30% of cases of secondary amenorrhoea. Functional hypothalamic amenorrhoea (FHA) is where there is no structural lesion present; it is commonly unrecognized. FHA is predominantly caused by signific weight loss or intense exercise, leading to a relative energy deficit or other factors such as stress or chronic illness. Presentation is usually with menstrual disturbance or infertility. Treatment is crucial to avoid long-term consequences such as infertility and osteoporosis, in addition to reducing psychological morbidity. Initial management is focused on resolving the precipitating cause (such as low weight, excessive exercise or stress). If symptoms are prolonged, other treatments involve hormone replacement, ovulation induction or assisted reproduction in those seeking pregnancy. Hormone replacement requires both oestrogen and a progestogen in order to preserve bone mass and prevent endometrial hyperplasia.

References

[1] G. Kovacs and P. Briggs, 'Basic physiology: The menstrual cycle'. In *Lectures in Obstetrics, Gynaecology and Women's Health*, Springer, 2015, pp. 3–7.

[2] M. G. Munro, H. O. Critchley, M. S. Broder et al., FIGO Working Group on Menstrual Disorders, 'FIGO classification system (PALM-COEIN) for causes of abnormal uterine bleeding in nongravid women of reproductive age', *Int J Gynaecol Obstet*, vol. **113**, no. 1, pp. 3–13, 2011.

[3] M. G. Munro, A. H. Balen, S. Cho et al., ‘The FIGO ovulatory disorders classification system’, *Hum Reprod*, vol. **37**, no. 10, pp. 2446–2464, 2022.

[4] R. MacGregor, V. Jain, S. Hillman et al., ‘Investigating abnormal uterine bleeding in reproductive aged women’, *BMJ*, vol. **378**, e070906, 2022.

[5] NICE/NG88, ‘Heavy menstrual bleeding: Assessment and management’. May 2021. Accessed: 29 Apr. 2024. [Online]. Available: www.nice.org.uk/guidance/ng88.

[6] J. R. Bull, S. P. Rowland, E. B. Scherwitzl et al., ‘Real-world menstrual cycle characteristics of more than 600,000 menstrual cycles’, *NPJ Digital Medicine*, vol. **2**, no. 1, 83, 2019.

[7] E. L. Billings, J. B. Brown, J. J. Billings et al., ‘Symptoms and hormonal changes accompanying ovulation’, *Lancet*, vol. **1**, pp. 282–284, 1972.

[8] K. Betts, ‘The Billings method of family planning: An assessment’, *Stud Fam Plann*, vol. **15**, no. 6, pp. 253–266, 1984.

[9] The Rotterdam ESHRE/ASRM-Sponsored PCOS Consensus Workshop Group, ‘Revised 2003 consensus on diagnostic criteria and long-term health risks related to polycystic ovary syndrome (PCOS)’, *Hum Reprod*, vol. **19**, pp. 41–47, 2003.

[10] R. S. Legro, M. E. Lujan, M. Costello and A. Dokras, ‘International, evidence-based guideline for the assessment and management of polycystic ovary syndrome 2023’. In *ASRM 2023 Scientific Congress & Expo*, 17 Oct., ASRM, 2023.

[11] W. C. Duncan, ‘A guide to understanding polycystic ovary syndrome (PCOS)’, *J Fam Plann Reprod Health Care*, vol. **40**, pp. 217–225, 2014.

[12] R. E. Roberts, L. Farahani, L. Webber et al., ‘Current understanding of hypothalamic amenorrhoea’, *Ther Adv Endocrinol Metab*, vol. **11**, 2042018820945854, 2020.

[13] J. C. Stevenson, S. Rozenberg, S. Maffei et al., ‘Progestogens as a component of menopausal hormone therapy: The right molecule makes the difference’, *Drugs in Context*, vol. **9**, 2020.

Chapter

2 Management of Children and Adolescents with Gynaecological Problems in Primary Care

Jane Dickson and Nana Anim-Addo

Key Points

- Vaginal discharge is the most common complaint in prepubertal girls and is often a symptom of vulvovaginitis.
- Examination under anaesthetic is indicated for blood-stained vaginal discharge in children.
- Safeguarding processes should be implemented if there is any suspicion of sexual abuse; for example, diagnosis of sexually transmitted infection.
- Vaginal examinations are rarely necessary for menstrual symptoms in adolescents.
- Treatment of precocious puberty and primary amenorrhoea/delayed puberty should be undertaken by a specialist, such as a paediatric endocrinologist/adolescent gynaecologist.
- Pregnancy may be the cause of menstrual dysfunction and a thoughtful enquiry should be made about sexual activity.
- Gynaecological symptoms may be 'functional'; that is, presentation for other causes of anxiety such as abuse or bullying.
- Dysmenorrhoea in adolescents may be the first presenting sign of endometriosis.
- A risk assessment must be undertaken in sexually active young people.
- Female genital mutilation must be reported to the police in an under 18-year-old girl.

Box 2.1: Vaginal Discharge

Vaginal discharge is the most common gynaecological complaint for a prepubertal girl (see Table 2.1). Non-specific bacterial vulvovaginitis is the most frequent cause of symptoms and may be very distressing, particularly if recurrent. Itching and soreness may be associated with discharge and are commonly empirically treated as thrush, although candida is an uncommon cause [1, 2, 3]. Prepubertal girls are predisposed to vaginal discharge because:

- the anus is anatomically very close to the vagina, predisposing to cross-contamination of flora
- the vulval and vaginal skin is thin and atrophic due to low prepubertal oestrogen levels
- neutral vaginal pH predisposes to infectious colonisation. An acidic pH provides microcidal protection.

Although often challenging to obtain, a good history from both parent and child is highly advantageous in narrowing down a cause. A large proportion of cases can often be treated with improved hygiene alone. An additional benefit of involving young children in their consultation is building trust, understanding and rapport ahead of physical examination. Examination needs to be done sensitively and gently; it can often be a frightening experience for a young child. The child should either be sitting on a parent's lap or on a couch in a 'frog-leg' position. The labia should be gently parted enough to visualize the introitus and a swab can be taken from the posterior fourchette (the smallest swab available should be used). If examination would cause too much distress, there is bloody discharge or a foreign body is suspected, then referral should be made to secondary care for vaginoscopy under general anaesthetic.

In vulvovaginitis, the discharge may be clear, yellow, green and malodorous and there may be accompanying itch, soreness or dysuria; rarely there is associated vaginal bleeding. If bleeding is present, other more serious conditions must be excluded, such as sexual abuse, foreign body, tumours and precocious puberty. Non-specific mixed bacterial vulvovaginitis is the commonest cause of discharge and this may relate to poor hygiene, particularly contamination from the anus on wiping. Treatment of this and other bacterial causes is with an antibiotic to which the organism(s) is sensitive. Candida is a rare cause of prepubertal discharge, unless there is

Table 2.1 Causes of vaginal discharge in girls

Hormonal	Oestrogen related, e.g. newborn female
Bacterial	Non-specific mixed vaginal flora, e.g. anaerobes, coliforms, staphylococci Group A beta-haemolytic streptococci *Haemophilus influenzae* Shigella
Viral	Varicella Measles Rubella
Fungal	Candida
Other infections	Threadworms Sexually transmitted infections, e.g. chlamydia, gonorrhoea, trichomoniasis
Foreign bodies	E.g. paper, coins, small toys
Vulval dermatitis	Soap Bubble bath Sand Prolonged contact of urine/faeces with skin Irritants, e.g. perfume, dye, detergents
Structural problems	Labial adhesions Vaginal agenesis Urethral prolapse Ectopic ureter
Vaginal tumours	Embryonal rhabdomyosarcoma Mesonephric carcinoma Clear-cell adenocarcinoma

a precipitating factor such as wearing nappies, antibiotics or diabetes mellitus; moreover, associations have been suggested with sexual abuse [3]. If the symptom is predominantly itch, especially at night, a diagnosis of threadworms should be considered. History may be enough to lead to the diagnosis; otherwise a 'sticky tape test' can be performed by pressing sticky tape over the anus which may identify worms or eggs.

Vulval skin conditions may rarely present with discharge – itch and soreness are more usual features. Atopic eczema and lichen sclerosis may be present in children and the management of these conditions would include emollients and topical steroids.

Management of Vulvovaginitis and Vaginal Discharge

- Antibiotics can be used when a specific pathogen is identified.
- Mebendazole is the treatment of choice if threadworms are identified.
- If there is a sexually transmitted organism present or there is any suspicion of abuse, then safeguarding procedures should be implemented immediately.
- Simple hygiene, such as front-to-back wiping. The British Association of Dermatology has a very good patient information leaflet – 'Vulvitis in Childhood' [4].
- Avoid perfumed soap, bubble bath, lotions and shampoo.
- Emollients such as Hydromol ointment may be helpful.
- Loose-fitting cotton underwear and no pants at night.
- Avoid constipation, soiling and bedwetting.
- Examination under anaesthetic for unexplained vaginal bleeding or suspicion of a retained foreign body.

Case Scenario 2.1: Ellie

Ellie is a happy and chatty child. On direct questioning she says that her 'front bottom' is sore. Her mother has noticed yellow discharge for about a week. On examination, in 'frog-leg' position, she has vulval erythema and yellow discharge. A swab shows mixed organisms including coliforms. Treatment would be with a broad-spectrum antibiotic with advice about appropriate vulval hygiene and front-to-back wiping.

Puberty and Amenorrhoea

Case Scenario 2.2: Charlotte

Charlotte is a 15-year-old who has not yet had a period. She has small breasts and no pubic hair. She has not been sexually active. She is very clever and is thriving at school.

Normal Puberty and Menarche

Normal puberty follows a very set pattern, as it depends on activation of the hypothalamic-pituitary-gonadal (HPG) axis, which initiates a cascade of changes. The foundation of the information we have on pubertal development in young girls was gathered from a longitudinal study by Marshall and Tanner published in 1969, looking at white British girls of the Harpenden Growth Study [5]. From this information, the Tanner stages, also known as the Sexual Maturity Mating, were developed (Table 2.2 and Figure 2.1) [2].

Normally breast development begins at around age 10, followed by pubic hair 6 months later. There is then an increase in height. Tanner stage 4 pubic hair and stage 3–4 breast development occurs, and these usually immediately precede menstruation. Menstruation is closely related to bone age and the average age for menarche is between 12 and 13 years. Girls of African origin have an earlier average age of menarche; this is proposedly due to higher insulin responses to glucose and subsequently higher levels of IGF1 which accelerates development [6].

Table 2.2 Tanner staging

Stage	Pubic hair	Breast development
1.	Prepuberty	Prepuberty
2.	Narrow border along the labia majora	Small mound and areola start to grow
3.	Becoming darker and curlier – spreading to mons	Further increase and loss of contour of separation between breast and areola
4.	Increasing, but still just at mons	Areola and nipple form secondary mound
5.	Spreads to adult female triangle pattern	Adult breast appearance

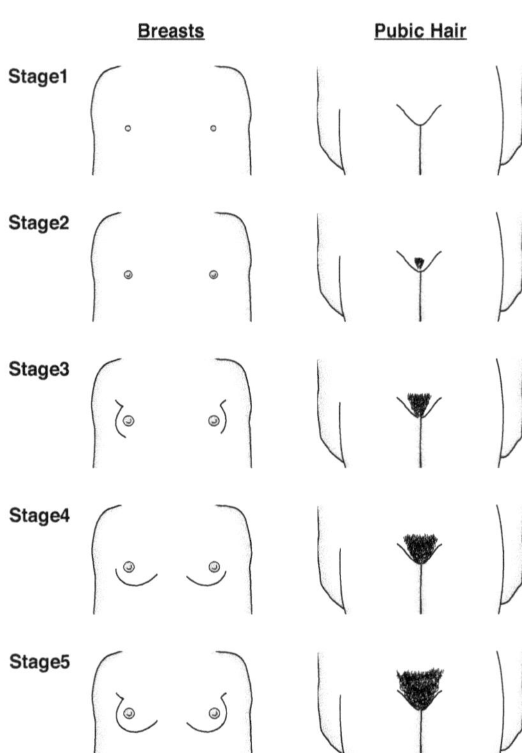

Figure 2.1 Tanner staging of puberty.

Factors which influence the timing of puberty and menstruation include:

- genetic factors
- nutrition
- exercise
- general health
- racial differences.

Amenorrhoea

Amenorrhoea is the absence of periods. It is *primary* amenorrhoea if there have never been any periods and *secondary* amenorrhoea if periods were present but have stopped for three cycles or for six or more months in the absence of pregnancy. See Table 2.4 for investigations for amenorrhoea in primary care.

Primary Amenorrhoea

Primary amenorrhoea with the absence of development of secondary sexual characteristics should be investigated at 13 years old. In the presence of secondary sexual characteristics, it should be investigated at 15 years old (Table 2.3) [7].

Constitutional Delay

Constitutional delay is often familial and occurs when bone age is less than chronological age. Menstruation will occur when bone age catches up with chronological age. Patients should be followed up and careful consideration should be given to the social consequences of this problem, such as difficulties with peers.

Chronic Disease

Any systemic disease can impair development and delay menstruation. Treatment of the disease will usually resolve the situation. Conditions associated include diabetes mellitus, hypothyroidism, chronic renal disease, cystic fibrosis, congenital cardiac disease, coeliac disease and Crohn's.

Table 2.3 Causes of primary amenorrhoea [7,8]

Constitutional	Constitutional delay
Systemic	• Chronic disease, e.g. cystic fibrosis, Crohn's, cardiac disease • Weight loss • Endocrine, e.g. thyroid disease
Hypothalamic-pituitary dysfunction	• Hypothalamic (hypogonadotropic hypogonadism), e.g. intense exercise, idiopathic, anorexia nervosa • Intracranial pathology, e.g. brain tumours, head injury, hydrocephalus • Pituitary, e.g. hypopituitarism, hyperprolactinaemia • Laurence–Moon–Bardet–Biedl syndrome (LMBBS) • Prader–Willi syndrome • Kallman syndrome
Gonadal dysfunction	• Premature ovarian failure • Turner syndrome • Gonadal dysgenesis, e.g. Swyer syndrome • Polycystic ovarian syndrome
Anatomical abnormalities	• Müllerian agenesis, e.g. Rokitansky syndrome • Complete androgen insensitivity syndrome • Absent or imperforate vagina

Table 2.4 Investigations for amenorrhoea in primary care

Clinical examination	Body mass index Pubertal staging Indications of endocrine disease, e.g. hirsutism Signs of Turner syndrome
Investigations	Pregnancy test Follicle-stimulating hormone, luteinising hormone, oestradiol Prolactin Thyroid function tests Testosterone Sex hormone binding globulin Karyotype

Hypothalamic-Pituitary Dysfunction

The commonest hypothalamic-pituitary causes are idiopathic or related to extreme exercise/weight loss. Conditions that compress the pituitary or hypothalamus will lead to reduced LH and FSH production, and may produce symptoms such as galactorrhoea, headaches and visual disturbances. Some rare syndromes, which may lead to dysfunction, include:

- Laurence–Moon–Bardet–Biedel – autosomal recessive condition associated with obesity, retinitis pigmentosa, learning disability, polydactyly and hypogonadism.
- Prader–Willi – a loss of function genetic disorder of chromosome 15 resulting in hypotonia, learning disability, characteristic facies, polyphagia and obesity.
- Kallmann – hypogonadotropic hypogonadism genetic disorder which results in agenesis of olfactory bulbs and anatomical defects of the hypothalamus, which leads to anosmia and lack of secondary sexual development.

Ovarian Dysfunction and Failure

Ovarian dysfunction may present as primary or secondary amenorrhoea. Premature ovarian failure is an extremely distressing diagnosis as it confers loss of fertility.

Causes of Premature Ovarian Failure

- idiopathic
- chemotherapy
- radiotherapy
- metabolic disease, such as galactosaemia
- autoimmune conditions, such as Addison's disease
- infections, such as mumps
- chromosomal anomalies, such as Turner syndrome.

Turner Syndrome

The premature ovarian failure associated with Turner syndrome relates to gonadal dysgenesis. Turner syndrome occurs in 1 in 2,000–3,000 live female births and is related either to the classic karyotype 45X0 or a mosaic form such as 45X/46XX or 45X/46XY. The ovaries have a 'streak' appearance – it is thought that normal numbers of oocytes develop until the fifth month in utero, but they then degenerate rapidly so that very few are present by birth. Spontaneous menstruation may occur, especially when there is mosaicism, but premature ovarian failure usually results. With early diagnosis and karyotyping, fertility preservation may be an option; 2% of women with Turner syndrome conceive spontaneously.

The physical appearance of those with Turner syndrome may vary markedly, but there are typical features more generally associated with the X0 karyotype. Those features may include:

- short stature
- webbing of the neck
- cubitus valgus
- lymphoedema of hands or feet
- widely spaced nipples
- cardiac or renal abnormalities
- coarctation of the aorta
- autoimmune hypothyroidism.

Diagnosis may be made in infancy if there are typical features or as a result of investigation of short stature in childhood. Amenorrhoea is often the presentation in adolescence. Levels of LH and FSH are high and oestradiol levels low. Chromosomal analysis should be performed. Presence of a Y chromosome fragment means that the gonads should be removed because there is a risk of malignancy.

Swyer Syndrome

Swyer syndrome is 46XY gonadal dysgenesis. It is due to a gene mutation, usually of the SRY gene. The external physical appearance is often of a tall female. There is no testosterone so the internal female genitalia develop, but there are intra-abdominal dysgenetic testes present rather than ovaries. These testes have up to a 40% chance of malignancy so should be removed as soon as the condition is discovered. As in Turner syndrome, the FSH and LH levels are high. Because a uterus is present, childbearing may be possible with egg donation and fertility treatment.

Anatomical Abnormalities

Anatomical abnormalities may account for primary amenorrhoea when secondary sexual characteristics are present. The uterus may be absent when the Müllerian duct has failed to develop, such as is the case in complete androgen insensitivity syndrome and Mayer–Rokitansky–Küster–Hauser syndrome. Absent or imperforate vagina may also present as primary amenorrhoea but is actually cryptomenorrhoea (i.e. menstruation is occurring but not being seen, *kryptós* being the Greek for hidden).

Complete Androgen Insensitivity Syndrome (CAIS)

In CAIS a child has the karyotype 46XY and is phenotypically female. It is an X-linked recessive condition. Puberty is often delayed with normal breast development but sparse pubic and axillary hair, and they may be taller than average. In utero, there are normal testes producing testosterone and Müllerian inhibitory factor. This means that the structures derived from the Müllerian duct – that is, the uterus and upper vagina – degenerate and so are absent, but normal external female genitalia develop.

Diagnosis may be made in infancy due to the presence of gonads in the inguinal area or later as a consequence of primary amenorrhoea. Investigation will reveal normal LH and FSH levels, high testosterone and low oestradiol. Some testosterone is aromatized into oestradiol, notably by adipose tissue, the presence of which allows breast development. Treatment involves gonadectomy as the intra-abdominal testes have a higher malignancy potential (best performed after puberty to allow for normal breast development), vaginal reconstruction surgery and long-term oestrogen replacement therapy.

Mayer–Rokitansky–Küster–Hauser Syndrome (MRKH)

This syndrome occurs in 1 in 5,000 female births and there is a 46XX genotype and normal female appearance. There is failure of development of the Müllerian duct, which means there is no uterus or upper vagina, but normal ovaries are present. There is usually a short blind-ending vagina and 30–40% of cases have associated urinary abnormalities such as renal agenesis, ectopic or horseshoe kidney and abnormal collecting ducts [7]. Levels of LH, FSH and oestradiol will all be normal.

The most important aspects of treatment are psychological support and the creation of a vagina so that penetrative sexual intercourse may be achieved. This would initially be with vaginal dilators, but surgical treatment may be necessary where this fails. It is feasible for these women to have their own genetic children using their ova and a surrogate mother. However, this can be quite a challenging process emotionally, physically and financially. The surrogate will be the child's legal parent at birth and any prior surrogacy agreement is not enforceable by UK law.

Cryptomenorrhoea

There is cyclical pain in association with amenorrhoea and this is due to an obstruction, usually in the vagina. The commonest cause for this is an imperforate hymen – there may be an abdominal mass with pressure symptoms, such as urinary retention. A blue bulging membrane can be seen on parting the labia. This is treated with a simple incision. Other rare causes include a transverse vaginal septum and cervical agenesis.

Treatment of Delayed Puberty/Menarche

Treatment is best undertaken by a specialist such as a paediatric endocrinologist or adolescent gynaecologist. Usually very low-dose oestrogen is given initially. Later, treatment will usually involve either combined hormonal contraception (CHC) (as hormone replacement) or conventional hormone replacement therapy.

Secondary Amenorrhoea

Secondary amenorrhoea may occur in adolescents and the most likely causes are:

- pregnancy
- polycystic ovarian syndrome
- premature ovarian failure
- pituitary disorders
- hypothalamic disorders.

Polycystic Ovarian Syndrome (PCOS)

PCOS (see Chapter 14) is classically related to obesity and there may be signs of raised androgens presenting as acne or hirsutism. There may be oligomenorrhoea or secondary amenorrhoea (very rarely primary amenorrhoea). Initial management is with weight loss and exercise. CHC is often very effective. CHC causes sex hormone binding globulin levels to increase and this 'mops up' androgens. This leads to cycle regulation and reduction in androgen-related side effects. Any CHC may be used, such as pills, patch or vaginal ring, but some preparations may be particularly helpful. A drospirenone-containing combined pill such as Yasmin®, Yiznell® or Lucette® may be more beneficial due to the anti-androgen effects of drospirenone. It is important to remember these preparations confer a slightly higher VTE risk of 9–12 compared to 5–7 incidence per 10,000. Co-cyprindiol-containing preparation is also of benefit as cyproterone is an anti-androgen. First-line use is not recommended due to adverse side effects including VTE risk [9]. PCOS is linked with insulin resistance and metformin may have a beneficial effect on menstrual regulation, but this would be part of specialist rather than primary care management [8,10].

Precocious Puberty

This is puberty occurring before the age of eight in girls and nine in boys. In 74% of cases in girls it is idiopathic. It may be gonadotrophin dependent; that is, when the HPG axis is prematurely activated. It may also be gonadotrophin independent, where there are raised sex steroids, such as congenital adrenal hyperplasia, adrenal or ovarian tumours or McCune–Albright syndrome [2,7].

Adrenarche marks the onset of the adrenal glands secreting sex hormones. In premature adrenarche there is an isolated raised androgen level leading to pubic hair, body odour and acne. It is important to rule out other causes of raised androgens, such as congenital adrenal hyperplasia or a virilizing tumour, but otherwise it does not cause long-term problems. It may be related to insulin resistance and a later development of PCOS. In either case, these children should be referred to a paediatric endocrinologist for further investigations and management.

Case Scenario 2.3: Charlotte

Charlotte needs to be investigated as she has primary amenorrhoea and is 15 years old. She has a normal body mass index and minimal androgen-dependent secondary sexual characteristics, such as pubic and axillary hair. Investigations show her to have a very high testosterone level and normal LH and FSH levels. Her chromosomes demonstrate a 46XY pattern and she has no internal female genitalia on ultrasound scan. She has a diagnosis of complete androgen insufficiency syndrome and treatment will involve psychological support, gonadectomy, oestrogen replacement therapy, self-dilation therapy or surgical vaginoplasty, if desired.

Menstrual Dysfunction

Case Scenario 2.4: Safia

Safia is 14 years old. Her periods began when she was 11. She has extremely painful periods, which are often associated with diarrhoea. She misses at least two days of school every month because of her pain.

Heavy Menstrual Bleeding

Heavy or painful menstruation is the commonest reason for an adolescent to be referred to a gynaecologist. Adolescents may have irregular cycles for the first four years following menarche. Cycles in this situation are often anovulatory, which results in heavy dysfunctional bleeding – the endometrium becomes thick and unstable under the influence of unopposed oestrogen. Girls with regular periods are more likely to be ovulating; increased fibrinolysis and prostaglandins are thought to be responsible for heavy bleeding in these situations.

Approximately 1 in 10 adolescent girls will require treatment for heavy menstrual bleeding. Despite the fact that different management options may be preferred, the National Institute for Health and Care Excellence (NICE) heavy menstrual bleeding guidance still applies [11]. Initial assessment should include a full blood count and when simple treatment is not effective, consider conditions such as Von Willebrand disease and idiopathic thrombocytopenic purpura. Vaginal examination is not usually required if there are no related symptoms, as it is unlikely to add value to the assessment.

Periods may present additional problems to young women with learning disabilities as there may be problems related to the use of sanitary wear, such as soiling and cyclical behavioural problems. Also, if epileptic, seizures may heighten either premenstrually or during periods. In these situations, menstrual control may be even more important to quality of life.

Treatment Options

- The Mirena® intrauterine system is the first-line treatment, but this may not be practical in young women who have never been sexually active. The uterine cavity length needs to be at least 6 cm. In young woman with special needs, insertion could be considered under general anaesthetic [12]. The Kyleena® intrauterine device is smaller, lasts for five years and is not currently licensed for the management of heavy menstrual bleeding, but may well have some benefits in this area.
- Antifibrinolytics, such as tranexamic acid 1 g tds, are helpful to reduce menstrual flow. These may be used in conjunction with non-steroidal anti-inflammatory drugs, such as ibuprofen 400 mg tds or mefenamic acid 500 mg tds, which are also helpful in reducing menstrual pain because of anti-prostaglandin action.
- CHC is a safe treatment option provided there are no absolute contraindications, such as thrombophilia. Options include the combined oral contraceptive pill and the combined contraceptive patch such as Evra®. The patch is particularly useful for young women with learning disabilities as it can be placed on parts of the body where it is difficult to remove, such as the shoulder. CHC can be used either cyclically or continuously in a tailored manner. This means using pills or patches continuously and taking a break of four to seven days when there have been three consecutive days of breakthrough bleeding.
- Continuous progestogens such as Desogestrel should be a first-line option for heavy menstrual bleeding where COC is not wanted or contraindicated [13], and intrauterine contraception is not accepted.
- Progestogen-containing injectables may be considered in this group, such as Depo-Provera® or Sayana Press®. These are given every 13 weeks and have a high likelihood of resulting in amenorrhoea. However, careful consideration needs to be given before use because of potential risk to bone mineral density in those who have not achieved peak bone mass. When there are considerable risk factors for osteoporosis, such as immobility, oral steroid uses, nicotine use or low body mass index, progestogen-containing injectables are best avoided.
- The progestogen-containing contraceptive implant Nexplanon® may sometimes be tried, but bleeding irregularity is a very common side effect.
- Cyclical progestogen, such as norethisterone 5 mg tds given 21 days each cycle (D5–26), is an option, but may cause considerable androgenic side effects, such as acne or hirsutism.

Norethisterone should be used with caution as a small proportion of the drug is aromatised to Ethinylestradiol. Therefore when prescribing therapeutic norethisterone it should be seen as a combination-like product with the same associated VTE risks. For those with high VTE risk, medroxyprogesterone 10 mg tds is a safer choice [14].

Dysmenorrhoea

Menstrual pain may be disabling in adolescents and is more usually associated with ovulatory rather than anovulatory cycles. It often develops 6–12 months after the onset of menstruation and is known as primary dysmenorrhoea as it is not related to pathology. Prostaglandins are responsible, causing uterine spasms and other related symptoms, such as diarrhoea and pain radiating to thighs and nausea. Non-steroidal anti-inflammatory agents, such as ibuprofen 400 mg or mefenamic acid 500 mg tds, are helpful for this type of pain. Alternatively, some of the agents used for heavy menstrual bleeding, such as CHC, may be useful.

In adolescents, where pain does not resolve with simple measures, pathology should be considered. Endometriosis is the commonest cause of secondary dysmenorrhoea. It has been estimated that it may be responsible for chronic pelvic pain in as many as 73% of adolescents, where pain is unresponsive to treatment. In these situations, laparoscopy may be necessary: endometriosis may be seen as clear or white foci rather than the typical brown lesions of older women, but treatment options are the same for both groups.

Rarely, dysmenorrhoea may be caused by anatomical anomalies. If menstrual flow is partly obstructed, accumulated blood may cause pain; the treatment of this would be surgical.

Adolescent girls may be sexually active, so enquiry into this needs to be sensitively explored and is often best done in the absence of the parent. Both pregnancy and sexually transmitted infections can result in problems with pain and bleeding. Untreated sexually transmitted infections can progress to pelvic inflammatory disease; this should be treated as soon as suspected to avoid long-term complications such as adhesions, chronic pelvic pain and infertility.

Case Scenario 2.5: Safia

Safia's periods have been heavy and painful since they became regular. She has no problems when she is not menstruating and has never been sexually active. She has no other symptoms of note and has no family history of bleeding problems. The most likely problem is primary dysmenorrhoea. She does not require other investigation initially and treatment options include mefenamic acid and CHC.

Legal and Ethical Issues

Sexual Abuse

Sexual abuse should be considered in many gynaecological presentations, such as genital soreness, genitourinary injuries, vaginal discharge, recurrent dysuria, sexually transmitted infections and pregnancy. Additionally, there are non-gynaecological symptoms where abuse should be considered, such as faecal soiling, rectal bleeding, enuresis and generalised abdominal pain. A young person's behaviour may change to indicate distress or anxiety; for example, self-harm, an eating disorder or there may be inappropriate sexualised behaviour when abuse has occurred. Where there are any concerns, local safeguarding processes must be implemented expediently.

Consent and Child Sexual Exploitation

Approximately 30% of young people have sexual intercourse before the age of 16. Many relationships are healthy and consensual; nonetheless, a risk assessment should be undertaken to ensure that there is no child sexual exploitation. Firstly, there should be assessment of competency (Fraser guidelines relate specifically to sexual and reproductive health, for example contraception, STIs and abortion, whereas Gillick competence applies to wider aspects of medical care and consent).

Child sexual exploitation is a complex form of abuse and it can be difficult for those working with children to identify and assess. The indicators for child sexual exploitation can sometimes be mistaken for 'normal adolescent behaviours'. It requires knowledge, skills, professional curiosity and an assessment which analyses the risk factors and personal circumstances of individual children to ensure that the signs and symptoms are interpreted correctly and appropriate support is given. Even where a young person is old enough to legally consent to sexual activity, the law states that consent is only valid where they make a choice and have the freedom and capacity to make that choice. If a child feels they have no other meaningful choice, are under the influence of harmful substances or are fearful of what might happen if they don't comply (all of which are common features in cases of child sexual exploitation), consent cannot legally be given, whatever the age [15,16].

Risk factors include vulnerabilities, such as learning or physical disability, living in care, mental health problems, addictions of child or parents, lack of support networks and past history of abuse or exploitation. The Child Sexual Exploitation Risk Questionnaire (CSERQ4) (Table 2.5) has been developed by the National Safeguarding Team of NHS

Table 2.5 Child Sexual Exploitation Risk Questionnaire (CSERQ4)

		Yes	No
1	Have you ever stayed out overnight or longer without permission from your parent(s) or guardian?		
2	How old is your boyfriend/girlfriend or the person(s) you have sex with? Age of partner ______ Age of client/patient ______ Age difference ______ If age difference is 4 or more years then tick 'YES'		
3	Does your boyfriend/girlfriend or the person(s) you have sex with stop you from doing things you want to do?		
4	Thinking about where you go to hang out, or to have sex. Do you feel unsafe there or are your parent(s) or guardian worried about your safety?		

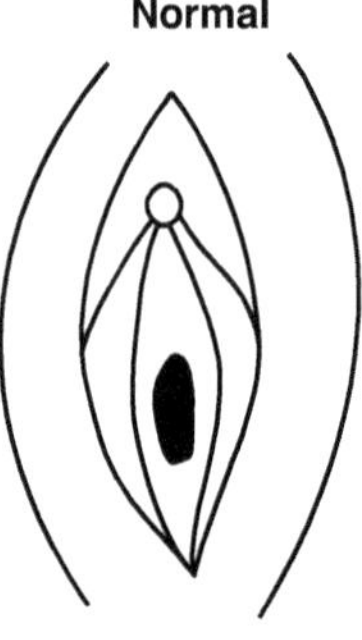

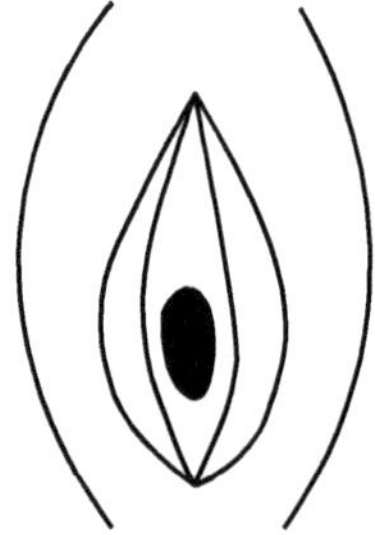

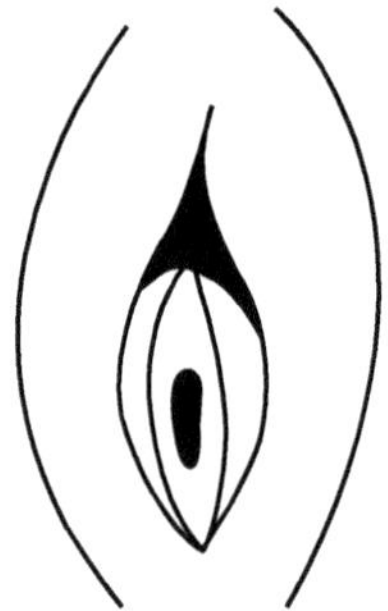

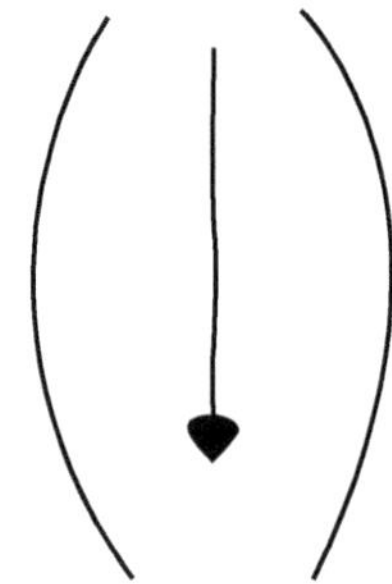

Type 4 – Other harmful procedures e.g. pricking, cutting, piercing

Figure 2.2 World Health Organization female genital mutilation classification.

Wales for healthcare professionals who have time-limited contact with young people to quickly identify those at risk of sexual exploitation [17]. If a child answers yes to any of these questions or demonstrated any vulnerabilities, safeguarding procedures should be initiated.

Female Genital Mutilation

Female genital mutilation (FGM) is defined as partial or total removal of the external female genitalia for non-medical reasons (Figure 2.2). It is illegal in the UK to perform, arrange or assist in arranging for this procedure to be performed in the UK or outside the country. If suspected, confirmed or disclosed in a girl under the age of 18, it is a mandatory requirement in England and Wales for this to be reported to the police on 101 (most local safeguarding structures now interact directly with the police). FGM is most often carried out on girls between infancy and the age of 15.

FGM is practised across 29 countries in Africa with the highest prevalence in northeast Africa, in which type 3 (infibulation) is practised almost exclusively. Somalia, Guinea, Djibouti and Egypt all have a prevalence of FGM over 90%. FGM is also practised outside of Africa, notably in Yemen, Iraqi Kurdistan, Indonesia and Malaysia, and to a lesser extent in India, Pakistan, the United Arab Emirates and Colombia. In many countries it is practised by traditional practitioners using crude instruments; however, in some countries, such as Egypt, the majority of procedures are undertaken by healthcare professionals. The reasons given for the procedure are complex and vary from region to region but include 'custom', 'rite of passage', 'cleansing' and 'status'. Short-term complications include haemorrhage, urinary retention, infection and death. Long-term complications include scarring, urinary and gynaecological problems, and sexual and psychological dysfunction [16,18].

If FGM is identified in an adult, it is important to record that advice has been given that the procedure is illegal and make enquiries about intentions for female children. Risk factors include status of family, family history of FGM, family from a high-prevalence area and any talk of a 'special holiday' – the long summer holidays are the most high-risk time. If there are any concerns, then safeguarding procedures should be followed.

Increasingly, young women present with concerns about their labial appearance. Female genital cosmetic surgery may be prohibited under the FGM act, unless it is necessary for physical or mental health. It is very important for GPs to provide reassurance.

Notably, genital piercing has become popular in the UK, and although there is a distinct difference between FGM and female genital piercing for decorative purposes, they are subject to the same legislation. Genital piercing would be classed as type 4 FGM and if this has been performed in a child under 18 years, it is an offence and triggers the same safeguarding procedures.

References

[1] L. Hayes and S. M. Creighton, 'Prepubertal vaginal discharge', *Obstet Gynecol*, vol. **9**, no. 3, pp. 159–163, Jul. 2007, https://doi.org/10.1576/toag.9.3.159.27335.

[2] A. Garden, M. Hernon and J. Topping, *Paediatric and Adolescent Gynaecology for the MRCOG and Beyond*. Cambridge University Press, 2008. https://doi.org/10.1017/CBO9781139871631.

[3] S. McGreal and P. Wood, 'Recurrent vaginal discharge in children', *J Pediatr Adolesc Gynecol*, vol. **26**, no. 4, pp. 205–208, Aug. 2013, https://doi.org/10.1016/j.jpag.2011.12.065.

[4] 'British Association of Dermatologists'. Accessed: 13 Apr. 2024. [Online]. Available: www.bad.org.uk/pils/vulvitis-in-childhood.

[5] W. A. Marshall and J. M. Tanner, 'Variations in pattern of pubertal changes in girls', *Arch Dis Child*, vol. **44**, no. 235, pp. 291–303, Jun. 1969, https://doi.org/10.1136/adc.44.235.291.

[6] O. Karapanou and A. Papadimitriou, 'Determinants of menarche', *Reprod Biol Endocrinol*, vol. **8**, p. 115, Sep. 2010, https://doi.org/10.1186/1477-7827-8-115.

[7] L. Michala and S. Creighton, 'Adolescent gynaecology', *Obstet Gynaecol Reprod Med*, vol. **24**, no. 3. pp. 74–79, Mar. 2014, https://doi.org/10.1016/j.ogrm.2014.01.001.

[8] K. Hoeger, K. Davidson, L. Kochman et al., 'The impact of metformin, oral contraceptives, and lifestyle modification on polycystic ovary syndrome in obese adolescent women in two randomised, placebo-controlled clinical trials', *J Clin Endocrinol Metab*, vol. **93**, no. 11, pp. 4299–4306, 2008.

[9] 'Scenario: Management – adolescents | Management | Polycystic ovary syndrome | CKS | NICE'. Accessed: 14 Apr. 2024. [Online].

Available: https://cks.nice.org.uk/topics/polycystic-ovary-syndrome/management/management-adolescents/#.

[10] A. B. Martha Hickey, 'Menstrual disorders in adolescence: Investigation and management', *Hum Reprod Update*, vol. **9**, no. 5, pp. 493–505, 2003.

[11] NICE Guideline, 'Recommendations | Heavy menstrual bleeding: assessment and management | Guidance | NICE', NG88. Accessed: 14 Apr. 2024. [Online]. Available: www.nice.org.uk/guidance/ng88/chapter/Recommendations#management-of-hmb.

[12] L. L. Bayer and P. J. A. Hillard, 'Use of levonorgestrel intrauterine system for medical indications in adolescents', *J Adolesc Health*, vol. **52**, no. 4, pp. S54–S58, Apr. 2013, https://doi.org/10.1016/j.jadohealth.2012.09.022.

[13] 'The British Society for Paediatric & Adolescent Gynaecology Guideline for the management of Heavy Menstrual Bleeding (HMB) in adolescents'. Accessed: 14 Apr. 2024. [Online]. Available: https://britspag.org/wp-content/uploads/2020/06/HMB-management-in-PAG-guideline-2020.pdf.

[14] D. Mansour, 'Safer prescribing of therapeutic norethisterone for women at risk of venous thromboembolism', *J Fam Plann Reprod Health Care*, vol. **38**, no. 3, pp. 148–149, Jul. 2012, https://doi.org/10.1136/jfprhc-2012-100345.

[15] 'Natsal-3 Reference Tables National Survey of Sexual Attitudes and Lifestyles (Natsal-3) Reference tables prepared by Soazig Clifton, Elizabeth Fuller and Dan Philo NatCen Social Research on behalf of the Natsal team', Accessed: 15 Apr. 2024. [Online]. Available: www.data-archive.ac.uk.

[16] K. Rogstad, A. Thomas, O. Williams et al., 'UK national guideline on the management of sexually transmitted infections and related conditions in children and young people (2009)', *Int J STD AIDS*, vol. **21**, no. 4, pp. 229–241, 2010, https://doi.org/10.1258/ijsa.2009.009353.

[17] Legislation.gov.uk(i), 'Social Services and Wellbeing (Wales) Act 2014', UK Public General Acts. Accessed: 15 Apr. 2024. [Online]. Available: www.legislation.gov.uk/anaw/2014/4/contents.

[18] N. Low-Beer and S. Creighton, 'Female genital mutilation and its management', *RCOG Green-Top Guideline*, no. **53**, pp. 1–17, 2015. Accessed: 15 Apr. 2024. [Online]. Available: www.gov.uk/government/publications/safeguarding-women-.

Chapter

3 Contraceptive Choices in Primary Care

Joanna Speedie and Diana Mansour

Key Points

- The majority of women attend primary care for their contraception.
- Long-acting reversible methods of contraception (LARCs) have lower typical failure rates than methods requiring user input – a LARC should always be offered during a contraception consultation.
- Many contraceptive methods also have non-contraceptive benefits.
- Use of the UK medical eligibility criteria (UKMEC) reduces risk when prescribing contraception. Not all contraindications are discussed in this chapter; always refer to the UKMEC.
- There are few contraindications to progestogen-only contraception.
- Erratic menstrual bleeding is common in the first few months of progestogen-only contraception and, in some women, continues with ongoing use.
- All brands of the 52 mg levonorgestrel intrauterine device (LNG-IUD) can be used for contraception, management of heavy menstrual bleeding (HMB) and the progestogenic component of HRT; devices with a lower dose of levonorgestrel cannot be used as part of HRT.
- The copper-intrauterine device (Cu-IUD) is the most effective method of emergency contraception (EC) and should be offered to all women requesting EC.
- Condoms prevent STI transmission but have a high typical contraceptive failure rate.
- Sterilisation is permanent; reversal is not usually funded by the NHS.

Introduction

The third UK National Survey of Sexual Attitudes and Lifestyles [1] reported that 16% of British pregnancies are unplanned and a further 29% of women are ambivalent about pregnancy, despite contraception being free on the NHS. This chapter discusses contraception available in the UK.

Two studies have shown that healthcare professionals (HCPs) who are well educated in LARC options are more likely to discuss them, their patients are more likely to use LARC and rates of unplanned pregnancies are lower [2,3].

Combined Hormonal Contraception [4]

Case Scenario 3.1

Rebecca is 21 and has been seeing her boyfriend for one year. They use condoms and she has used oral EC twice recently. She wants to discuss contraception and start 'the pill', wondering if you could give her Yasmin®, which a friend takes.

Composition

Combined hormonal contraceptives (CHCs) contain oestrogen and progestogen (mostly synthetic, but natural in some newer pills) and come as a pill, patch or vaginal ring. Most CHCs contain ethinylestradiol at varying dosages, although some newer combined oral contraceptives (COCs) contain estradiol and estetrol, which are thought to have less metabolic impact. Since the launch of the COC 60 years ago, the oestrogen dose has decreased; most pills now contain less than 35 μg of ethinylestradiol, reducing oestrogenic side effects and cardiovascular risks.

CHCs contain different progestogens, which are grouped into 'generations' with different estimated venous thromboembolism (VTE) risks (Table 3.1).

Mode of Action

CHCs work by:

- inhibiting ovulation
- thickening cervical mucus
- causing endometrial atrophy
- altering tubal motility and secretion.

Table 3.1 Types of progestogen in CHCs

Generation	Progestogen type	Example of CHC
First	Norethisterone®	Norimin®
Second	Levonorgestrel Norgestimate	Microgynon 30® Cilique®
Third	Desogestrel Gestodene	Marvelon® Femodene®
Fourth	Cyproterone acetate Drospirenone	Dianette® Yasmin®
Non-oral progestogens	Norelgestromin Etonogestrel	Evra patch® Nuvaring®
Unclassified	Dienogest Nomegestrol acetate	Qlaira® Zoely®

Effectiveness

CHC effectiveness is 0.3% in the first year of use with perfect use and 9% with typical use (all forms of CHC) [5]. Efficacy is not affected by broad-spectrum antibiotics but is reduced by enzyme-inducing drugs and by some other drug interactions.

Regimens

Traditionally, women would take CHC for 21 days then have a hormone-free interval (HFI) for seven days, during which they would have a withdrawal bleed (Table 3.2). Tailored CHC use, which reduces or avoids a monthly bleed, has grown in popularity – the monthly bleed has no health benefits.

CHC Advantages [4]

- Lighter and less painful bleeding.
- Used to treat HMB [6] and endometriosis [7].
- Reduced risk of ovarian, endometrial and colorectal cancers.
- Improve acne, especially preparations containing cyproterone acetate or drospirenone. Maximum benefit is seen after 12 months of use.
- May reduce premenstrual and polycystic ovarian syndrome symptoms, particularly preparations containing drospirenone.

Disadvantages and Risks [4]

- Temporary early hormonal side effects include breast tenderness, nausea and bloating. The vaginal ring may increase discharge. About 10% of patch users report a local skin reaction.

Table 3.2 Different CHC regimes

Regime	Period of CHC use	HFI
Standard	21 days	7 days
Shortened HFI	21 days	4 days
Tricycling	9 weeks	4–7 days
Flexible extended	Continuous use for at least 21 days then if problematic bleeding occurs for 3–4 days, take an HFI	4 days
Continuous	Continuous	None

Table 3.3 VTE risk with CHCs

Exposure	Risk per 10,000 women per year
Background risk in women of reproductive age	2
CHC containing levonorgestrel, norethisterone, norgestimate	5–7
Vaginal ring or patch	6–12
CHC containing drospirenone, desogestrel, gestodene, cyproterone acetate	9–12
Pregnancy	29
Postpartum	300–400

- Menstrual headaches/migraines can occur during the HFI when circulating hormones fall.
- Nuvaring® (but not the newer vaginal ring SyreniRing®) requires a cold chain and can only stay at room temperature for four months.
- Small increased risk of myocardial infarction and stroke and approximately double the risk of VTE; the absolute risk is very low (Table 3.3). The risk is highest in the first three months of use and when restarted after a hormone-free break of at least one month.
- Small increased risk of breast cancer, depending on duration of use. This is similar to a never-user by 10 years after stopping. The risks of using CHC probably outweigh the benefits for women who are known carriers of a gene mutation associated with breast cancer [8].
- May increase the risk of cervical cancer after five years of use; reverts to that of a non-user 10 years after discontinuation.

Table 3.4 UKMEC criteria

UKMEC category	Definition
UKMEC 1	A condition for which there is no restriction for the use of the contraceptive method.
UKMEC 2	A condition for which the advantages of using the method generally outweigh the theoretical or proven risks.
UKMEC 3	A condition where the theoretical or proven risks usually outweigh the advantages of using the method. The provision of a method requires expert clinical judgement and/or referral to a specialist contraceptive provider, since use of the method is not usually recommended unless other more appropriate methods are not available or not acceptable.
UKMEC 4	A condition which represents an unacceptable health risk if the contraceptive method is used.

- Effectiveness may be reduced after bariatric surgery; this varies with the type of surgery. It is also reduced for four weeks after initiation or dose change of tirzepatide.

Contraindications

The UKMEC [8] assigns each contraindication a number to define the risk associated with any given contraceptive (Table 3.4) and should be consulted for a full list of contraindications.

CHCs have more contraindications than other forms of contraception, but they are safe for most women. Absolute contraindications (UKMEC 4) include smoking ≥ 15 cigarettes/day when aged ≥ 35, migraine with aura, current breast cancer, ischaemic heart disease, cerebrovascular disease, a personal history of VTE, decompensated cirrhosis and hepatocellular adenoma/carcinoma [7].

Starting and Switching

Please refer to Tables 3.7 and 3.8 at the end of the chapter for starting and switching advice for all methods discussed in this chapter.

A CHC containing 30 mg ethinylestradiol with levonorgestrel is usually the first-choice pill for women and should be taken daily.

Diarrhoea and Vomiting

If vomiting occurs within three hours of taking a COC, another pill should be taken as soon as possible, with the next pill taken at its normal time.

For those with severe diarrhoea lasting more than 24 hours, the COC should be continued with extra precautions until the diarrhoea ends, and for another seven days. If vomiting or diarrhoea occurs in the last week of the packet, omit the seven-day gap.

The vaginal ring and patch avoid first-pass metabolism and are therefore unaffected.

Missed CHC Rules [9]

During the HFI, follicular development returns, with 20% of women having ovarian follicles larger than 10 mm diameter on the seventh day. During the first week of pill-taking these follicles are suppressed and ovarian quiescence returns. If the COC is restarted after a gap of more than seven days, ovulation may occur.

For details of what actions to take when CHC has been used incorrectly, see Figures 3.1, 3.2 and 3.3.

Follow-Up

A 12-month supply can be given at initiation or review [4]; annual review is required, at which blood pressure and body mass index (BMI) should be checked. CHCs should be discontinued immediately if an absolute contraindication develops. Only three months' supply of Nuvaring® can be supplied at one time because of the cold chain requirement.

Progestogen-Only Pill [10,11]

Case Scenario 3.2

Tara has been using a COC for six months; she reports new migraines with visual aura, an absolute contraindication, but she wants to continue with oral contraception.

Composition

Traditional POPs contain either norethisterone or levonorgestrel. Newer POPs contain desogestrel (DSG) or drospirenone (DRSP). The DRSP POP contains 24 active pills followed by 4 placebo pills.

Guidance on actions after incorrect use of combined oral contraception
(monophasic ethinylestradiol COC without placebo pills only)

Late restarting after HFI

≥9 completed days since last active pill was taken
(see page 4 for **how to calculate days**)

Consider EC if UPSI has taken place during or after the HFI

- Take the most recent missed pill as soon as possible
- Continue the remaining pills at the usual time
- Condoms should be used or sex avoided until pills have been taken for 7 consecutive days
- Consider follow up pregnancy test

1 missed pill (48 to <72 hours since last pill in current pack was taken)

1 pill missed in week 1 after HFI
(the first pill after the HFI must have been taken correctly; if not, see above box on late restarting)

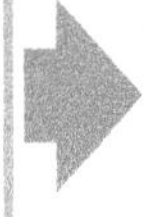

EC not required*

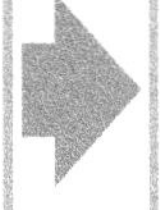

- Take the missed pill as soon as possible
- Continue the remaining pills at the usual time
- No additional contraceptive precaution required*

* if consistent, correct use earlier in week 1 and the 7 days prior to the HFI

1 pill missed in week 2 or week 3 after HFI
(or subsequent consecutive weeks of continuous pill-taking)

EC not required**

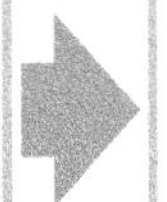

- Take the missed pill as soon as possible
- Continue the remaining pills at the usual time
- No additional contraceptive precaution required**

**if consistent, correct use in the previous 7 days

2 or more missed pills (≥72 hours since last pill in current pack was taken)

2–7 pills missed in week 1 after HFI
(the first pill after the HFI must have been taken correctly; if not, see above box on late restarting)

Consider EC if UPSI has taken place during the HFI or week 1

- Take the most recent missed pill as soon as possible
- Continue the remaining pills at the usual time
- Condoms should be used or sex avoided until pills have been taken for 7 consecutive days
- Consider follow up pregnancy test

2–7 pills missed in week 2 or week 3 after HFI
(or subsequent consecutive weeks of continuous pill-taking)

EC not required**

- Take the most recent missed pill as soon as possible
- Continue the remaining pills at the usual time
- If 2 or more pills missed in the 7 days prior to a scheduled HFI, omit the HFI
- Condoms should be used or sex avoided until pills have been taken for 7 consecutive days[a]

**if consistent, correct use in the previous 7 days

>7 consecutive pills missed in any week of pill taking

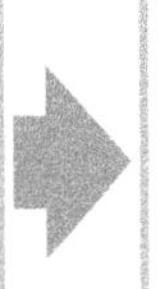

Consider EC

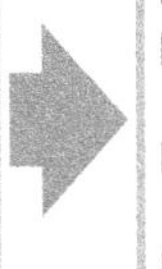

- Manage as new start contraception
- Consider immediate pregnancy test
- Quick start new COC packet (or consider other effective contraception)
- Condoms should be used or sex avoided until pills have been taken for 7 consecutive days
- Consider follow up pregnancy test

Figure 3.1 Missed COC rules. Source: Reproduced with permission of the CoSRH.
[a] Overcautious, but a back-up in case of subsequent incorrect use

Guidance on actions after incorrect use of the combined vaginal ring

Late restarting ring after scheduled HFI

Situation		EC		Action
≥8 completed days since ring was removed for scheduled HFI (see page 4 for **how to calculate days**)	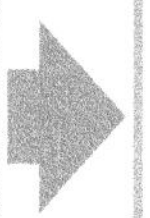	Consider EC if UPSI has taken place during or after the HFI		▶ Insert ring as soon as possible ▶ Keep ring in until scheduled ring removal day ▶ Condoms should be used or sex avoided until ring has been used for 7 consecutive days ▶ Consider follow up pregnancy test

Unscheduled ring removal for <48 hours

Situation		EC		Action
In week 1 after HFI	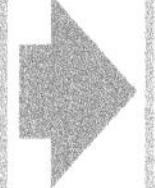	EC not required*		▶ Insert ring as soon as possible. ▶ Keep ring in until scheduled ring removal day ▶ No additional contraceptive precaution required*
In weeks 2 or 3 after HFI (or a subsequent week of correct consecutive ring use in an extended regimen)	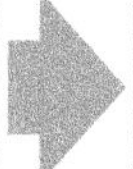	EC not required**	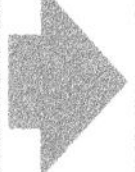	▶ Insert ring as soon as possible. ▶ Keep ring in until scheduled ring removal day ▶ No additional contraceptive precaution required**

* if correct use earlier in week 1 and the 7 days prior to the HFI

** if correct use in the previous 7 days

Unscheduled ring removal for ≥48 hours

Situation		EC		Action
In week 1 after HFI	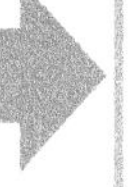	Consider EC if UPSI has taken place during the HFI or week 1	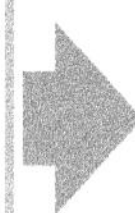	▶ Insert ring as soon as possible ▶ Keep ring in until scheduled ring removal day ▶ Condoms should be used or sex avoided until new ring has been used for 7 consecutive days ▶ Consider follow up pregnancy test
In weeks 2 or 3 after HFI (or a subsequent week of correct consecutive ring use in an extended regimen)[b]		EC not required if correct use in the previous 7 days		▶ Insert ring as soon as possible. ▶ Keep ring in until scheduled ring removal day ▶ If unscheduled removal ≥48 hours occurred in the week prior to a scheduled HFI, omit the HFI ▶ Condoms should be used or sex avoided until new ring has been used for 7 consecutive days[a]

Accidental continued use of the same ring beyond 3 weeks

Situation		EC		Action
Use of the same ring for >21 days and ≤28 days		EC not required if ring was correctly used from day 21 to day 28		▶ Start HFI (if scheduled) and insert new ring at end of HFI **OR** insert new ring ▶ No additional contraceptive precaution required if ring was consistently in situ from day 21 to day 28 of use
Use of the same ring continued for >4 and ≤5 weeks		EC not required if ring was correctly used for the last 7 days		▶ Omit HFI ▶ Insert new ring as soon as possible ▶ Condoms should be used or sex avoided until new ring has been correctly used for 7 consecutive days[a]
Use of the same ring continued for >5 weeks	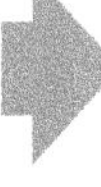	Consider EC if UPSI has taken place during week 5 or later		▶ Consider immediate pregnancy test ▶ Omit HFI ▶ Insert new ring as soon as possible ▶ Condoms should be used or sex avoided until new ring has been used for 7 consecutive days ▶ Consider follow up pregnancy test

Figure 3.2 Missed patch rules. Source: Reproduced with permission of the CoSRH.

[a] Overcautious, but a back-up in case of subsequent incorrect use

[b] Theoretically this could apply to up to 7 consecutive days unscheduled ring removal, but evidence is lacking

Guidance on actions after incorrect use of the combined transdermal patch

Late restarting patch after scheduled HFI

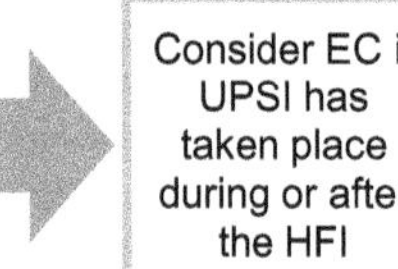
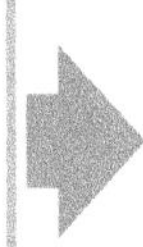

Situation	EC	Actions
≥8 completed days since last patch was removed for scheduled HFI (see page 4 for how to calculate days)	Consider EC if UPSI has taken place during or after the HFI	▶ Attach new patch as soon as possible ▶ Keep new patch on until scheduled removal day ▶ Condoms should be used or sex avoided until new patch has been used for 7 consecutive days ▶ Consider follow up pregnancy test

Unscheduled patch detachment for <48 hours or continued use of same patch for up to 48 additional hours

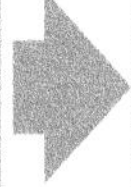

Situation	EC	Actions
In week 1 after HFI	EC not required*	▶ Attach new patch as soon as possible ▶ Keep new patch on until scheduled removal day ▶ No additional contraceptive precaution required*

* if correct use earlier in week 1 and the 7 days prior to the HFI

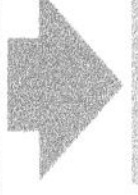

Situation	EC	Actions
In weeks 2 or 3 after HFI (or a subsequent week of correct consecutive patch use in an extended regimen)	EC not required**	▶ Attach new patch as soon as possible ▶ Keep new patch on until scheduled removal day ▶ No additional contraceptive precaution required**

** if correct use in the previous 7 days

Unscheduled patch detachment for ≥48 hours or continued use of the same patch for ≥48 additional hours

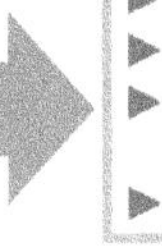

Situation	EC	Actions
In week 1 after HFI	Consider EC if UPSI has taken place during the HFI or week 1	▶ Attach new patch as soon as possible ▶ Keep new patch on until scheduled removal day ▶ Condoms should be used or sex avoided until new patch has been used for 7 consecutive days ▶ Consider follow up pregnancy test

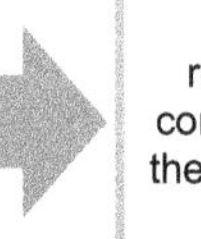
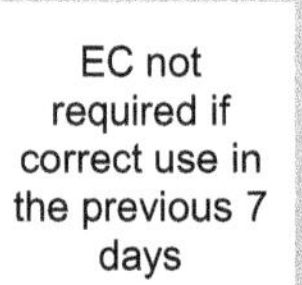

Situation	EC	Actions
In weeks 2 or 3 after HFI (or a subsequent week of correct consecutive patch use in an extended regimen)[b]	EC not required if correct use in the previous 7 days	▶ Attach new patch as soon as possible ▶ Keep new patch on until scheduled removal day ▶ If unscheduled removal ≥48 hours occurred in the week prior to a scheduled HFI, omit the HFI ▶ Condoms should be used or sex avoided until new patch has been used for 7 consecutive days[a]

Figure 3.3 Missed ring rules. Source: Reproduced with permission of the CoSRH.
[a] Overcautious, but a back-up in case of subsequent incorrect use
[b] Theoretically this could apply to up to 7 consecutive days unscheduled ring removal, but evidence is lacking

Mode of Action

POPs work by:

- thickening cervical mucus
- causing endometrial atrophy
- inhibiting ovulation in about 40% of women taking traditional POPs and in nearly all women using a DSG or DRSP POP.

Effectiveness

Efficacy is not affected by broad-spectrum antibiotics but is reduced by enzyme-inducing drugs and reduced for four weeks after initiation or dose increase of tirzepatide.

Advantages

- POPs can be used by most women, despite contraindications to CHC, with little effect on coagulation or metabolic parameters. The only absolute contraindication for all POPs is current breast cancer; DRSP should not be used with acute renal failure or severe renal insufficiency [7].

Table 3.5 Possible bleeding patterns with POP [10]

Individuals considering use of a traditional POP should be advised that bleeding pattern is unpredictable; but as a guide, over a 3-month period ending at about 12 months of use:

- Fewer than 1 in 10 (only about 2%) LNG POP users may be amenorrhoeic.
- About 8 in 10 LNG POP users may have normal frequency bleeding (3–5 bleeding/spotting episodes).
- About 1 in 10 LNG POP users may have frequent bleeding (6 or more bleeding/spotting episodes).
- Fewer than 1 in 10 LNG POP users may have prolonged bleeding (bleeding/spotting episode(s) lasting >14 days).

Individuals considering use of a DSG POP should be advised that bleeding pattern is unpredictable; but as a guide, over a 3-month period ending at about 12 months of use:

- About 4 in 10 DSG POP users may have normal frequency bleeding (3–5 bleeding spotting/episodes).
- About 2–3 in 10 DSG POP users may be amenorrhoeic.
- About 3 in 10 DSG POP users may have infrequent bleeding (<3 bleeding/spotting episodes).
- Fewer than 1 in 10 DSG POP users may have frequent bleeding (6 or more bleeding/spotting episodes).
- About 1 in 10 DSG POP users may have prolonged bleeding (bleeding/spotting episode(s) lasting >14 days).

Individuals considering use of a DRSP POP should be advised that bleeding pattern is unpredictable; they may or may not have 'scheduled' bleeding/spotting during the 4-day HFI and they may or may not have 'unscheduled' bleeding/spotting at other times. Both scheduled and unscheduled bleeding/spotting may reduce in frequency over the first year of use. Over a 3-month period at around 6–9 months of use:

- The total number of days of bleeding/spotting (scheduled plus unscheduled) may be similar to the number of days of bleeding/spotting with the DSG POP.
- About 2–3 in 10 DRSP POP users may be amenorrhoeic.
- Fewer than 1 in 10 DRSP POP users may have frequent bleeding.
- Fewer than 1 in 10 DRSP POP users may have bleeding episode(s) lasting >14 days.

EP = extra precautions (e.g. condoms or avoidance of intercourse); PT = pregnancy test; UPSI = unprotected sexual intercourse. CHC guidance here is for the patch, vaginal ring and for monophasic pills which contain ethinylestradiol – for other regimes, please follow manufacturer's recommendation.

Source: Reproduced with permission from CoSRH.

- POPs can be used when breastfeeding and until menopause; they do not mask menopausal symptoms.

Disadvantages

- Altered vaginal bleeding (see Table 3.5) and temporary hormonal side effects including acne.
- Small increased risk of developing breast cancer, but the absolute increase is small.
- Effectiveness may be reduced after bariatric surgery; this varies with the type of surgery.

Diarrhoea and Vomiting [10,11]

If vomiting occurs within two to four* hours of taking a POP, another pill should be taken as soon as possible, with the next pill taken at its normal time.

If there is severe watery diarrhoea soon after taking the POP, another pill should be taken. Depending on when the replacement pill was taken, the woman may need to follow missed pill rules.

*For traditional POP = 2 hours.
For DSG/DRSP POP = 3–4 hours

Missed POP Rules [10]

The window for a missed pill is 3 hours (traditional), 12 hours (DSG) or 24 hours (DRSP). If that is exceeded, take the missed pill as soon as possible, continue the packet as normal and use extra protection for the next 48 hours (or 7 days with DRSP). With DRSP, the four placebo pills should be omitted if any of the last seven active pills have been missed.

EC is needed if there has been unprotected sex after the time of the missed pill until contraceptive effectiveness has resumed. In addition, for DRSP users, EC will be required if pills are missed on days 1–7 of the packet and unprotected sex has occurred during the four placebo pills.

Progestogen-Only Injectable Contraception [12]

Case Scenario 3.3

Laura is 25 years old and requesting contraception; she doubts that she'd remember a pill. Her periods are heavy and painful; she'd be happy if they stopped.

Composition

The UK injectable contraceptive contains depo medroxyprogesterone acetate (DMPA), which can be given as an intramuscular (Depo-Provera®) or subcutaneous (Sayana Press®) injection.

Mode of Action

Injectable contraception works by:

- inhibiting ovulation
- altering the cervical mucus
- inducing endometrial atrophy.

Effectiveness

Failure rate in the first year is 0.2% with perfect use and 6% with typical use [5]. Efficacy is not affected by diarrhoea, vomiting, broad-spectrum antibiotics or enzyme-inducing drugs.

Advantages

- Long-acting, effective and non-user-dependent.
- Helps heavy/painful periods, with many having infrequent or no periods at one year.
- May decrease the risk of endometrial and ovarian cancer.
- Reduced functional ovarian cysts and fibroids.

Disadvantages and Risks [12]

- About 50% have no periods by one year of use – some may not like this.
- Some women will gain weight, particularly if aged under 18 with a starting BMI of ≥ 30 kg/m^2. Gaining ≥ 5% of baseline weight in the first six months is predictive of further weight gain.
- Anovulation decreases oestradiol levels, resulting in a 4–6% loss of bone mineral density (BMD). This is largely recovered when the injection is stopped and is usually not clinically relevant. In women with osteoporotic risk factors, a careful discussion of the risks and benefits should be documented, with any decision to use an injectable clearly justified. Women should come for review if they develop new risk factors. In young women who have not yet reached their peak BMD and in women aged over 45 years, use of the injection is UKMEC 2.
- It can take up to one year for normal fertility and menstruation to return after DMPA use. The average return to fertility is 5.5 months.
- Injection site reactions are more common with the subcutaneous injectable, with a range of 1.6–21% reported; this may be greater with self-administration than with HCP administration.
- Hormonal side effects include acne, headaches, mood changes and vaginitis.
- An initial adverse effect on lipid levels settles within two years.
- There is a weak link between DMPA use of more than five years and cervical cancer. This risk diminishes with time on cessation.
- Small increased risk of breast cancer, and the 2025 UKMEC update highlighted an increased risk of VTE.

Contraindications

The only absolute contraindication is current breast cancer. Injectables are UKMEC 3 with multiple risk factors for cardiovascular disease or VTE.

Administration

- Intramuscular DMPA is given every 13 weeks into the gluteus maximus or ventrogluteal region. The deltoid should be used if the woman has obesity to ensure intramuscular administration.
- Subcutaneous DMPA is injected every 13 weeks into the subcutaneous fat of the anterior thigh or abdomen over 5–7 seconds.

Overdue DMPA Injections

A DMPA injection is overdue after 14 weeks. A further dose can be administered if there has been no unprotected sex since the injection expired, but the woman should use additional protection for the next seven days.

If she has had unprotected sex since the injection expired, assess the need for EC. It is unclear if ulipristal acetate will be effective if a DMPA injection has only recently expired, so levonorgestrel is the preferred choice. The injection should be restarted as soon as possible, and extra precautions used for seven days. A pregnancy test is advised three weeks after the last unprotected sex. If ulipristal acetate is given, DMPA should be avoided for five days.

Follow-Up

Women should always be asked about general health and any side effects. A one-year supply of Sayana Press® can be given upfront once the woman is confident to self-administer. Osteoporotic risk factors should be assessed at least every two years.

Progestogen-Only Subdermal Implant [13]

Case Scenario 3.4

Jane is 18 years old. She gave birth six weeks ago and is using condoms for contraception. She got pregnant on the pill and wants the most reliable form of contraception.

Composition

Nexplanon®, containing 68 mg of etonogestrel, is the only implant available in the UK.

Mode of Action

Implants work by:

- inhibiting ovulation
- altering the cervical mucus
- inducing endometrial atrophy.

Effectiveness

Implants are the most effective reversible method of contraception with a typical failure rate of 0.05% in the first year of use [5]. Efficacy is not affected by diarrhoea, vomiting or broad-spectrum antibiotics, but is reduced by enzyme-inducing drugs.

Advantages

- Very effective LARC with no user input needed.
- Safe to use when breastfeeding.
- May improve painful periods.
- No effect on lipid or carbohydrate metabolism or BMD.

Disadvantages and Risks

- Menstrual bleeding can be erratic, with about 40% of women experiencing regular bleeding, 30% infrequent bleeding, 20% no periods and 10% frequent bleeding. Up to 20% of women will experience 14 days of bleeding, which can be regular, infrequent or frequent. Bleeding patterns can change during the duration of use.
- Hormonal side effects include acne and headaches.
- Small increased risk of breast cancer.
- Insertion and removal risks include:
    - scarring
    - bruising
    - infection
    - deep insertion
    - non-insertion
    - damage to blood vessels or nerves.

Contraindications

The only absolute contraindication is current breast cancer.

Extended Use

Limited evidence suggests that failure is uncommon during the fourth year of use, but routine use for over three years is not currently recommended. If a woman presents for an implant to be replaced that has been in situ for between three and four years, a pregnancy test should be done if necessary and the implant replaced. Extra precautions will be needed for seven days. If the implant has been present for over four years, the same applies but EC should also be offered if appropriate.

Follow-Up

Routine follow-up is not needed. Women should return if they have side effects or cannot feel the implant.

Levonorgestrel Intrauterine Device [14]

Case Scenario 3.5

Samira is 42 years old, has four children and has completed her family. She has been using condoms for contraception. Recently her periods have become heavier.

Composition

There are five levonorgestrel intrauterine devices (LNG-IUDs) available in the UK – see Table 3.6 for further information.

Mode of Action

LNG-IUD works by:

- inducing endometrial atrophy
- altering the cervico-uterine mucus

Table 3.6 Key differences between LNG-IUDs

	Mirena®	Benilexa®	Levosert®	Kyleena®	Jaydess®
Composition	52 mg levonorgestrel	52 mg levonorgestrel	52 mg levonorgestrel	19.5 mg levonorgestrel	13.5 mg levonorgestrel
Licensed indications	Contraception Heavy menstrual bleeding Progestogen component of HRT	Contraception Heavy menstrual bleeding	Contraception Heavy menstrual bleeding	Contraception	Contraception
Licensed duration of use for contraception	8 years	8 years	8 years	5 years	3 years
Licensed duration of use for HRT	4 years	Not licensed	Not licensed	N/A	N/A
Device dimensions	32 mm × 32 mm	32 mm × 32 mm	32 mm × 32 mm	28 mm × 30 mm	28 mm × 30 mm
Inserter tube diameter	4.4 mm	4.8 mm	4.8 mm	3.8 mm	3.8 mm

- inhibiting ovulation in some women (<25% with 52 mg LNG-IUDs).

Effectiveness

The first-year failure rate for 52 mg LNG-IUDs is 0.2% for perfect and typical use [5] and the failure rate for Jaydess® and Kyleena® during licensed use is around 0.3% [14]. Efficacy is not affected by diarrhoea, vomiting, broad-spectrum antibiotics or enzyme-inducing drugs.

Advantages

- The 52 mg LNG-IUD decreases menstrual blood loss by up to 90% and reduces dysmenorrhoea. After one year, 20% of women have no periods, compared with 12% of Kyleena® users and 6–9% of Jaydess® users. It is the most effective medical treatment for heavy menstrual bleeding [6] and can relieve pain from endometriosis and adenomyosis [7].
- The 52 mg LNG-IUD may reduce the size of small fibroids and can treat endometrial hyperplasia [15]; it may reduce the incidence of endometrial cancer [16,17].
- When used alongside oestrogen, a 52 mg LNG-IUD can be used for premenstrual symptoms or as the progestogen component of HRT. Only Mirena® has a licence for endometrial protection, but the College of Sexual and Reproductive Healthcare (CoSRH) supports the use (for five years) of any 52 mg LNG-IUD for this purpose [14].

Disadvantages

- Prolonged, frequent and irregular vaginal bleeding are all common in the first 90 days of use. Bleeding tends to settle with duration of use.
- Hormonal side effects include breast tenderness, mood swings and acne in the first few months.
- If the LNG-IUD fails, the proportion of pregnancies that are ectopic is higher than when no LNG-IUD is used.
- Association with ovarian cysts which are usually asymptomatic and tend to resolve.
- Fitting can be painful.
- Perforation risk is <2 per 1,000 insertions and increased in women who are postpartum or breastfeeding.
- Expulsion (5%), usually in the first three months.
- Possible increased risk of failure with a malpositioned device.
- Pelvic infection (<1%), in the first three weeks post-insertion, usually due to a pre-existing undetected STI.
- Approximately 18% of women will have non-visible threads, which may be due to colposcopy (if cut too short), the device moving within the uterus, expulsion, perforation or pregnancy. This percentage can be up to 30% when the device is fitted within 48 hours of a vaginal birth and 50% when fitted at the time of a caesarean section.
- Small increased risk of breast cancer.

Contraindications

Absolute contraindications include current breast cancer, cervical cancer awaiting treatment, endometrial cancer, postpartum or postabortion sepsis, current symptomatic pelvic infection, unexplained vaginal bleeding and gestational trophoblastic disease with elevated β HCG levels.

When to Replace/Stop

- If pregnancy is not desired, women should avoid sex or use a barrier method for seven days before LNG-IUD removal, with alternative contraception started immediately after removal. Alternatively, the new method can be started seven days before the LNG-IUD is removed. If a device is being removed and replaced, sex should be avoided (or a barrier method used) for seven days before this procedure, in case the old device is removed and a new one cannot be fitted. This also applies to the copper-intrauterine device.
- Any 52 mg LNG-IUD fitted after the age of 45 years can be used for contraception until 55 years of age, but if it is also being used as the progestogenic component of HRT, then it must be replaced at five years.
- Women under 45 years presenting with an LNG-IUD that is overdue for change can have the device replaced immediately if no unprotected sex has occurred in the last 21 days and a pregnancy test is negative. Extra protection is needed for seven days following the fit.
- If an LNG-IUD is overdue for change and there has been unprotected sex in the last 21 days, replacement should be delayed until a pregnancy can be excluded; that is, a negative pregnancy test at least 21 days after the last unprotected sex. The POP is an ideal bridging method to fill this gap.

Follow-Up

Routine follow-up at 4–6 weeks is necessary only when the LNG-IUD is fitted within 48 hours of a vaginal birth or at the time of a caesarean section. Other women should check their threads at four to six weeks post-insertion and seek medical help if they cannot feel them. This also applies to the copper-intrauterine device.

Copper-Intrauterine Devices [14]

Case Scenario 3.6

Samantha is 32 years old. She has tried various pills, the injection and implant, but discontinued all of them because of 'hormonal side effects'. She wants an effective, non-hormonal option.

Composition

Copper-intrauterine devices (Cu-IUDs) come in different shapes and sizes. The most effective Cu-IUDs contain more than 300 mm^2 of copper. Devices are licensed for use for between 5 and 10 years. When a Cu-IUD containing more than 300 mm^2 of copper is fitted over the age of 40, it can be left in until after the menopause – 2 years after the last menstrual period (LMP) if it occurs before 50 years of age, otherwise 1 year.

Mode of Action

Cu-IUDs work by:

- their toxic effect on eggs and sperm
- inhibiting sperm motility
- causing a foreign body reaction in the endometrium.

Effectiveness

The failure rate in the first year of use is 0.8% with typical use and 0.6% with perfect use [5]. Efficacy is not affected by diarrhoea, vomiting, broad-spectrum antibiotics or enzyme-inducing drugs.

Advantages

- Effective and immediately reversible.
- Works immediately.
- Non-hormonal.
- Most effective EC method.
- Inexpensive.
- No increase in cancer; may reduce incidence of endometrial cancer [16,17].

Disadvantages and Risks

- Possible worsened menstrual blood loss, intermenstrual bleeding and dysmenorrhoea, with longer periods.
- Fitting can be painful.

- Risks of perforation, expulsion, malposition, infection and non-visible threads are similar to the LNG-IUD.

Contraindications

Absolute contraindications include cervical cancer awaiting treatment, endometrial cancer, postpartum or postabortion sepsis, current symptomatic pelvic infection, unexplained vaginal bleeding and gestational trophoblastic disease with elevated β HCG levels.

Condoms, Caps, Diaphragms and Fertility Awareness [18,19]

Barrier methods have high failure rates but do protect against STIs. The failure rate for male condoms is 2% with perfect use and 18% with typical use [5]. Latex, non-latex and polyisoprene condoms are available in the UK. Couples should be educated on correct use, including avoidance of oil-based lubricants, which can damage condoms.

Cervical caps plus spermicide have failure rates of 12% with typical use and 9% for perfect use in nulliparous women – this increases to 24% and 20%, respectively, in parous women. Diaphragms with spermicide are associated with failure rates of 12% with typical use and 6% with perfect use [5]. Caps and diaphragms should be used with spermicide and inserted into the vagina prior to sex. They should remain in place for at least 6 hours following sex but should be removed no later than 48 hours. Both devices should be fitted by a health professional, and the woman may need a different size if she has a baby or changes weight.

Fertility awareness is only appropriate for women having regular cycles. There are several indicators which predict ovulation, including working out the fertile phase after keeping a menstrual calendar for at least three months, measuring basal body temperature at the beginning of each day to detect a rise of 0.2–0.4°C after ovulation and examining the cervical mucus daily to identify the changes over the month. Using all three methods perfectly can result in failure rates of 1–9%, but the typical failure rate is 24% [5]. Some women use fertility awareness apps. Others may choose fertility monitors which can detect concentrations of oestrogen metabolites and luteinizing hormone in the urine – the monitor will advise the woman when it is and is not safe to have sex and may have been designed to help women who were trying to conceive to let them know the most fertile times to have sex.

Emergency Contraception [20]

Case History 3.7

Leanne is 36 years old and has a new partner. She is currently on day 13 of her cycle and has had several episodes of unprotected sex this month. Her menstrual cycles range from 27 to 31 days. She is requesting EC and would like to discuss STI screening and ongoing contraception.

Copper-Intrauterine Device

A Cu-IUD can be inserted up to five days after the first episode of unprotected sex in the cycle, or up to five days after the earliest expected date of ovulation, if cycles are regular enough to calculate this. It is the most effective method of EC, with success rates of over 99%. If a woman chooses a Cu-IUD for EC but it cannot be immediately fitted, she should also be offered oral EC, in case she does not return for fitting or changes her mind about having a Cu-IUD.

Levonorgestrel

One dose of levonorgestrel (LNG) 1.5 mg can be taken up to 72 hours after unprotected sex (ineffective if used after this time) and used multiple times per cycle, if necessary. It can be given with multiple episodes of unprotected sex in the cycle.

This is a very safe option with no absolute contraindications. It delays or stops ovulation prior to the luteinising hormone (LH) surge but is less effective when taken close to ovulation and ineffective once the LH surge has started. Approximately 0.6–2.6% of women who take LNG will still become pregnant. Side effects include nausea and vomiting.

Contraception can be 'quick started' immediately and additional precautions taken until the method is effective.

LNG EC may be less effective in women who weigh more than 70 kg or have a BMI over 26 kg/m^2; these women should take 3 mg or use ulipristal at the usual dose. Women taking liver enzyme-inducing drugs also need 3 mg. In both these scenarios, a Cu-IUD is preferred.

LNG is safe in breastfeeding women.

Ulipristal Acetate

Ulipristal acetate (UPA) (30 mg) can be taken up to 120 hours after unprotected sex and can be used more than once in a cycle. UPA should be avoided in women with severe asthma controlled by oral steroids and those using liver-enzyme inducers.

UPA is a progesterone receptor modulator which stops or delays ovulation. It is less effective after the LH surge and ineffective after ovulation. Approximately 1–2% of women who take UPA will still become pregnant.

Its action may be altered by hormonal contraception, therefore initiation of a new hormonal method should be delayed for 5 days after taking UPA and additional contraception, then used for 48 hours to 7 days, depending on the method. The effectiveness of UPA could be affected if a woman has used progestogen in the preceding week and it should therefore be avoided in such situations.

UPA is safe in breastfeeding women - CoSRH guidance changed in 2025 and there is now no need to express and discard after taking UPA [21]. The side-effect profile is similar to levonorgestrel 1.5 mg.

Male Sterilisation [22]

Case History 3.8

Colin is 41 years old and married with three children. Both he and his wife feel their family is complete and he is requesting a vasectomy.

Pre-procedure

Vasectomy is a permanent procedure and reversal is not usually funded by the NHS. Special caution should be taken with men who are young, who have not fathered children or who suffer from mental health issues – these factors are associated with increased regret.

The Procedure

Generally, vasectomies are carried out under local anaesthesia as an outpatient. The minimally invasive procedure makes a puncture wound in the scrotum through which the vas deferens can be identified and divided.

Post-procedure

Men should rest, wear supportive underwear and avoid sex for 48 hours. Simple analgesia is advised. Semen analysis should be performed 12 weeks post-procedure to confirm that there are no sperm present. If azoospermia is found, no further semen samples are needed. If sperm continue to be identified, repeat semen samples are needed. If motile sperm are still noted seven months post-procedure, a repeat procedure is advised. Alternative contraception should be continued until semen analysis reveals no sperm.

Complications

- Bleeding (<20%).
- Haematoma formation.
- Infection (<2%).
- Failure (0.15%).
- Chronic scrotal pain at three months post-procedure (~10%).

Female Sterilization [22]

Case History 3.9

Jill is 29 years old and pregnant with her fifth baby. She is struggling to cope financially and mentally. All of her children have been born by caesarean section. She wants to be sterilised at the time of her caesarean; she is adamant that she does not want more children.

Table 3.7 When to stop contraception post-sterilisation

Method of contraception used	When to stop following female sterilization	Special instructions
CHC	After 7 days	If sterilisation performed on day 1 following the HFI, continue CHC for another 7 days or omit the HFI and continue CHC for 7 days
POP	After 7 days	-
Implant	At any time	-
LNG-IUD	After 7 days	-
Cu-IUD	After 7 days	-

For switching methods of contraception, see Table 3.8.

Table 3.8 Switching methods of contraception [23]

Initial method	Switch to traditional or DSG POP	Switch to DRSP POP	Switch to CHC	Switch to implant	Switch to DMPA	Switch to LNG-IUD	Switch to Cu-IUD
No method – having menstrual cycles.	• Day 1–5 of cycle (day 1 only for estradiol or estetrol combined pill or DRSP POP) – start new method, no EP (extra precautions) needed. • Any other time in cycle and reasonably sure that she isn't pregnant, start new method with EP as below. • Any other time in cycle, with UPSI since start of LMP – as below but consider bridging method until next period before starting DMPA, and do not start LNG-IUD until next period comes. Cu-IUD can be used as EC if criteria met. Consider also the need for emergency contraception and a pregnancy test 3 weeks after the last UPSI.						
	2 days.	7 days.					No EP.
No method – amenorrhoeic, with negative PT today and no UPSI in the last 21 days.	Start new method with 2 days EP.	Start new method with 7 days EP.					Start new method, no EP needed.
No method – amenorrhoeic, with negative PT today, but has had UPSI in the last 21 days.	• Consider the need for EC. • Consider bridging contraception before starting DMPA in this situation, but if it is the only option, start as below. • Do pregnancy test at least 21 days after last UPSI.						
	Start new method with 2 days EP.	Start new method with 7 days EP.				Do not start until proven to not be pregnant.	Do not start until proven to not be pregnant, or using under the criteria for EC.
CHC used correctly: • **Week 2–3 of traditional use.** • **Subsequent weeks of continuous or tailored use.** • **Day 1 of HFI**	Start new method, no EP needed.						
CHC used correctly – day 2 of HFI and no UPSI since start of HFI.	Start new method, no EP needed.					Start new method, 7 days EP.	Start new method, no EP needed.
CHC used correctly – day 3–7 of HFI and no UPSI since start of HFI.	Start new method with 2 days EP.	Start new method with 7 days EP.					Start new method, no EP needed.

CHC used correctly – day 3–7 of HFI with UPSI since start of HFI.	Restart/continue CHC until 7 days of active pills or the patch/ring has been used, then start new method with no EP needed.		Start new method and also restart/ continue CHC until 7 days of active pills or the patch/ring has been used.		Start new method, no EP needed.
CHC used incorrectly – no UPSI in the last 21 days and negative PT today.	Start new method with 2 days EP.	Start new method with 7 days EP.			Start new method, no EP needed.
CHC used incorrectly – UPSI in the last 21 days and negative PT today.	• Consider the need for EC. Pregnancy test needs to be done at least 21 days after last UPSI. • Consider bridging contraception before starting DMPA in this situation, but if it is the only option, start as below.				
	Start new method with 2 days EP.	Start new method with 7 days EP.		Do not start until proven to not be pregnant.	Start if criteria for EC met (all UPSI in last 5 days), otherwise do not start until proven not to be pregnant.
Implant in place for up to three years.	Start new method, no EP needed.				
Implant in place for 3–4 years, negative PT and no UPSI in the last 21 days.	Start new method with 2 days EP.	Start new method with 7 days EP.			Start new method, no EP needed.
Implant in place for 3–4 years, negative PT but with UPSI in the last 21 days.	As row above but also advise home PT at 21 days after last UPSI.				
Implant in place for >4 years, negative PT today and no UPSI in the last 21 days.	Start new method with 2 days EP.	Start new method with 7 days EP.			Start new method, no EP needed.
Implant in place for >4 years, negative PT today but with UPSI in the last 21 days.	• Consider the need for EC. Pregnancy test needs to be done at least 21 days after last UPSI. • Consider bridging contraception before starting DMPA in this situation, but if it is the only option, start as below.				
	Start new method with 2 days EP.	Start new method with 7 days EP.		Do not start until proven to not be pregnant.	Start if criteria for EC met (all UPSI in last 5 days), otherwise do not start until proven not to be pregnant.
DMPA with last injection <14 weeks ago.	Start new method, no EP needed.				

Table 3.8 (cont.)

Initial method	Switch to traditional or DSG POP	Switch to DRSP POP	Switch to CHC	Switch to implant	Switch to DMPA	Switch to LNG-IUD	Switch to Cu-IUD
DMPA with last injection >14 weeks ago and no UPSI which is >14 weeks since last injection, or UPSI which is >14 weeks since the last injection, but not in the last 21 days, with negative PT today.	Start new method with 2 days EP.	Start new method with 7 days EP.					Start new method, no EP needed.
DMPA with last injection >14 weeks ago and UPSI within the last 21 days, with negative PT today.	• Consider the need for EC. Pregnancy test needs to be done at least 21 days after last UPSI. • Consider bridging contraception before starting DMPA in this situation, but if it is the only option, start as below.						
	Start new method with 2 days EP.	Start new method with 7 days EP.				Do not start until proven to not be pregnant.	Start if criteria for EC met (all UPSI in last 5 days), otherwise do not start until proven not to be pregnant.
Traditional POP used correctly.	Start new method, no EP needed.	Start new method with 7 days EP.					Start new method, no EP needed.
DSG POP used correctly.	Start new method, no EP needed.						
DRSP POP during the HFI (days 25–28 of the last packet) or days 1–7 of the new packet, with no UPSI since the start of the HFI.	Start new method with 2 days EP.	NA.	Start new method with 7 days EP.				Start new method, no EP needed.
DRSP POP during the HFI (days 25–28 of the last packet) or days 1–7 of the new packet, but with UPSI since the start of the HFI.	Restart or continue DRSP POP until 7 days of active pills taken, then start new method with no EP needed.	NA.	Restart or continue DRSP POP until 7 days of active pills taken, then start new method with no EP needed.	Start new method immediately and also restart/continue DRSP POP until 7 consecutive active pills have been taken.			
DRSP POP, days 8–24 of packet.	Start new method, no EP needed.	NA.	Start new method, no EP needed.				
Any POP used incorrectly, negative PT today and no UPSI in the last 21 days.	Start new method with 2 days EP.	Start new method with 7 days EP.					Start new method, no EP needed.

Any POP used incorrectly, negative PT today but with UPSI in the last 21 days.	• Consider the need for EC. Pregnancy test needs to be done at least 21 days after last UPSI. • Consider bridging contraception before starting DMPA in this situation, but if it is the only option, start as below.			
	Start new method with 2 days EP.	Start new method with 7 days EP.	Do not start until proven to not be pregnant.	Start if criteria for EC met (all UPSI in last 5 days), otherwise do not start until proven not to be pregnant.
Any LNG-IUD in situ for the CoSRH recommended time for contraception.	Start new method with 2 days EP.	Start new method with 7 days EP.	Start new method, no EP needed, but advise no UPSI for 7 days before change, in case old device is removed and new one cannot be fitted – if this is not adhered to, delay device change for 7 days.	
Any LNG-IUD in situ for longer than the CoSRH recommended time for contraception, negative PT today but with UPSI in the last 21 days.	• Consider the need for EC. Pregnancy test needs to be done at least 21 days after last UPSI. • Consider bridging contraception before starting DMPA in this situation, but if it is the only option, start as below.			
	Start new method with 2 days EP.	Start new method with 7 days EP.	Do not start until proven to not be pregnant. (can start with 7 days EP if no UPSI in last 21 days and PT negative today).	Start if criteria for EC met (all UPSI in last 5 days), otherwise do not start until proven not to be pregnant. Can start with no EP if no UPSI in last 21 days and PT negative today.
Cu-IUD in situ for the CoSRH recommended time for contraception, or in situ for longer than this but within the first 5 days of the cycle (day 1 only if changing to estradiol or estetrol combined pill and DRSP POP). If device in date but later in cycle than this, use EP for 2 days if changing to traditional/ DSG pill and 7 days for all other methods except insertion of a new Cu-IUD.	Start new method, no EP needed.		Start new method, no EP needed, but advise no condomless sex for 7 days before change, in case old device is removed and new one cannot be fitted – if this is not adhered to, delay device change for 7 days. Do not start LNG-IUD after first 5 days of cycle if pregnancy cannot be excluded.	

Table 3.8 (cont.)

Initial method	Switch to traditional or DSG POP	Switch to DRSP POP	Switch to CHC	Switch to implant	Switch to DMPA	Switch to LNG-IUD	Switch to Cu-IUD
Cu-IUD in situ for longer than the CoSRH recommended time for contraception and after day 5 of the cycle. Negative PT today and no UPSI in the last 21 days or since the LMP.	Start new method with 2 days EP.	Start new method with 7 days EP.					Start new method, no EP needed. If UPSI in last 7 days, defer change until no UPSI for 7 days, in case old device is removed and new one cannot be fitted.
CU-IUD in situ for longer than the CoSRH recommended time for contraception and after day 5 of the cycle. Negative PT today but with UPSI, since the LMP, in the last 21 days.	• Consider the need for EC. • Consider bridging contraception before starting DMPA in this situation, but if it is the only option, start as below. • Pregnancy test at home at least 21 days after last UPSI.						
	Start new method with 2 days EP.	Start new method with 7 days EP.				Do not start until proven to not be pregnant.	Start if criteria for EC met (all UPSI in last 5 days or before 5 days after ovulation), otherwise do not start until proven not to be pregnant.
Ulipristal EC in the last 5 days.	Do not start any hormonal contraception for 5 days after UPA-EC.						Start if criteria for EC met (all UPSI in last 5 days or before 5 days after ovulation), otherwise do not start until proven not to be pregnant.
Ulipristal EC more than 5 days ago or at any time after levonorgestrel EC.	Start new method with 2 days EP.	Start new method with 7 days EP.				Do not start until proven to not be pregnant.	Start if criteria for EC met (all UPSI in last 5 days or before 5 days after ovulation), otherwise do not start until proven not to be pregnant.

Pre-procedure

Sterilisation is a permanent procedure and its reversal involves major surgery, which is not usually funded by the NHS. Some experience heavier periods following surgery, as hormonal contraceptives (which tend to lighten periods) have been stopped.

Effective contraception is advised up until the day of surgery, with a pregnancy test performed on that day. If unprotected sex has occurred in the prior three weeks, the procedure should be delayed until a pregnancy can confidently be excluded.

The Procedure

Sterilisation is usually performed via laparoscopy, with the fallopian tubes occluded using rings, clips or by excising part of the tube. Risks include damage to the bladder, bowel and blood vessels, along with any complications associated with general anaesthesia. The failure rate is 0.5%.

Stopping Contraception at the Time of Sterilisation

See Table 3.7.

References

[1] 'The National Survey of Sexual Attitudes and Lifestyles'. Accessed: 6 Aug. 2024. [Online]. Available: www.natsal.ac.uk.

[2] C. C. Harper, C. H. Rocca, K. M. Thompson et al., 'Reductions in pregnancy rates in the USA with long-acting reversible contraception: A cluster randomised trial', *The Lancet*, vol. **386**, pp. 562–568, 2015.

[3] H. F. Peipert, T. Madden, J. E. Allsworth et al., 'Preventing unintended pregnancies by providing no-cost contraception', *Obstet Gynaecol*, vol. **120** (suppl. 6), pp. 1291–1297, 2012.

[4] CoSRH, 'Combined hormonal contraception'. 2023. Accessed: 6 Aug. 2024. [Online]. Available: https://www.cosrh.org/Common/Uploaded%20files/documents/fsrh-guideline-combined-hormonal-contraception-october-2023.pdf.

[5] NICE CKS, 'Contraception – assessment'. Jan. 2024. Accessed: 6 Aug. 2024. [Online]. Available: https://cks.nice.org.uk/topics/contraception-assessment.

[6] NICE, 'NG88. Heavy menstrual bleeding: Assessment and management'. May 2021. Accessed: 6 Aug. 2024. [Online]. Available: www.nice.org.uk/guidance/ng88.

[7] NICE CKS, 'Endometriosis'. Oct. 2023. Accessed: 6 Aug. 2024. [Online]. Available: https://cks.nice.org.uk/topics/endometriosis.

[8] CoSRH, 'UK medical eligibility criteria for contraceptive use'. Accessed: 6 Aug. 2024. [Online]. Available: https://www.cosrh.org/Public/Public/Standards-and-Guidance/uk-medical-eligibility-criteria-for-contraceptive-use-ukmec.aspx.

[9] CoSRH, 'CEU Guidance: Recommended actions after incorrect use of combined hormonal contraception (e.g. late or missed pills, ring and patch)'. Accessed: 6 Aug. 2024. [Online]. Available: https://www.cosrh.org/Common/Uploaded%20files/documents/fsrh-ceu-recommended-actions-after-incorrect-use-of-chc-march-2020-amended-jul-2021-.pdf.

[10] CoSRH, 'Progestogen-only pills'. Jul. 2023. Accessed: 6 Aug. 2024. [Online]. Available: www.fsrh.org/Public/Public/Documents/ceu-guideline-progestogen-only-pills.aspx.

[11] CoSRH, 'CEU statement: Drospirenone progestogen-only pill'. Jan. 2024. Accessed: 6 Aug. 2024. [Online]. Available: https://www.cosrh.org/Common/Uploaded%20files/documents/fsrh-ceu-statement-drsp-pop-janu24.pdf.

[12] CoSRH, 'Progestogen-only injectable'. Jul. 2023. Accessed: 6 Aug. 2024. [Online]. Available: https://www.cosrh.org/Common/Uploaded%20files/documents/progestogen-only-injectable-december-2014-amended-11july2023.pdf.

[13] CoSRH, 'Progestogen-only implant'. Jul. 2023. Accessed: 6 Aug. 2024. [Online]. Available: https://www.cosrh.org/Common/Uploaded%20files/documents/fsrh-guideline-progestogen-only-implants.pdf.

[14] CoSRH, 'Intrauterine contraception'. Jul. 2023. Accessed: 6 Aug. 2024. [Online]. Available: https://www.cosrh.org/Common/Uploaded%20files/documents/fsrh-clinical-guideline-intrauterine-contraception-mar-23-amended.pdf.

[15] RCOG, 'Management of endometrial hyperplasia (Green-Top Guideline no. 67)'. Feb. 2016. Accessed: 6 Aug. 2024. [Online]. Available: www.rcog.org.uk/guidance/browse-all-guidance/green-top-guidelines/management-of-endometrial-hyperplasia-green-top-guideline-no-67.

[16] A. S. Felix, M. M. Gaudet, C. La Vecchia et al., 'Intrauterine devices and endometrial cancer risk: A pooled analysis of the Epidemiology of Endometrial Cancer Consortium', *Int J Cancer*, vol. **136**, no. 5, E410-22, 2015.

[17] N. Minalt, A. Caldwell, G. M. Yedlicka et al., 'Association between intrauterine device use and endometrial, cervical, and ovarian cancer: An

expert review', *Am J Obstet Gynecol*, vol. **229**, no. 2, pp. 93–100, 2023.

[18] CoSRH, 'Barrier methods for contraception and STI prevention'. Oct. 2015. Accessed: 7 Aug. 2024. [Online]. Available: https://www.cosrh.org/Common/Uploaded%20files/documents/ceuguidancebarriermethodscontraceptionsdi.pdf.

[19] CoSRH, 'Fertility awareness methods'. Jun. 2015. Accessed: 7 Aug. 2024. [Online]. Available: https://www.cosrh.org/Common/Uploaded%20files/documents/ceuguidancefertilityawarenessmethods.pdf.

[20] CoSRH, 'Emergency contraception'. Jul. 2023. Accessed: 7 Aug. 2024. [Online]. Available: https://www.cosrh.org/Public/Documents/ceu-clinical-guidance-emergency-contraception-march-2017.aspx.

[21] CoSRH, 'Using emergency contraception during breastfeeding'. Oct. 2023. Accessed: 7 Aug. 2024. [Online]. Available: https://www.cosrh.org/Common/Uploaded%20files/documents/FSRH-Statement-Ulipristal-Acetate-and-Breastfeeding.pdf.

[22] CoSRH, 'Clinical guideline: Male and female sterilisation'. Sep. 2014. Accessed: 7 Aug. 2024. [Online]. Available: https://www.cosrh.org/Public/Documents/cec-ceu-guidance-sterilisation-cpd-sep-2014.aspx.

[23] CoSRH, 'Guidance: Switching or starting methods of contraception'. Apr. 2023. Accessed: 12 Aug. 2024. [Online]. Available: https://fsrhlearning.learningpool.com/course/view.php?id=277 (available to CoSRH members only).

Chapter 4

Managing Contraception Problems in Primary Care

Fiona Sizmur

Key Points

- Stopping and switching methods of contraception leaves women at risk of pregnancy.
- All women starting contraception should be offered easy access to advice if they experience any problems and should be encouraged to maintain their current method until starting an alternative.
- Acceptable bleeding patterns vary between individuals, whose expectation and tolerance of unscheduled bleeding as a side effect of contraception may vary. Tolerance of different bleeding patterns should inform contraceptive choice.
- Investigation and exclusion of pathology is essential in the management of unscheduled bleeding.
- It is important to record any new onset or changed headache, particularly for women using combined hormonal methods.
- Headache in the hormone-free interval can be managed effectively without stopping the method.
- All combined hormonal contraceptives reduce acne.

Contraception is primarily used for the prevention of pregnancy, but the choice of contraception may also consider non-contraceptive benefits. Experience of unacceptable side effects, concerns over media reports, change in lifestyle or the need for greater reliability may all prompt a desire to switch methods. This is often preceded by a period of stopping the current method and hence a risk of conception. A cohort study found that these so-called stoppers and switchers are at high risk of unplanned pregnancy [1].

Women who start a new method should be made aware of possible side effects and have easy access to advice on how to manage these. The importance of continuing with the current method until advice is received may help to reduce unplanned pregnancies. This chapter discusses management of some of the more frequent problems encountered when using contraception.

Case Scenario 4.1

Lucy is a 17-year-old college student and national-level athlete. She came to see you eight months ago because of frequent heavy periods, which were interfering with her studies and sport; you started her on a desogestrel (DSG) progesterone-only pill (POP). She had attended surgery in the past for her acne and is currently using a topical preparation, Duac® gel (benzoyl peroxide/clindamycin). She takes no other regular medication but was issued some sumatriptan before her GCSEs, in case she got a recurrence of her previous migraine during the exams. She never needed to use it.

The POP had induced amenorrhoea, until two months ago, when she started experiencing painful bleeds every two to three weeks.

Unscheduled Bleeding

Progestogens (P) and oestrogens (E) affect ovarian sex steroid production via central mechanisms, have a direct action on the ovary and may also directly affect the endometrium.

Prolonged exposure to a low-dose progestogen, such as is used in the POP, implant, levonorgestrel intrauterine device (LNG-IUD) and depo medroxyprogesterone acetate injection (DMPA), causes an increase in superficial vascular fragility within the endometrium. Different progestogens have differing effects on local mediators of endometrial function, causing dysregulation of endometrial breakdown and repair cycles, thereby increasing endometrial instability.

In contrast, high-dose progestogens, used therapeutically in the management of menorrhagia, cause pseudo-decidualisation of the endometrium and reduced bleeding.

The exact mechanisms of breakthrough bleeding are not fully understood, and it is impossible to predict with certainty the bleeding pattern from contraceptive hormones in any individual woman.

Unscheduled bleeding (UB) is a common problem with progestogen-only methods, particularly during the first three months; it usually settles without treatment. Anyone reporting symptoms should be assessed for the risk of sexually transmitted infections (STIs). One small study of combined oral contraceptive (COC) users suggested that chlamydia infection was three times more likely in the presence of UB compared to a control group without bleeding, but who had either recently changed sexual partners or reported vaginitis [2]. Gonorrhoea is a rarer cause of UB. Establish if Lucy has been, or is currently, sexually active, whether she uses condoms and whether she has had a recent partner change. This will allow appropriate sexual health screening as well as assessment of contraceptive needs.

Consider also other causes such as missed pills, pregnancy, gynaecological pathology and interactions with prescribed or over-the-counter medications. Non-adherence with pill taking, drug interactions (e.g. enzyme inducers) or reduced absorption due to bariatric surgery, tirzepatide or some eating disorders may cause UB and increase the risk of pregnancy.

There is little evidence supporting the long-term benefits of any option to treat UB in contraceptive users, but pragmatic measures, discussed later in the chapter, may assist some women [3].

Progestogen-Only Pill [4]

There are three types of POP available, all with variable and often unpredictable bleeding patterns. Definitions of scheduled and UB differ between studies, making comparisons of data difficult, but most women generally report improvement in bleeding patterns over time.

Users of the original levonorgestrel (LNG) or norethisterone (NET) pills (rarely prescribed now) tended to experience more regular bleeds and less infrequent bleeding or amenorrhoea. Those using DSG may initially experience frequent irregular bleeding but have higher long-term rates of amenorrhoea. Prolonged bleeding occurs in up to 10% of users of any POP.

Users of drospirenone (DRSP) may experience less unscheduled or prolonged bleeding but may or may not experience scheduled bleeds in the hormone-free interval (HFI). Total bleeding days are similar to other types of POP, but some women prefer a predictable bleed.

Women may be concerned breakthrough bleeding reduces pill effectiveness; they can be reassured that there is no evidence of this, assuming good adherence and no concerns regarding absorption.

The type and dose of progestogen, route of administration, endogenous circulating estradiol levels and ovulation can all affect bleeding patterns, so changing the type of POP may help, although there is little strong evidence. Some studies have noted lower bleeding-related cessation of the DRSP pill compared to the DSG pill [5]. Double-dose DSG has been reported to be beneficial in the management of heavy menstrual bleeding (HMB) in adolescents; there is no evidence for using it in the management of UB, but anecdotally this is often done [6].

Combined Hormonal Contraception

Oestrogen produces a more stable endometrium by stimulating stromal proliferation, and therefore UB is less common with combined hormonal contraception (CHC) than progestogen-only methods, but it still affects up to 20% of users in the first three months and is one of the commonest reasons for discontinuation [3]. It usually settles with time, so an early change of method should be discouraged.

Suggestions for managing this include the following.

- Change the E dose – 20 mcg pills have reportedly higher rates of UB compared to 30 and 35 mcg preparations, but comparative studies are difficult due to differing progestogens. There is no proven benefit to increasing the ethinylestradiol dose from 30 to 35 mcg.
- Change the E or P type. There is little evidence that any progestogen is superior to any other in terms of bleeding patterns [7], but women report an absence of withdrawal bleeds in some cycles with newer progestogens such as nomegestrel acetate. This progestogen has high receptor selectivity, producing a thin decidualised endometrium with atrophied glands. The absence of a withdrawal bleed isn't predictable, and this may not be

acceptable to all women. While newer oestrogen combinations give favourable bleeding patterns, this may be as much related to the reduction in HFI as to the type of progestogen [8].

- Change the regime. Regimes with a shorter HFI are associated with shorter, lighter bleeding episodes and less UB [9].

Extended CHC use decreases the number of bleeding days in the long term when compared to traditional cyclical use, although there may be initial higher rates of UB, leading to early discontinuation. Such regimes include scheduled extended pill-taking (e.g. bi/tricycling) followed by a seven-day or shorter HFI, as well as unscheduled extended pill-taking, or patient tailored regimes. There is some evidence that the combined vaginal ring offers better cycle control than oral methods [9].

Depot Injection, IUDs and Implant

Altered bleeding is common in users of the intramuscular or subcutaneous depot injection and may cause discontinuation in up to 25% of women in the first year [10]. For those who persist, around half will experience amenorrhoea by 12 months [11].

Frequent bleeding or spotting is common in the first few months of LNG-IUD use but decreases over time. Amenorrhoea becomes more prevalent over time, with rates at one year being approximately 6–9% for the 13.5 mg device, 12% for the 19.5 mg device and 20% for the 52 mg device. By five years, rates of amenorrhoea are 23% for 19.5 mg devices and 42% for 52 mg devices. Around 20% of women experience UB in the first few months of copper intrauterine device (Cu-IUD) use; this usually improves [12].

The bleeding pattern in the first three months of implant use is broadly predictive of future bleeding patterns, although 50% of women with prolonged or frequent bleeding at three months may still improve [13,14].

Options to manage UB include the following.

- Addition of short-term E, for example using the combined contraceptive pill on a cyclical or continuous basis, can reduce UB for those using the implant or depot. The effect ceases once it is stopped. It may also be a pragmatic option for management of UB in intrauterine device (IUD) users. This use is unlicensed [3].
- NSAIDs, such as mefenamic acid or naproxen, used for short courses, are effective at reducing bleeding through inhibition of inflammatory endometrial prostaglandins Some benefit has been shown for depot, implant and IUD users [3,12,15,16].
- Tranexamic acid, an antifibrinolytic used to manage HMB, may also be a short-term therapeutic option [3].

It is good practice to counsel patients regarding the side effects of their chosen method, but studies comparing intensive to routine counselling prior to starting the implant and other long-acting reversible contraception (LARC) methods have shown little or no benefit in continuation rates [17]. Awareness of women's preferences and tolerance of bleeding patterns is useful when discussing contraception and it is worth exploring these at the initial consultation, particularly when considering different cultures [18,19]. Surveys have shown that almost equal numbers of women express preference for monthly bleeds or less frequent bleeds, as well as no bleeding [20].

Case Scenario 4.2

Lucy explains that she has never been sexually active. You note a history of migraines with aura, raising concerns about oestrogen use. After considering her options, she decides to try the etonogestrel implant, but she is concerned that it might worsen her acne or headaches.

Acne

Hormones undoubtedly influence acne. Oestrogens suppress luteinising hormone-driven androgen production and increase sex hormone-binding globulin; this decreases free androgen levels and improves acne, as well as reducing hirsutism.

The effect of progestogens is less clear. Levonorgestrel and norethisterone may activate the androgen receptor, worsening acne. Desogestrel and norgestimate are less active, and drospirenone blocks androgens from binding to the receptor, so combined pills with differing progestogens may have variable effects on the skin. Some studies have shown cyproterone acetate and drospirenone-containing COCs to be superior for acne, but a large Cochrane review showed that all COCs reduce acne lesions, with the effects of the oestrogen outweighing the effects of the progestogen [21]. It may take three to four months to see any benefit; during this period, therapies such as topical retinoids and antibiotics may help.

Acne has been reported as a transient side effect of the LNG-IUD in the first few months after fitting; less than 3% of women discontinue the device because of this [12].

Lucy should be advised that acne can occur as a new side effect, but that in patients with pre-existing acne, improvement is much more common than deterioration, and that only around 1% of users discontinue the implant due to acne [13].

Headache

Headache is common, with or without contraceptive use – this is an important consideration when assessing studies looking at the effect of hormones on headache. Migraine with aura (but not migraine without aura) is associated with a twofold increased risk of ischaemic stroke, although the absolute risk is very low in healthy, non-smoking women. Women using CHC should be questioned at each visit regarding any change in nature or new onset of headache.

Initial exacerbation of headache in the early months of using CHC and progestogen-only methods appears to resolve with continued use, although two studies have reported an increase in headaches over time with DMPA. The incidence of headache is not related to the oestrogen dose, progestogen type or method of hormone delivery.

The HFI is a risky time for increased headache, triggered by the withdrawal of oestrogen. Management is simple and can be achieved with continuous use of CHC (pill, patch or ring) in an extended or tailored regime, or by using oestrogen supplementation, for example 2 g oestrogen gel daily in the HFI. The latter is not mentioned in current CoSRH guidelines on CHC [22,23]. Switching women to a desogestrel pill has been found to improve oestrogen-related headache and menstrual migraine [25,26].

Case Scenario 4.3

Lucy explains that she has not had any migraines since before her GCSEs and wonders if she will be OK to have the combined pill now.

Evidence suggests that migraine with aura is a marker of an individual at an increased risk of ischaemic stroke, and even a distant history or single episode is associated with an increased risk. Given the availability of alternative and effective progestogen-only contraception, it would be prudent to avoid combined methods, as the risks will still outweigh the benefits [27]. The risk-to-benefit ratio may change for women using CHC for medical as well as contraceptive indications; such decisions should be made on an individual basis, with full discussion of all options and well-documented informed consent that considers other risk factors such as smoking and body mass index (BMI).

Case Scenario 4.4

Lucy is seen again two years later. She has been amenorrhoeic since about three months after implant insertion. She is now in a sexual relationship and has started to have frequent light periods again. She is also worried that the implant is affecting her sex drive and feels different in her arm.

Low Libido

Low sexual desire is the commonest sexual problem among women, with a prevalence of around 20–30% in women of reproductive age [28,29]. Oestrogens in CHC can cause a varying overall drop in total and free testosterone levels [30]. Androgen insufficiency may cause decreased libido, but sexual desire is affected by a complex interaction of physical, emotional and environmental factors; studies show that reduced testosterone levels do not always correlate with low libido.

Heterogeneity of studies and the complex nature of factors influencing sexual desire make comparison of the effect of pill type on libido difficult. A more androgenic pill might theoretically help in cases of low libido, but this isn't borne out in clinical practice.

The following points may be useful during a consultation about low libido in a patient on hormonal contraception.

- Asking about specific symptoms which may influence sexual enjoyment. Use of a 20 mcg pill may be associated with more vaginal dryness than higher-dose pills [9].
- Women experiencing breast tenderness may benefit from a less oestrogenic pill or one with a lower oestrogen dose; if breast tenderness

occurs mainly during the HFI, then extended pill-taking may help [9].

- Estradiol valerate used in combination with dienogest has been demonstrated to improve desire. In addition, a 24/4 pill regime may have a better effect than traditional 21/7 regimes.
- Most studies report no change in libido while taking hormonal contraception and indeed many studies suggest an increase [31]. For those experiencing problems, it may be worth reflecting on the complex nature of sexual desire and other influencing factors aside from the hormonal ones.

Case Scenario 4.5

After excluding all other causes of bleeding, you examine the implant and notice a 'dimple' midway along the implant.

Implants

Broken, Bent and Impalpable Implants

The in vitro release rate from damaged implants is only slightly increased, compared to undamaged implants, and contraceptive efficacy is unlikely to be affected. The decision to replace the implant, ensuring that it is all removed, is therefore a matter of clinical judgement and personal preference for the woman.

If the implant is impalpable, refer to a specialist with experience in this field and access to real-time ultrasound [13]. Exclude any risk of pregnancy and provide ongoing contraception while this is arranged.

Implant Site Reactions

Implant site reactions such as pain, bruising, irritation and itching are common and usually present in the first few days or weeks after insertion. Reassurance or the use of antihistamines are usually sufficient. Infections are uncommon, but usually require antibiotics, and removal of the implant. Since the introduction of barium sulphate into the device, allergic reactions have also been reported; they can present in a similar way to infection. Severe pain, paraesthesia, numbness or loss of motor function in the hand or fingers require prompt referral to specialist services to consider the possibility of nerve damage [13].

Case Scenario 4.6

Lucy requests that her implant is removed and decides to use an LNG-IUD to manage her periods and provide contraception. She attends surgery for an uneventful fitting but returns eight weeks later, unable to feel the threads. She has been experiencing irregular bleeding and cramping abdominal pain. Chlamydia screening taken during fitting was negative. At pelvic examination, the coil threads cannot be visualised.

Intrauterine Devices

Lost Threads [12]

When the threads of an IUD cannot be seen or palpated, they have either been drawn into the uterus/cervical canal or the device has migrated or been expelled. Management should start with a pregnancy test and referral for a pelvic ultrasound to look for the IUD.

Pregnancy Test Negative

- Advise about ongoing contraception and emergency contraception if needed.
- Consider if the pregnancy test was done too early and may be a false negative, in which case arrange a repeat at least three weeks after the last intercourse.
- If this is not the case, and pregnancy can be reliably excluded, an experienced practitioner may attempt to locate the threads within the cervical canal using a thread retriever.
- If ultrasound confirms the device to be correctly within the uterus, the patient can be reassured and the device left until due for removal.
- If ultrasound cannot locate the IUD and there is no definite evidence of expulsion, a plain abdominal X-ray with pelvic views should be arranged, looking for an extrauterine device. If this confirms an uncomplicated perforation, the patient should be provided with alternative contraception and referred for elective laparoscopic removal of the device. Reinsertion may be offered following a minimum of six weeks after perforation.
- If X-ray does not identify the device, expulsion can be assumed and reinsertion offered if wanted.

Pregnancy Test Positive

- The absolute risk of ectopic pregnancy is greatly reduced by the use of an IUD compared to no contraception, but if it fails, the proportion of pregnancies which are ectopic is greater than if the pregnancy were to occur without an IUD in place.
- In some studies, half the pregnancies that occurred with an IUD in place were ectopic and therefore an urgent scan to localise the pregnancy is essential.
- Removal of the device before 12 weeks of gestation reduces the risk of miscarriage.

Malpositioned Devices [12]

There is no definite evidence as to whether an IUD which is displaced from the uterine fundus provides similar or reduced contraceptive efficacy when compared to one in the correct place. Theoretically, the efficacy of an LNG-IUD may be less affected by position due to its primary effect of local progestogen release. There is also evidence that devices can move within the uterine cavity, both upwards and downwards, particularly in the initial months after insertion.

Consensus opinion from the CoSRH Guideline Development Group [12] is that contraceptive effect cannot be guaranteed for non-fundal devices, especially if over 2 cm from the fundus on ultrasound measurement, or if the IUD lies fully or partially within the cervical canal.

Clinical judgement and documented informed consent should be used when deciding whether to remove or replace the device. Replacement should be considered if there are symptoms that may be related to malposition, such as pain or bleeding. Delaying removal of partially expelled devices may be sensible if there is a recent pregnancy risk and the woman is asymptomatic. Removal of partially embedded devices is usually straightforward and only required if the woman is symptomatic.

Infection/Pelvic Inflammatory Disease [12]

The risk of pelvic infection is low (<1%), with the risk being greatest in the first 21 days after fitting.

A diagnosis of pelvic inflammatory disease (PID) should be considered, and empirical antibiotic treatment offered, in any sexually active woman with recent onset bilateral pelvic pain associated with tenderness on bimanual examination, after exclusion of pregnancy. Testing for gonorrhoea and chlamydia is recommended; a positive result supports the diagnosis, but absence of proven infection does not exclude PID, which is a clinical diagnosis. Making a definitive diagnosis is difficult and therefore a low threshold for treatment is recommended, with broad-spectrum antibiotics covering STIs as well as aerobic and anaerobic bacteria isolated in the genital tract [32].

Women should be reviewed after 48–72 hours and may retain the IUD if symptoms are improving. If there is no improvement, consider removal of the IUD but balance this against pregnancy risk and consider if there is a need for oral emergency contraception.

Actinomyces-Like Organisms [12]

Actinomyces israelii is a commensal of the genital tract. Actinomyces-like organisms (ALOs) are now rarely reported on cervical screening samples since the move towards primary HPV screening and liquid-based cytology. If ALO are reported and the woman is asymptomatic, colonisation rather than infection is most likely, and the device may be left in place. *Actinomyces* pelvic infection is rare, but if a woman with known ALOs presents with pelvic pain, consider removal of the device and liaise with microbiology regarding treatment.

References

[1] K. Wellings, N. Brima, K. Sadler et al., 'Stopping and switching contraceptive methods: Findings from Contessa, a prospective longitudinal study of women of reproductive age in England', *Contraception*, vol. **91**, no. 1, pp. 57–66, 2015.

[2] J. E. Krettek, S. I. Arkin, P. Chaisilwattana et al., 'Chlamydia trachomatis in patients who used oral contraceptives and had intermenstrual spotting', *Obstet Gynecol*, vol. **81**, no. 5, pp. 728–731, 1993.

[3] CoSRH, 'Problematic bleeding with hormonal contraception'. Jul. 2015. Accessed: 27 Feb. 2024. [Online]. Available: https://www.cosrh.org/Common/Uploaded%20files/documents/ceuguidanceproblematicbleedinghormonalcontraception.pdf.

[4] CoSRH, 'Progestogen only pills'. Jul. 2023. Accessed: 27 Feb. 2024. [Online]. Available: https://www.cosrh.org/Public/Documents/ceu-guideline-progestogen-only-pills.aspx.

[5] P. A. Regidor, E. Colli, and S. Palacios, 'Overall and bleeding-related discontinuation rates of a new oral contraceptive containing 4 mg

drospirenone only in a 24/4 regimen and comparison to 0.075 mg desogestrel', *Gynecol Endocrinol*, vol. **37**, no. 12, pp. 1121–1127, 2021.

[6] R. C. Burton and C. E. Williams, 'Double-dose desogestrel: Is it effective in adolescent menstrual dysfunction?', *J Pediatr Adolesc Gynecol*, vol. **34**, no. 5, pp. 662–665, 2021.

[7] T. A. Lawrie, F. M. Helmerhorst, N. K. Maitra et al., 'Types of progestogens in combined oral contraception: Effectiveness and side-effects', *Cochrane Database Syst Rev*, vol. **5**, CD004861, 2011.

[8] D. Mansour, C. Westhoff, U. Kher et al., 'Pooled analysis of two randomized, open-label studies comparing the effects of nomegestrol acetate/ 17betaestradiol and drospirenone/ethinyl estradiol on bleeding patterns in healthy women', *Contraception*, vol. **95**, pp. 390–397, 2017.

[9] CoSRH, 'Combined hormonal contraception'. Oct. 2023. Accessed: 27 Feb. 2024. [Online]. Available: https://www.cosrh.org/Common/Uploaded%20files/documents/fsrh-guideline-combined-hormonal-contraception-october-2023.pdf.

[10] J. Villavicencio and R. H. Allen, 'Unscheduled bleeding and contraceptive choice: increasing satisfaction and continuation rates', *Open Access J Contracept*, vol. **7**, pp. 43–52, 2016.

[11] CoSRH, 'Progestogen-only injectable'. Jul. 2023. Accessed: 27 Feb. 2024. [Online]. Available: https://www.cosrh.org/Common/Uploaded%20files/documents/progestogen-only-injectable-december-2014-amended-11july2023.pdf.

[12] CoSRH, 'Intrauterine contraception'. Jul. 2023. Accessed: 27 Feb. 2024. [Online]. Available: https://www.cosrh.org/Common/Uploaded%20files/documents/fsrh-clinical-guideline-intrauterine-contraception-mar-23-amended.pdf.

[13] CoSRH, 'Progestogen-only implant'. Jul. 2023. Accessed: 27 Feb. 2024. [Online]. Available: https://www.cosrh.org/Common/Uploaded%20files/documents/fsrh-guideline-progestogen-only-implants.pdf.

[14] D. Mansour, L. Bahamondes, H. Critchley et al., 'The management of unacceptable bleeding patterns in etenogestrel-releasing contraceptive implant users', *Contraception*, vol. **83**, pp. 202–210, 2011.

[15] P. Phaliwong and S. Taneepanichskul, 'The effect of mefenamic acid on controlling irregular uterine bleeding second to Implanon use', *J Med Assoc Thai*, vol. **87** (suppl. 3), pp. S64–68, 2004.

[16] S. N. Upawi, M. F Ahmad, M. A. Abu et al., 'Management of bleeding irregularities among etonogestrel implant users: Is combined oral contraceptives pills or nonsteroidal anti-inflammatory drugs the better option?', *J Obstet Gynaecol Res*, vol. **46**, no. 3, pp. 479–484, 2020.

[17] W. Modesto, M. V. Bahamondes, L. Bahamondes, 'A randomized clinical trial of the effect of intensive versus non-intensive counselling on discontinuation rates due to bleeding disturbances of three long-acting reversible contraceptives', *Hum Reprod*, vol. **29**, no. 7, pp. 1393–1399, 2014.

[18] G. S. Merki-Feld, N. Breitschmid, B. Seifert et al., 'A survey on Swiss women's preferred menstrual/ withdrawal bleeding pattern over different phases of reproductive life and with use of hormonal contraception', *Eur J Contracept Reprod Health Care*, vol. **19**, no. 4, pp. 266–275, 2014.

[19] A. F. Glasier, K. B. Smith KB, Z. M. van der Spuy et al., 'Amenorrhea associated with contraception: An international study on acceptability', *Contraception*, vol. **67**, pp. 1–8, 2003.

[20] C. B. Polis, R. Hussain, A. Berry, 'There might be blood: A scoping review on women's responses to contraceptive-induced menstrual bleeding changes', *Reprod Health*, vol. **15**, 114, 2018.

[21] A. O. Arowojolu, M. F. Gallo, L. M. Lopez et al., 'Combined oral contraceptive pills for treatment of acne', *Cochrane Database of Syst Rev*, vol. **7**, CD004425, 2012.

[22] E. A. MacGregor, 'Contraception and headache', *Headache*, vol. **53**, no. 2, pp. 247–276, 2013.

[23] V. De Leo, V. Scolaro, M. C. Musacchio et al., 'Combined oral contraceptives in women with menstrual migraine without aura', *Fertil. Steril.*, vol. **96**, pp. 917–920, 2011.

[24] A. G. Edlow and D. Bartz, 'Hormonal contraceptive options for women with headache: A review of the evidence', *Rev Obstet Gynecol.*, vol. **3**, no. 2, pp. 55–65, 2010.

[25] R. E. Nappi, G. S. Merki-Feld, E. Terreno et al., 'Hormonal contraception in women with migraine: Is progestogen-only contraception a better choice?', *J Headache Pain*, vol. **14**, no. 1, 66, 2013.

[26] G. S. Merki-Feld, N. Caveng, G. Speiermann et al., 'Migraine start, course and features over the cycle of combined hormonal contraceptive users with menstrual migraine: Temporal relation to bleeding and hormone withdrawal: a prospective diary-based study', *J Headache Pain*, vol. **21**, no. 1, 81, 2020.

[27] CoSRH, 'UK medical eligibility criteria for contraceptive use'. Sept. 2019. Accessed: 27 Feb. 2024. [Online]. Available: https://www.cosrh.org/Public/Public/Standards-and-Guidance/uk-medical-eligibility-criteria-for-contraceptive-use-ukmec.aspx and change date to 2025.

[28] S. L. West, A. A. D'Aloisio, R. P. Agans et al., 'Prevalence of low sexual desire and hypoactive sexual desire disorder in a nationally representative sample of US women', *Arch Intern Med*, vol. **168**, no. 13, pp. 1441–1449, 2008.

[29] J. Zheng, R. M. Islam, R. J. Bell et al., 'Prevalence of low sexual desire with associated distress across the adult life span: An Australian cross-sectional study', *J Sex Med*, vol. **17**, no. 10, pp. 1885–1895, 2020.

[30] Y. Zimmerman, M. J. Eijkemans, H. J. Coelingh et al., 'The effect of combined oral contraception on testosterone levels in healthy women: A systematic review and meta-analysis', *Hum Reprod Update*, vol. **20**, no. 1, pp. 76–105, 2014.

[31] Z. Pastor, K. Holla, and R. Chmel, 'The influence of combined oral contraceptives on female sexual desire: A systemic review', *Eur J Contracept Reprod Health Care*, vol. **18**, pp. 27–43, 2013.

[32] BASHH, '2018 United Kingdom national guideline for the management of pelvic inflammatory disease'. Accessed: 27 Feb. 2024. [Online]. Available: https://www.bashh.org/resources/6/pid_2019/.

Chapter

5 Management of Vaginal Discharge in Primary Care

Catherine Armitage

Key Points

- Physiological and infective causes (non-STI) are the most common reasons for altered vaginal discharge in the reproductive years.
- A sexual history is crucial, regardless of the age of the woman – symptoms cannot exclude STIs.
- A woman's self-diagnosis of *Candida* or bacterial vaginosis (BV) may not be reliable – take a full history of the symptoms.
- Empirical treatment runs the risk of over-diagnosis of *Candida* – have a low threshold for examination.
- Narrow-range pH paper is a useful tool in near-patient assessment.
- Test for multiple possible diagnoses when undertaking genital examination, with a low threshold for repeat examination/testing in recurrent/persisting symptoms.
- Remember trichomonas as a possible differential.
- Take care not to label a patient as having recurrent *Candida* or BV – ensure that it is appropriately diagnosed on testing.
- Genital dermatoses, including contact dermatitis, and herpes simplex ulceration are commonly and mistakenly attributed to vulvovaginal candidiasis. Consider a woman's vulval care routine in case of exogenous triggers for symptoms.
- Most cases of vaginal discharge can be diagnosed and managed in primary care; establish if the local sexual health service has a clinician who has an interest in recurrent *Candida* and BV. This may be more appropriate than gynaecological referral for recurrent symptoms.

Case Scenario 5.1: Emma

Emma is 19 and is a first-year student at the local university, having been registered with you since the preceding September. She has had a vaginal discharge for four days; it is white and sometimes thick. This is the third such episode since September – after speaking to her sister and looking online during the last two episodes, she thought that it was thrush, so used some over-the-counter treatments – the discharge resolved. She thinks that this is a third episode and wants some treatment and to stop the symptoms recurring; this is her first consultation about it.

Introduction

Vaginal discharge is an extremely common presentation in primary care. It is normal for women of reproductive age to have some degree of discharge [1]. The characteristics may vary, depending on the stage of the menstrual cycle. In the follicular phase, before ovulation, the mucus goes from thick (non-fertile) to thinner and more slippery (fertile). As oestrogen levels fall and progesterone levels increase in the luteal phase, after ovulation, the mucus becomes thicker and is hostile to sperm.

From the onset of puberty, increasing oestrogen levels lead to colonisation of the vagina with lactobacilli. Lactobacilli metabolise glycogen and produce lactic acid, making the vaginal environment acidic, with a pH of ≤4.5. Other commensals include anaerobic bacteria, alpha-haemolytic streptococci and coagulase-negative staphylococci. Some commensal organisms result in altered discharge if they proliferate – including *Candida albicans*, *Staphylococcus aureus* and *Streptococcus agalactiae*. The possible causes of vaginal discharge are shown in Figure 5.1.

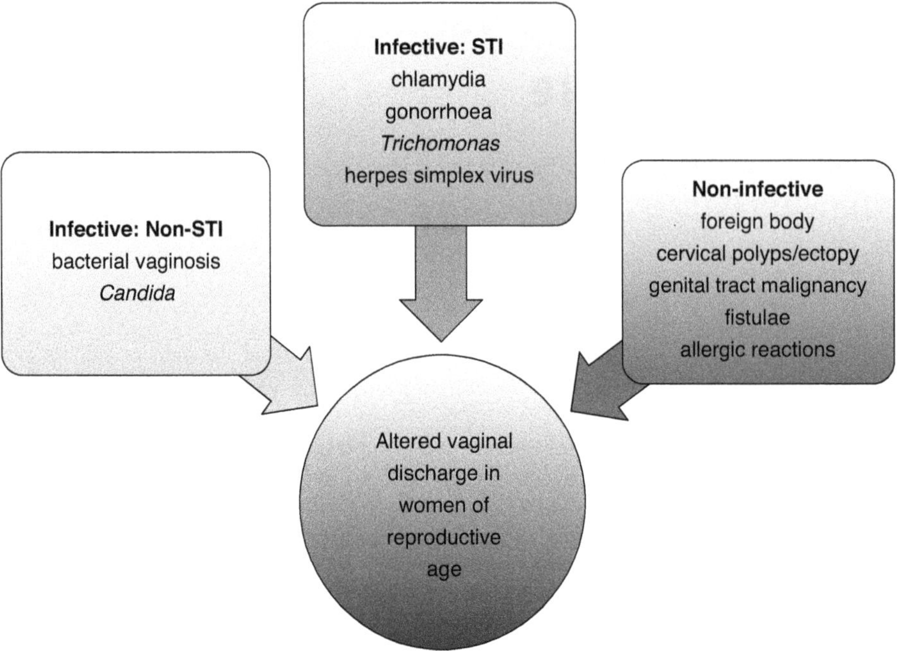

Figure 5.1 Altered vaginal discharge in women of reproductive age.

What Are the Commonest Causes of Altered Vaginal Discharge in Women of Reproductive Age?

The most common causes are physiological, BV and *Candida*, but STIs and non-infective causes should be considered.

Bacterial Vaginosis

BV is the commonest cause of abnormal discharge in women of reproductive age [2], affecting between 5% and 50% of individuals at various ages [3].

In BV, the vaginal pH is above 4.5. Lactobacilli may be present, but the vaginal flora is altered and includes anaerobic bacteria. *Gardnerella vaginalis*, *Prevotella* species, *Mycoplasma hominis* and *Mobiluncus* species have been cultured. There is debate as to whether BV is an imbalance only in vaginal flora or whether it starts as an STI – the current position is that it is not an STI but has some characteristics of STIs, such as being associated with recent change of sexual partner, with the presence of an STI and with receiving oral sex. Other associations include Afro-Caribbean ethnicity, vaginal douching, smoking and the presence of an intrauterine device. An increased incidence of BV has been described in women who have sex with women. BV has also been described in women who have never had sex. There may be an increase in users of copper intrauterine devices (Cu-IUDs), but the evidence is limited and conflicting. Evidence relating to users of levonorgestrel intrauterine devices (LNG-IUDs) is too limited to make any link [3].

Clinical features include a malodorous vaginal discharge, not typically associated with itch or discomfort. Approximately 50% of women are asymptomatic. Genital examination reveals a white discharge, typically thin, coating the walls of the vagina and vestibule. Inflammation is not usually noted.

Despite BV not being an STI, the prevalence is high in women with pelvic inflammatory disease (PID). In pregnancy, BV is associated with second trimester miscarriage, premature rupture of membranes, preterm delivery and postpartum endometritis [2].

Diagnosis

A diagnosis of BV in sexual health services is made based on a combination of symptoms, signs and Gram staining of vaginal sampling.

Amsel's criteria require at least three of the following four to be present:

1. Thin white homogenous discharge.

2. Clue cells on microscopic examination of sample from discharge (not Gram stained).
3. A pH of vaginal fluid >4.5.
4. Release of fishy odour on addition of 10% potassium hydroxide – less frequently used now.

Gram-stained microscope slides can be evaluated with the Hay/Ison criteria or the Nugent score. The Hay/Ison criteria are:

1. Normal – lactobacilli predominate.
2. Intermediate – mixed flora.
3. BV – predominant *Gardnerella/Mobiluncus*.

The British Association for Sexual Health and HIV (BASHH) recommend the Hay/Ison criteria for use in genitourinary medicine services [2]. The Nugent score is based on the relative proportions of bacterial morphotypes to give a score between 0 and 10. Greater than 6 is BV.

Isolation of *Gardnerella vaginalis* on high vaginal swab is insufficient to diagnose BV, as it can be cultured from the vagina in 30–50% of asymptomatic women who do not meet all the diagnostic criteria. Using narrow-range pH paper along with a history can guide immediate management while waiting for test results to come back.

Management

A woman with BV should avoid vaginal douching (intravaginal cleansing with liquids) and perfumed products around the genitalia and in the bath. These can create an imbalance in pH and so encourage the development of BV.

Treatment is indicated for symptomatic women and possibly for women undergoing some surgical procedures, including uterine instrumentation.

Recommended regimens are [2,4]:

1. Metronidazole 400 mg BD for five to seven days.
2. Metronidazole 2 g single dose.
3. Intravaginal metronidazole gel (0.75%) OD for five days.
4. Intravaginal clindamycin cream (2%) OD for seven days.

All have clearance rates of about 70–80% at four weeks – the 2 g single dose may be slightly less effective. Advice on side effects, and to avoid alcohol with metronidazole, should be given, whatever the route of administration.

Treatment with probiotics or lactic acid preparations have not been shown to be effective.

BV in Pregnancy and Breastfeeding

Results of clinical trials investigating BV screening in pregnancy have been conflicting. Symptomatic women should be treated in the same way as non-pregnant women. There is insufficient evidence to recommend routine treatment for asymptomatic pregnant women, though women with additional risk factors for preterm birth may benefit from treatment before 20 weeks' gestation [2]. Metronidazole is present in breast milk and can alter taste – single high doses such as the 2g single dose should be avoided in pregnancy and breastfeeding.

Some studies support screening for BV before surgical termination of pregnancy to reduce subsequent endometritis or PID [2,4].

Recurrent BV

Recurrent BV has no formal definition; some studies have used a definition of three or more episodes of symptomatic BV per year [5] or repeated cases of BV after treatment [6]. Studies looking at treatments have included administration of twice-weekly metronidazole gel over a 16-week period and the use of probiotics. Lactic acid gel and acetic acid gel have not been adequately evaluated in well-designed randomized controlled trials. Assessment of a woman with recurrent BV should include details of her vulval care routine and sexual history. A symptom diary of up to three months may help to identify triggers.

Appropriately detailed discussion of BV should occur, supported by written information. Dialogue should include treatments and risks of recurrence. UK guidelines do not (as of early 2026) recommend screening male partners, but the American guidelines were updated in October 2025 and suggest that partner therapy is considered [16]. Testing for STIs is recommended for any woman with genital symptoms, and in women diagnosed with BV, due to the links between BV and STIs.

Candida

Vulvovaginal candidiasis (VVC) is common in the reproductive years – it is a symptomatic inflammation of the vagina and/or vulva caused by superficial fungal infection. The prevalence of VVC is not known but it is diagnosed in 5–15% of women who attend sexual health/sexual and reproductive health clinics [8].

Symptoms could include vaginal discharge (typically non-offensive), discomfort/itch, dysuria and superficial dyspareunia. Signs of severe VVC could include extensive vulval erythema, fissuring, oedema and excoriation, along with discharge.

No symptom or sign is pathognomonic for VVC, so laboratory testing is useful, as many women might have other conditions such as allergy or genital dermatoses. Up to two-thirds of women who have self-diagnosed acute VVC do not actually have the condition [9,10].

Acute VVC is defined as a first or single isolated presentation, with signs and symptoms of acute VVC and *Candida* species on testing [7]. VVC is attributed to *Candida albicans* in 80–89% of cases, with *C. glabrata*, *C. tropicalis*, *C. krusei*, *C. parapsilosis* and *Saccharomyces cerevisiae* making up the remainder. Up to 20% of women during reproductive years may be colonised with *Candida* species but have no signs or symptoms: they do not require treatment [8]. *Candida* occurs most commonly when there is oestrogen in the vagina; that is, between puberty and the menopause and during pregnancy. *Candida* overgrowth can be triggered by antibiotic use, immunosuppression and diabetes mellitus. An estimated 75% of women will have at least one lifetime episode of VVC, and 40–45% will have two or more episodes [7].

There is limited and contradictory evidence on the risk of VVC in users of combined hormonal contraceptives. Users of the combined vaginal ring have reported more vaginal discharge and irritation compared to other combined hormonal contraceptive users, but there is no evidence of an increase in inflammatory cells [8].

In genitourinary medicine settings, sampling from the anterior fornix and vaginal walls is taken and assessed by Gram stain and plating on fungal media, such as Sabouraud's agar. Microscopy is the primary laboratory investigation for acute VVC. Culture is no longer recommended as a primary laboratory investigation for acute VVC [7]. BV and *Candida* can be diagnosed simultaneously on microscopy. The pH is not altered in *Candida* and so would be less than 4.5; narrow-range pH paper is therefore helpful to differentiate *Candida* from BV in primary care.

Management [7]

Management includes advice on vulval care routines such as use of bland emollients as a soap substitute and skin conditioner, along with avoiding perfumed products and potential irritants.

All topical and oral azole therapies give a clinical and mycological cure rate of over 80% in uncomplicated acutely symptomatic women, so the choice of regime is a matter of personal preference, availability and affordability.

Treatment regimes include the following.

- A single dose of 150 mg fluconazole, or two doses on days 1 and 4.
- A 500 mg clotrimazole intravaginal pessary, or two doses on days 1 and 4.

Women may have vulval symptoms due to other conditions and may have colonisation with *Candida* which is not necessarily contributing to the symptoms.

There is no evidence to support test of cure or the treatment of male partners in either episodic or recurrent VVC.

Candida in Pregnancy

Asymptomatic colonisation and symptomatic episodes are more common during pregnancy. Topical treatments are indicated, with no single optimal regimen. Longer courses may be needed. Oral therapy must be avoided in pregnancy and breastfeeding [7], but there is no documented association with adverse pregnancy outcomes.

Recurrent *Candida*

Approximately 6% of women in the reproductive years with a primary episode of VVC will develop recurrent VVC [7]. The diagnosis is based on at least four documented episodes of symptomatic *Candida* in a year, with at least partial resolution between episodes. Positive microscopy, or a moderate/heavy growth of *C. albicans*, should be documented on at least two occasions when symptomatic, although microscopy is generally not available in primary care. Recurrent *Candida* is usually due to *C. albicans* but is attributed to host factors rather than a more virulent strain. The triggers already outlined apply, and a link between recurrent *Candida* and allergy has also been observed (see Table 5.1).

Testing for *Candida* may be useful as non-*albicans* types are resistant to azole therapies. Blood tests for diabetes, full blood count, HIV and ferritin may pick up an underlying cause such as diabetes or immunosuppression.

Combined oral contraceptive pills have not been conclusively shown to be linked with recurrent *Candida* – the quality of evidence is mixed. The Cu-IUD is a possible risk factor for acute and recurrent VVC; there is mixed evidence, but it is possible for *Candida* to adhere to a Cu-IUD and produce a biofilm.

Table 5.1 Summary of the symptoms and signs of the commonest infective causes of vaginal discharge [11]

	Bacterial vaginosis	Vulvovaginal candidiasis	Trichomoniasis
Notes	Commonest cause of abnormal vaginal discharge. Not sexually transmitted	Perceived by women to be more common than it actually is. Not sexually transmitted	An STI – diagnosis should be made with a reliable method as there will be implications for partner(s)
Discharge	Homogeneous (thin and watery)	Variable – often thick, lumpy and white	Variable – may be frothy
Odour	Malodour	No malodour	Malodour
Associated symptoms (not all may be present)	Usually none (unless accompanied by *Candida*)	Itch/soreness, dysuria, superficial dyspareunia	Itch/soreness, dysuria, lower abdominal pain
Typical signs (not all may be present)	Discharge coats the vagina and vestibule No vaginal/vulval inflammation (unless accompanied by *Candida*)	May look normal or any of vaginal inflammation, vulval inflammation, fissures, oedema, satellite lesions	May look normal or frothy discharge, vulvitis, vaginitis, cervicitis – 'Strawberry cervix' often quoted but actually rare: <2%
Vaginal pH (take from lateral wall of vagina). Normal = 3.5–4.5	>4.5	≤4.5, i.e. normal	>4.5

Women with recurrent VVC wishing to try alternative contraception should be advised that the evidence supporting an association is weak and conflicting [3].

Treatment for recurrent *Candida* involves induction with fluconazole 150 mg every 72 hours for 3 doses, followed by maintenance of 150 mg fluconazole once weekly, lasting at least 6 months. Approximately 90% of women will remain disease-free at 6 months and 40% at 12 months. There are no trials addressing the optimal duration of suppressive therapy, no evidence to support the use of probiotics and insufficient evidence for any dietary recommendations [7]. Cetirizine 10 mg once daily for six months may lead to remission in women who fail to respond to the maintenance regimen with fluconazole [7].

The majority of non-*albicans* types are *C. glabrata* – this is susceptible to azoles but has a higher minimum inhibitory concentration when being tested for sensitivity to treatment. Nystatin pessaries are the only licensed alternative to azole therapy. Other unlicensed treatments such as boric acid, amphotericin B and flucytosine have been suggested as alternatives – it is advisable to seek advice from the local genitourinary medicine service if considering these alternatives.

Trichomonas Vaginalis

Trichomonas vaginalis (TV) is associated with altered vaginal discharge; testing is not always available in primary care so it is worth checking the situation in your area. It is sexually transmitted via the intravaginal or intraurethral route. There is evidence that trichomonas infection may enhance HIV transmission [13].

Ten to 50% of women are asymptomatic; up to 70% of symptomatic women have discharge. The discharge can be variable in consistency; only 30% of those with discharge have the classically described frothy yellow discharge. Only 2% of women have a 'strawberry cervix' appearance on naked-eye assessment [12].

In genitourinary medicine services, TV can be diagnosed on wet-mounted microscopy/point of care testing – flagellated protozoa can be seen swimming in the saline mount. It can also be diagnosed on culture and nucleic acid amplification technique (NAAT) testing. NAAT testing is the test of choice if resources allow. The pH is greater than 4.5. Those complaining of vaginal discharge or vulvitis, or who have been found to have evidence of vulvitis and/or vaginitis on examination, should be tested for TV. The first-line treatment is metronidazole, 400–500 mg twice daily for seven days. Metronidazole 2 g as a single oral dose is an alternative. Sexual partners need simultaneous treatment, with abstinence from sexual intercourse for at least one week after the index case and their partner/s have completed treatment and follow-up [12]. Vaginal discharge is not cited as a symptom of *Mycoplasma genitalium*, despite being associated with urethral discharge in males [14].

So, what about Emma? At this point she should not be labelled as having recurrent *Candida* as she does not meet the diagnostic criteria, having never been formally tested before.

Assessment of a Woman with Altered Vaginal Discharge

History

Establish the duration of symptoms, consistency of discharge, malodour and itch, triggers/relievers, and patterns of symptoms (e.g. relationship to the menstrual cycle), along with the use of over-the-counter treatments. Past medical history, sexual history/risk assessment and contraceptive use should be routinely sought (see Box 5.1).

Questioning should also cover symptoms which may suggest an STI or other pathology, such as altered bleeding, dysuria, abdominopelvic pain and superficial/deep dyspareunia. The absence of these symptoms does not exclude an STI.

Box 5.1 Core components of a sexual history [15]

- Symptoms/reasons for attendance
- Last sexual intercourse/contact, sex of her partner(s), anatomic sites of exposure, condom use, symptoms/suspicion of infection in partner
- Previous sexual partner details, as for last sexual contact
- Note total number of partners in past three months if more than two
- History of testing/diagnosis of STIs
- Last menstrual period and menstrual pattern, contraceptive history and cervical cytology history.
- History of HPV vaccination
- Pregnancy and gynaecology history
- Blood-borne virus risk assessment and vaccination history for those at risk
- Past medical and surgical history
- Medication history/drug allergies
- Agree method of giving results
- Establish competency

Consider also:

- Gender-based/intimate partner violence/ safeguarding in relation to children and vulnerable adults
- Alcohol and recreational drug history

Examination

A woman should be offered genital examination when symptomatic. This is particularly relevant when she has symptoms affecting the upper reproductive tract, has risk factors for STIs or is pregnant, postpartum or after termination of pregnancy or instrumentation of the uterus. Bloody discharge, uncertain symptoms or recurrent symptoms/symptoms that have not responded to treatment should also prompt examination [15].

If a woman is at low risk of STIs and declines examination, she could be treated based on history, using the presence of itch or malodour as a guide, but this is inevitably flawed as self-diagnosis is not reliable, BV can co-exist with STIs and BV can be due to a retained foreign body such as a tampon or condom – this should be discussed with the woman. Any woman who is managed in this way should return if symptoms persist/recur, with a view to examination at the next consultation.

Consent for examination, including speculum assessment and bimanual examination if indicated (e.g. when there are symptoms indicating pathology of the upper genital tract), along with the types of tests taken, should be sought, and received, checking if the woman has had an internal examination in the past. Offer a chaperone and document acceptance or refusal.

Examination should include:

- assessment of external genitalia anatomy/ architecture, skin changes or excoriation. Lichen sclerosus, lichen planus, eczema, lichen simplex, including contact dermatitis, psoriasis and vulval intraepithelial neoplasia can all give genital symptoms, including discomfort and itch
- presence of discharge/blood at introitus and possibly pH testing of discharge
- inspection of the vaginal walls and cervix and any foreign body.

Endocervical or vulvovaginal sampling for gonorrhoea and chlamydia can be taken. High vaginal swabs should be taken from the vaginal walls for *Candida*, and the posterior fornix for BV and TV. Urine testing and pregnancy testing may be appropriate based on history. HIV and syphilis testing completes the package of STI testing, with testing for hepatitis B and C in addition based on blood-borne virus risk assessment.

The newer NAAT tests for gonorrhoea and chlamydia do not need incubation and once taken can last for 30 days. Getting samples to the laboratory quickly is therefore not an issue, and swabs can be taken on a Friday evening without any concern that the weekend's delay will impact on results. There is increasing availability of NAAT testing for TV, with some laboratories testing for gonorrhoea, chlamydia and trichomonas on the same sample.

In the case of Emma, a sexual history must be part of the assessment, but as she is under 25, she already falls into a higher-risk group for STIs. She should be examined with tests taken for infective causes, both STI and non-STI. Use of narrow-range pH paper can guide management at the time of the consultation while waiting for test results.

Management

Management depends on presentation. Treatment may be offered based on symptoms while waiting for test results. It is important to agree how and when results will be given. Use of bland emollients as a soap substitute and moisturiser is useful advice for most women with altered vaginal discharge. She could avoid potential irritants in toiletries, antiseptics, wipes and products marketed for feminine hygiene and avoid washing underwear in biological washing powder and fabric conditioners. There is insufficient evidence to recommend the use of tea tree oil [7]. Written information to support discussion is a helpful guide to ongoing self-care.

Conclusion

The commonest causes of altered vaginal discharge in women of reproductive age are physiological, BV and *Candida*, but other causes must be considered.

Sexual history and risk assessment should form part of the consultation. A low threshold for examination is encouraged, especially in those at higher risk of STIs and those with recurrent or persisting symptoms. Most cases can be managed in primary care, as a careful history and genital examination help make the diagnosis in most cases.

Patient Information

www.nhs.uk/conditions/thrush-in-men-and-women. Accessed: Feb. 2024.

Bacterial vaginosis – patient information leaflet: https://www.bashh.org/_userfiles/pages/files/resources/bv_pil_screen_edit.pdf. Accessed: Feb. 2024.

Trichomonas vaginalis – patient information leaflet: https://www.bashh.org/_userfiles/pages/files/resources/tv_pil_mobilepdf_04.pdf. Accessed: Feb. 2024.

Training for Clinicians

- Diploma of the College of Sexual and Reproductive Health (DCSRH). This is open to a variety of healthcare professionals in the UK and Ireland. Most of the learning can be carried out remotely and the applicant will be supported by a trainer. https://www.cosrh.org/Public/Public/Education-and-Training/diploma.aspx.
- Sexual and Reproductive Healthcare eLearning. This has been developed by the CoSRH in partnership with Health Education for England and is hosted on the eLearning for health (eLFH) website. https://www.elfh.org.uk/programmes/sexual-and-reproductive-healthcare/.<ie,129.180>
- British Association for Sexual Health and HIV STI Foundation (STIF) course and competency framework. – with a focus on management of STIs. This course is available at a variety of levels, depending on previous experience and education. www.stif.org.uk (all accessed 5 Mar. 2024).

References

[1] NICE CKS, 'Vaginal discharge'. Jan. 2019. Accessed: 23 Feb. 2024. [Online]. Available: https://cks.nice.org.uk/topics/vaginal-discharge.

[2] British Association for Sexual Health and HIV, 'UK national guideline for the management of bacterial vaginosis'. 2012. Accessed: 23 Feb. 2024. [Online]. Available: https://www.bashh.org/resources/21/bacterial_vaginosis_2012/.

[3] CoSRH, 'FSRH Clinical Guideline: Intrauterine contraception'. Jul. 2023. Accessed: 23 Feb. 2024. [Online]. Available: https://www.cosrh.org/Public/Documents/ceu-guidance-intrauterine-contraception.aspx.

[4] NICE CKS, 'Bacterial vaginosis'. Jul. 2023. Accessed: 23 Feb. 2024. [Online]. Available: https://cks.nice.org.uk/topics/bacterial-vaginosis.

[5] C. A. Muzny and J. D. Sobel, 'Understanding and preventing recurring bacterial vaginosis: Important considerations for clinicians', *Int J Womens Health*, vol. **15**, pp. 1317–1325, 2023.

[6] M. S. Coudray and P. Madhivanan, 'Bacterial vaginosis: A brief synopsis of the literature', *Eur J Obstet Gynecol Reprod Biol*, vol. **245**, pp. 143–148, 2020.

[7] British Association for Sexual Health and HIV, 'British Association for Sexual Health and HIV national guideline for the management of vulvovaginal candidiasis'. 2019. Accessed: 23 Feb. 2024. [Online]. Available: https://www.bashh.org/resources/22/vulvovaginal_candidiasis_2019/.

[8] NICE CKS, '*Candida* – female genital'. Oct. 2023. Accessed: 23 Feb. 2024. [Online]. Available: https://cks.nice.org.uk/topics/candida-female-genital.

[9] D. G. Ferris, C. Dekle and M. S. Litaker, 'Women's use of over-the-counter antifungal medications for gynecologic symptoms', *J Fam Pract*, vol. **42**, no. 6, pp. 595–600, 1996.

[10] J. McLellan, C. Heneghan, N. Roberts et al., 'Accuracy of self-diagnosis in conditions commonly managed in primary care: Diagnostic accuracy systematic review and meta-analysis', *BMJ Open*, vol. **13**, no. 1, e065748, 2023.

[11] RCGP/BASHH, 'Sexually transmitted infections in primary care'. 2013. Accessed: 23 Feb. 2024. [Online]. Available: https://www.bashh.org/_userfiles/pages/files/sexuallytransmittedinfectionsinprimarycare2013.pdf.

[12] NICE CKS, 'Trichomoniasis'. Nov. 2023. Accessed: 23 Feb. 2024. [Online]. Available: https://cks.nice.org.uk/topics/trichomoniasis.

[13] S. C. Masha, P. Cools, E. J. Sanders et al., '*Trichomonas vaginalis* and HIV infection acquisition: A systematic review and meta-analysis', *Sex Transm Infect*, vol. **95**, no. 1, pp. 36–42, 2019.

[14] British Association for Sexual Health and HIV, 'British Association for Sexual Health and HIV national guideline for the management of infection with Mycoplasma genitalium'. 2018. Accessed: 23 Feb. 2024. [Online]. Available: https://www.bashh.org/resources/19/mycoplasma_genitalium_2025/.

[15] British Association for Sexual Health and HIV, '2019 UK National Guideline for consultations requiring sexual history taking: Clinical effectiveness group British association for sexual health and HIV'. 2019. Accessed: 23 Feb. 2024. [Online]. Available: https://www.bashh.org/resources/38/sexual_history_taking_2019/.

[16] https://www.acog.org/news/news-releases/2025/10/acog-recommends-concurrent-sexual-partner-treatment-recurrent-bacterial-vaginosis-first-time#:~:text=Washington%2C%20D.C.%20%E2%80%94%20New%20guidance%20from,occurrence%20of%20symptomatic%20bacterial%20vaginosis.

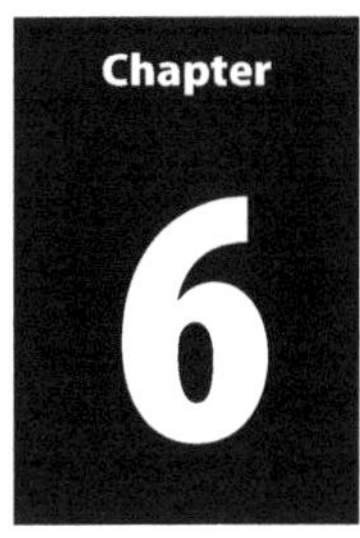

Sexually Transmitted Infections Managed in Primary Care

Richard Ma

Key Points

- Sexually transmitted infections (STIs) can be bacterial, viral, protozoal or due to infestations.
- Resistance patterns, latency and human sexual behaviour contribute to the prevalence of STIs.
- Diagnosis or suspicion of one STI should make us consider others, including blood-borne viruses such as HIV and hepatitis B and C.
- Newer technologies such as nuclear acid amplification techniques (NAATs) increase sensitivity and specificity and allow less invasive testing.
- STIs can explain common primary care symptoms, such as dysuria, pruritus, rash and abnormal vaginal bleeding.
- A sexual history will help to assess STI risk and inform appropriate examination and investigations.
- A sexual history should be taken sensitively, without judgement.
- Consider how sexual history-taking, STI and HIV testing could be part of routine clinical care in your setting.
- Treatment as Prevention (TasP) for those with HIV, and Pre-Exposure Prophylaxis (PrEP) for those who do not have HIV, can reduce the risk of onward transmission and acquisition of HIV, respectively.

Epidemiology of Sexually Transmitted Infections

According to the UK Health Security Agency (UKHSA, formerly Public Health England), there were 364,750 diagnoses of STIs in England in 2024; a decrease of 8.8% compared to 2023. Cases of chlamydia and gonorrhoea decreased from 2023 to 2024 and are now similar to pre-pandemic levels.

STIs can cause anxiety and embarrassment, as well as risking onward transmission to sexual partners. Left untreated, some STIs can have long-term complications such as pelvic infections, arthritis, dementia, epididymo-orchitis, sub-fertility and neonatal infections. Long-term untreated HIV and hepatitis can cause malignancy and be life-limiting.

STIs can be transmitted horizontally (through condomless sexual intercourse) and vertically (maternal–fetal transmission). Most do not survive long in vitro and their inefficient transmission means they require close bodily contact to do so, yet STI transmission continues. This is probably explained by three factors: latency, resistance and human sexual behaviour.

Infections such as herpes, genital warts and HIV have long latent periods before symptoms develop. The longer the latency, the longer the potential infectivity, so early access to testing, diagnosis and treatment might reduce STI transmission. People often cite confidentiality concerns as a reason for late presentation.

Some STIs are resistant to some treatments; HIV has different resistance patterns that respond to different anti-retroviral therapies (ARTs) and co-infection with more than one strain of HIV can make effective treatment difficult. The UK is now seeing cases of gonorrhoea that are resistant to common first-line antibiotics. This demonstrates the importance of antibiotic stewardship.

STIs do not always present with genital symptoms; extragenital sites such as skin, eyes, brain and joints may be affected. For example, syphilis can present acutely with genital ulcers, but at later stages presents with dermatological (rash), cardiovascular (aortitis) and cerebral (dementia) manifestations. Reiter's syndrome – now known as sexually acquired reactive arthritis (SARA) – presents with arthritis, conjunctivitis and urethritis, and can be caused by an STI; the commonest association is with chlamydia, identified in up to two-thirds of cases.

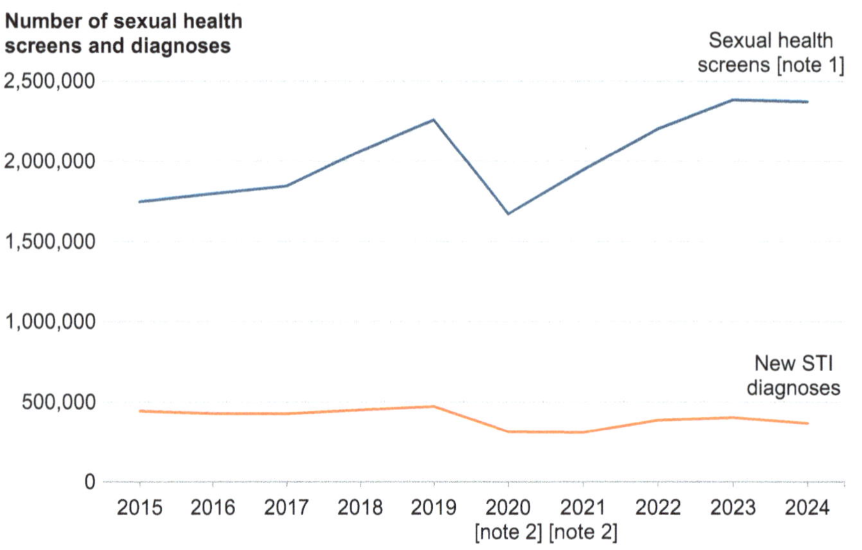

Figure 6.1 Number of sexual health screens and STI diagnoses, 2015 – 2024.

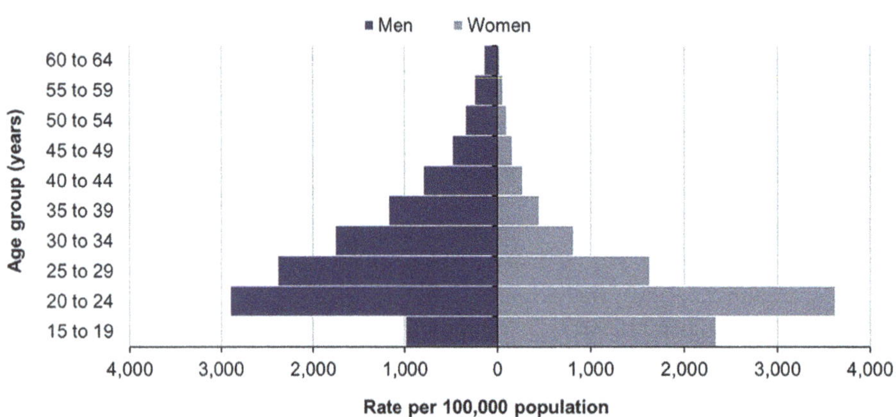

Figure 6.2 Rates of new STI diagnoses by gender and age group: England, 2022.

Sexual Behaviour and STI Transmission

Human sexual behaviour facilitates STI transmission; for this reason, opportunistic health promotion and prevention advice should be offered routinely in sexual health consultations. Increased diagnoses over time might also be explained by changes in sexual behaviour and partnerships, resulting in more opportunities for sex. According to the third British National Survey of Sexual Attitudes and Lifestyles (NATSAL-3), young people aged between 16 and 24 were most likely to report two or more sexual partners of the opposite sex in the past year; the average number of opposite-sex partners has increased among people aged 16–44 in the last three decades (Figure 6.3) [2,3,4,5]. NATSAL is among the largest surveys of sexual behaviour in the world; as of January 2026, the fourth survey has not yet been published.

Managing STIs: Basic Principles

STIs can be broadly divided by their causative organism: bacterial, protozoal, viral and infestations. Table 6.1 lists common STIs and their infective agents. Table 6.2 is a summary of their clinical manifestations, diagnosis and treatment and refers

Table 6.1 Classification of sexually transmitted infections

Organism	Infective agent	Condition
Bacterial	*Neisseria gonorrhoeae*	Gonorrhoea
	Chlamydia trachomatis	Chlamydia
	Treponema pallidum	Syphilis
	Mycoplasma genitalium	Mycoplasma
Protozoal	*Trichomonas vaginalis*	Trichomoniasis
Viral	Herpes simplex 1 and 2	Herpes
	Human immunodeficiency virus	HIV/AIDS
	Hepatitis A virus HAV, hepatitis B virus HBV, hepatitis C virus HCV	Hepatitis A, B and C, respectively
	Human papilloma virus (types 6 and 11)	Genital warts
	Molluscum contagiosum virus	Molluscum contagiosum
Infestations	*Sarcoptes scabiei*	Scabies
	Phthirus pubis	Pubic lice

This is the third Natsal survey that has been carried out in Britain: the first survey was undertaken in 1990–1991 and the second survey in 1999–2001.

Over the 1990s, we saw an increase in the number of opposite-sex partners people reported, and more people reporting same-sex experience. Over the last decade, we have only seen further increases for women, so the gender gap is narrowing.

Average (mean) number of opposite-sex partners, lifetime (people aged 16–44)

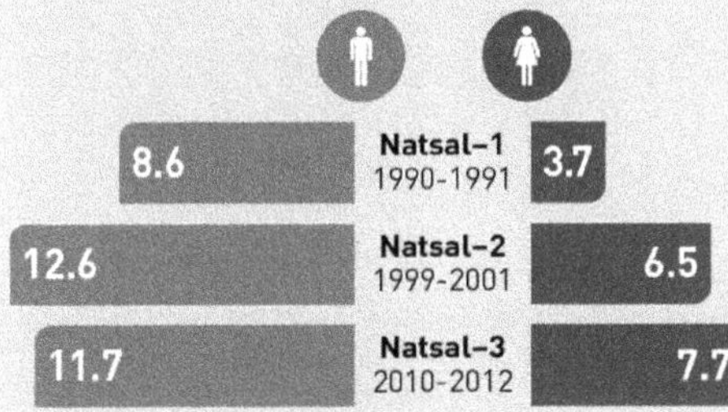

Figure 6.3 Results of the British National Survey of Sexual Attitudes and Lifestyles (NATSAL) surveys, 1–3.

to clinical guidelines from the British Association for Sexual Health and HIV (BASHH) [6].

NAATs are much more sensitive and specific than tests which use microscopy and culture. Sampling can be less invasive and more acceptable for patients; for example, a urine test from men or self-taken vulvovaginal swab from women. Other NAATs available include those for herpes virus, trichomonas and syphilis (*Treponema pallidum*). For all STIs, prompt diagnosis and treatment (sometimes empirical treatment before microbiological results are available) are needed to reduce infectiousness. Partner notification and safer sex advice reduce onward transmission and reinfection.

There has been interest in *Mycoplasma genitalium* recently. Although it is strongly associated with non-gonococcal urethritis (NGU), the majority of people with *M. genitalium* in the genital tract do not develop disease. There is some association between *M. genitalium* infection in women with postcoital bleeding and cervicitis, endometritis and pelvic inflammatory disease (PID) [7].

Case History 6.1: Pelvic Pain

Annabelle is a 24-year-old woman who presents to you with lower abdominal pain, pain on having sex and abnormal vaginal discharge. She had an intrauterine device (IUD) fitted three weeks ago on day three of her normal menstrual cycle. She was using condoms until the IUD was fitted.

What differential diagnoses will you consider?

Differentials include malposition of the IUD, PID, chlamydia, constipation and ectopic pregnancy. A sexual history will help to narrow these down.

She is unlikely to be pregnant (ectopic or otherwise) if she had a copper IUD fitted at day three of her normal menstrual cycle, but a pregnancy test is still sensible.

She is under 25, sexually active and has recently had an IUD fitted. Abnormal vaginal discharge and dyspareunia should alert you to a possible acute

Table 6.2 Summary of sexually transmitted infections

Infection	Symptoms and signs	Diagnosis	Treatment	Comments
Chlamydia	Asymptomatic in 80% of women. Abnormal vaginal discharge/bleeding. Dysuria. Pelvic pain Rectal and pharyngeal infections can be asymptomatic.	First catch urine (FCU) for men. Vulvovaginal swab (VVS) for women. Endocervical swabs are less sensitive than VVS. Tests from extragenital sites as indicated by sexual history – check what tests are available locally.	Doxycycline 100 mg BD 7/7 OR Azithromycin 1 g stat then 500 mg OD for 2/7 OR Erythromycin 500 mg BD 10–14/7 OR Ofloxacin 200 mg BD or 400 mg OD 7 days.	Partner notification. Abstain from sex during treatment and until partner(s) treated (and for 7 days after treatment if azithromycin is used). Rule out other STIs. Follow-up HIV test in 3 months. Use of fluroquinolones is associated with serious side effects including tendonitis or tendon rupture, muscle pain/ weakness, joint pain/swelling, peripheral neuropathy, and CNS/psychiatric effects. Consider carefully causative organisms, antimicrobial resistance factors and availability of alternative agents [20].
Gonorrhoea	Penile discharge/dysuria in over 90%. Abnormal vaginal discharge or dysuria. Pelvic pain. Rectal infections may cause anal discharge and pain or be asymptomatic. Pharyngeal infections are mostly asymptomatic.	NAAT as for chlamydia; many laboratories now test the same sample for both. Rectal and pharyngeal sites – check with local laboratory for tests. NAATs are more sensitive (>95%) than culture especially for oropharyngeal and rectal sites.	Ceftriaxone 500 mg IM stat if antimicrobial susceptibility not known or treat as per sensitivities if known.	As above. Refer to sexual health clinic for treatment, sensitivities and partner notification.
Mycoplasma	Usually asymptomatic in males and females. Males – discharge, dysuria and urethritis. Females – dysuria, cervicitis, postcoital bleeding, lower abdominal pain.	FCU in men, VVS in women, both sent for NAAT. Testing is recommended only for those with NGU, PID, cervicitis, postcoital bleeding, epididymitis and sexually acquired proctitis, and sexual partners. It is usually not available in primary care.	Doxycycline 100mg bd po 7/7 then EITHER azithromycin 1g po stat and 500mg po for 2/7, OR moxifloxacin 400mg po od 7/7. For complicated urogenital infection (PID, epididymo-orchitis) Moxifloxacin 400 mg orally OD for 14/7.	Only current partner(s) should be tested and treated if positive.
Trichomoniasis	Females – abnormal vaginal discharge, vulval soreness. Male – usually asymptomatic, but can cause urethral discharge and/or dysuria.	Microscopy and culture using specific culture medium. Some laboratories offer NAAT.	Metronidazole 400–500 mg PO BD 7/7 OR Metronidazole 2 g PO stat.	Partner notification. Abstain from sex during treatment and until partner(s) treated.
Syphilis	Primary syphilis: genital ulcer – can be sore or painless. Inguinal lymphadenopathy.	Dark ground microscopy of material from ulcer. Some laboratories offer NAAT of ulcer swab.	Benzathine penicillin G 2.4 MU IM stat OR Doxycycline 100 mg po BD 14–28 days OR	Refer to sexual health clinic for Treponemal tests remain positive for life so ask about previous treatment if a test is positive in primary care.

	Secondary syphilis: palmar/plantar rash, mucous patches, condylomata lata. Tertiary syphilis: aortitis, dementia.	Serology. This includes an antibody and/or enzyme immunoassay test for screening, then rapid plasma reagin (RPR) to assess disease activity or reinfection.	Ceftriaxone 500 mg IM daily for 10 days.	
Molluscum	Usually STI in adults. Small papules with central umbilication.	Clinical diagnosis	Expectant treatment; usually resolves in 12–18 months. Cryotherapy with liquid nitrogen or podophyllotoxin 0.5% could be used. Avoid squeezing molluscum spots as central plug carries the virus and can spread through auto-inoculation.	Rule out other STIs. Partner notification unnecessary.
Genital warts	Caused by HPV types 6 and 11, not caused by types 16 and 18 which cause cervical cancer. Perianal lesions common in both sexes even without history of anal sex.	Clinical diagnosis.	Cryotherapy. Podophyllotoxin. Imiquimod.	Rule out other STIs. Partner notification unnecessary unless reassurance about infectiousness and transmission is wanted.
Genital herpes	Painful genital ulcer, blisters or fissures. Febrile illness, dysuria and frequency. Inguinal lymphadenopathy. Majority of infections in adults are due to HSV-1. Prior infection with HSV-1 makes clinical manifestation of HSV-2 less severe. Recurrence rate for HSV-2 is four times that of HSV-1.	Swab ulcer for NAAT. Serology not helpful as sensitivity and specificity low and may not be related to recent symptoms.	Best started within 5 days of start of episode Preferred regimens: Aciclovir 400 mg TDS OR Valaciclovir 500 mg BD Alternative regimens: Aciclovir 200 mg 5× a day OR Famciclovir 250 mg TDS. All 5-day treatment and reduce severity and duration of episodes.	Rule out other STIs. Partner notification useful to reassure about infectiousness and transmission.
Scabies	Itching (worse at night and due to delayed sensitivity reaction, mite secretions and eggs) especially in finger webs, sides of fingers, axillary folds, wrists, penis and scrotum, buttocks and back of feet.	Clinical diagnosis – burrows in finger webs and wrists. Burrow ink test – apply black or blue ink to suspected papule and wipe off with alcohol to remove ink. A dark zigzagged line running across and away from lesion is a positive test.	Permethrin 5% cream, apply and wash off 8–12 hours later. Reapply after 1 week. Malathion liquid 0.5%, apply and wash off after 24 hours, reapply after 1 week. Bedding, clothing and towels used by individual, their close contacts and household should be washed at high 60°C. Post-scabies itch can continue up to 2 weeks after treatment. Treat with crotamiton 10%.	Rule out other STIs. Partner notification to check if has same symptoms. Repeated treatment causes skin irritation. Itch and rash improve within 2–4 weeks in most cases. In a third of individuals, itch can persist for between 4 weeks and 3 months.
Pubic lice	Itching in pubic area. Sometimes asymptomatic.	Clinical diagnosis. Adult lice can be visible to naked eye on hairs in pubic area and body hair.	Permethrin 1%, apply to damp hair and wash after 10 minutes. Malathion 0.5%. apply to dry hair and leave for 2–12 hours/overnight.	Rule out other STIs. Partner notification to check if has same symptoms.

infection, such as an STI, endometritis or pelvic infection. She had an STI check prior to the IUD fitting, which was normal, and she has had no recent change in sexual partners, so an acute STI such as chlamydia would be unlikely. A history excludes constipation as a cause.

Annabelle is apyrexial, her BP is 110/80 and the pulse rate is 70, regular. You note cervical excitation and left adnexal tenderness. Speculum examination revealed IUD threads of the expected length with white cervical discharge.

What would you include in your immediate management for Annabelle?

A diagnosis of PID seems likely from the history and examination. You should offer her antibiotics; the treatment regimen needs to cover chlamydia, anaerobes and gonorrhoea, which are possible causes. BASHH recommends the following [8]:

- Ceftriaxone 1,000 mg IM stat + doxycycline 100 mg BD PO 14/7 + metronidazole 400 mg BD PO 14/7 or
- Ofloxacin 400 mg BD PO 14/7 and metronidazole 400 mg BD PO 14/7.

Partner notification (including partner STI check) and abstinence from sex during treatment minimises reinfection risk. BASHH recommends follow-up at 72 hours, particularly if there are moderate or severe signs, and that a review at 2–4 weeks may be useful to ensure that symptoms have resolved and partner notification is complete.

There is no need to remove the IUD if the PID is adequately treated and her symptoms improve [9]. An ultrasound scan may be useful if you suspect malposition or migration of IUD, but this is unlikely if the threads are of the expected length.

Annabelle wants to know about the risk of infertility with PID. What would you tell her?

Chlamydia can cause PID as well as sub-fertility due to tubal scarring. However, the risks are minimised by prompt treatment, effective partner notification and use of barrier contraception to reduce future episodes. PID can occur in anyone of the female sex, whatever their gender identity; it should also be considered in a trans man with similar symptoms who uses a levonorgestrel IUD to cause amenorrhoea.

Case History 6.2: Genital Sores

Viktoria is a married 27-year-old woman. She presents to you with what she describes as 'painful lumps' on the labia for a couple of days.

What could she be describing?

It is often difficult to ascertain the diagnosis purely by the description, particularly in the early

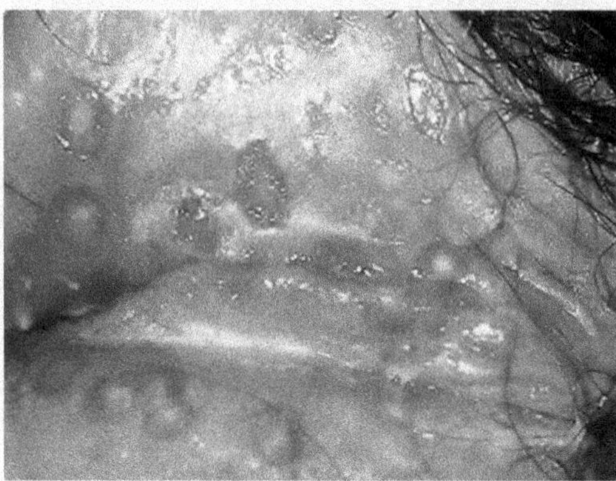

Figure 6.4 Herpes genitalis – female.

stages of infection. Genital warts and molluscum might be described as 'lumps' or 'a rash', but they are not usually painful. The description might also include herpetic blisters (Figure 6.2) or hair follicle infection or inflammation. Scabies infestation induces a hypersensitivity reaction and can present with itchy red genital papules. A sexual history and examination are needed for the diagnosis.

Viktoria has been married for two years and she has had three long-term partners. She has had one normal STI test in the past and she believes that she is at low risk of STIs. On examination, she has a small crop of blisters on the left labia majora and a couple of small ulcers. The left inguinal nodes are swollen.

What is the most likely diagnosis? What test would you do?

Herpes is best diagnosed by viral culture or NAAT of fluid from blisters/ulcers. Some laboratories also offer NAAT test for suspected syphilitic ulcers. Herpes swabs are often unavailable in primary care; suspected acute genital herpes will usually be seen on the same day in a sexual health clinic. A generic skin swab for microscopy, culture and sensitivities (MC&S) will not detect syphilis or herpes. Molluscum contagiosum usually presents with painless blisters with clear fluid and central umbilication; it can only be diagnosed clinically, but this presentation does not sound like molluscum.

Primary syphilis can be diagnosed using a swab from the ulcer sent either for NAAT testing or dark ground microscopy; the latter can only be done in sexual health clinics. Treatment for syphilis requires intramuscular injection of antibiotics and follow-up of blood markers; the patient should be referred to a sexual health clinic for treatment and follow-up if this is the suspected diagnosis.

There are two types of herpes viruses: HSV-1 and HSV-2. Not all cases of oro-labial herpes are caused by HSV-1 and not all cases of genital herpes are caused by HSV-2. Herpes virus is transmitted by close physical contact and the virus can be shed sporadically between outbreaks. Not everyone will have symptoms when they first acquire herpes and there is a long latency from exposure to symptoms; 80% of people with positive HSV serology are unaware that they have been infected. If symptoms occur, the first episode is usually more severe, becoming milder with subsequent outbreaks. Serology for HSV is type-specific and needs careful interpretation; sensitivity and specificity are both low. Antibody detection is not a reliable indicator of recent infection and may be from past asymptomatic infection. Oral antivirals should be given at the early stages of symptoms or if new blisters are still forming.

BASHH guidelines recommend any of the following regimens [10]:

- Aciclovir 200 mg five times a day PO or 400mg three times a day PO, both for five days.
- Valaciclovir 500 mg BD PO for five days.
- Famciclovir 250 mg TDS PO for five days.

Condoms might stop transmission between serodifferent partners. Asymptomatic shedding is more likely in the first 12 months after infection and is more common with HSV-2 than HSV-1. The Herpes Virus Association [11] produces useful information on how to explain and reassure people what this means for future sexual relations and pregnancy.

Case History 6.3: Fever, Tiredness and Rash

Mary is a 28-year-old woman who returned from Tanzania four weeks ago; she presents with low-grade fever, rash, jaundice and tiredness. She had malaria prophylaxis before her four-week trip to see family. She already had hepatitis A and typhoid injections five years ago.

What differential diagnoses might you consider?

Mary might be at risk of malaria and hepatitis A, despite travel vaccinations and malaria prophylaxis. Glandular fever, caused by the Epstein–Barr virus, can be a cause of flu-like illness and abnormal liver function tests. She may be at risk of hepatitis B and HIV – both have similar routes of infection.

Why would you raise the issue of HIV testing on this occasion?

Acute hepatitis could cause fever, jaundice and tiredness, whereas acute HIV infection might present with fever, flu-like illness and a rash. Some people might have none of these symptoms. HIV is prevalent in the adult population in sub-Saharan countries such as Tanzania; check if she or her partner have been at risk of exposure, through sexual contact, medical treatment or other risks such as tattoos. HIV and hepatitis B can both be transmitted sexually and through blood products. If your patient was born and grew up in a country where HIV is prevalent, offer them an HIV test if you suspect that they might be at risk [12].

You might feel that her symptoms suggest malaria and refer her urgently to your local hospital; many cases of acute HIV infection have been missed because other conditions were suspected, and HIV was not thought of [13]. If referring, consider testing for HIV as well; it may not be done in secondary care.

What might be the barriers to raising the issue of HIV testing on this occasion?

Asking about HIV risk and recommending testing should be done sensitively. Patients can be surprised or even offended by the suggestion. You might pre-empt such reactions by explaining why you are going to ask.

The following suggestions are taken from *HIV in Primary Care* published by Medfash [14]:

- You might be describing a common illness caused by viruses such as glandular fever or influenza. Some rare but important viruses may also be a cause, and this includes HIV. I am not sure if you might be at risk of HIV?
- I am not sure if you might be at risk of HIV, but this is one infection that can affect your immune system and give you these symptoms. May I ask you some questions to check if you could be at risk?
- You have travelled to/come from/grew up in a county where HIV is quite common. Do you know anyone who has been affected by HIV?

Reassure the patient about confidentiality; you should adhere to General Medical Council (GMC) guidance on confidentiality and when this can be breached, especially with respect to serious communicable diseases such as HIV, hepatitis and tuberculosis.

Life insurance has been available to people with HIV since 2009. The Association of British Insurers advise that GPs are required to inform insurers only if an applicant is HIV positive or has any STIs with long-term health implications. Insurance reports usually also ask if the results of any tests are awaited – this would include HIV. GPs are not required to notify insurers of negative HIV tests or any single episode of minor STIs. There are now travel and life assurance policies available for people with HIV who are stable on medications [15,16].

The most recent guideline on HIV testing from BASHH and the British HIV Association (BHIVA) [17] states that the only purpose of the pretest discussion is to establish informed consent and how the results would be communicated; a lengthy discussion is not necessary. However, a discussion might include:

- benefits of HIV testing
- what 'positive' or 'negative' test results mean
- if the test is negative, how they can continue to take steps to avoid HIV.

For somebody who might be at risk of HIV, or if you see someone who has a new diagnosis, you might wish to include in your discussion:

- HIV treatment is effective and will stop them from getting ill.
- They can take steps to prevent onward transmission.
- People with HIV can have healthy children if their HIV status is known early on in pregnancy.
- They will have more control over disclosing their status than if they find out while very ill with HIV infection.
- For people whose first language is not English, try saying 'your test result has come back and is HIV-positive, this means you have HIV', rather than saying your test is 'positive' which might be interpreted as 'good news'.

It is clearly devastating for someone to receive a positive HIV test result. They might have questions they wish to ask you, similar to anyone diagnosed with a life-threatening condition. However, there might be an extra dimension because of the infectious nature. Questions might include:

- What is going to happen to me?
- Do I need treatment?
- Can this be cured?
- What should I tell my current/future partners?
- My partner does not have HIV – will they catch it from me? How can I prevent this? Can they sue me if they catch HIV from me?
- Can I have a baby?
- Do I have to tell my employers? Will they sack me?

People who are diagnosed with HIV are offered antiretroviral therapy (ART) as soon as possible. This reduces the amount of virus in the body to a level that it cannot be detected using HIV viral load assays. When someone has an undetectable HIV viral load, they cannot pass on HIV to sexual partners during condomless sex ('U = U', Undetectable = Untransmissible). Starting ART soon after diagnosis therefore helps to prevent onward transmission of HIV; this is referred to as TasP [14]. People who do not have HIV but are at risk of acquiring it can be given PrEP from a sexual health clinic to protect themselves against HIV [18].

A number of charities offer advice, information, counselling and support for those who are newly diagnosed and want more information. These charities and HIV clinics encourage people with HIV to register with a GP.

- Terrence Higgins Trust: www.tht.org.uk.
- National AIDS Trust: www.nat.org.uk.
- Positively UK: www.positivelyuk.org.
- National AIDS Manual (NAM): www.aidsmap.com.

Many people diagnosed with HIV now will lead healthy normal lives with normal life expectancies because of highly effective ART. As people with HIV live longer, they may develop long-term conditions and have other primary care health needs related to ageing. The BHIVA Standards of Care for People Living with HIV specifically mention the contribution of general practice in the care of people living with HIV [19] and as GPs we may be able to offer or access the following:

- social welfare support
- psychological support
- contraception and preconceptual advice
- health promotion such as lifestyle advice
- cervical screening – women with HIV need annual screening, even if the tests remain normal
- health protection such as influenza and pneumococcal vaccinations.

Conclusions

STIs are common and some can be diagnosed and treated in primary care. Symptoms of some STIs can overlap with other conditions, so it is important to assess risk by considering factors such as age, lifestyle and sexual behaviour through sensitive sexual history-taking.

Although many STIs are easily treated, some have long-term implications for a person's current and future relationships, as well as other aspects of their lives. Through better awareness, we can equip ourselves with the skills and knowledge to support our patients, so that dealing with sexual health issues feels less like 'opening a can of worms'.

References

[1] UKHSA, 'Sexually transmitted infections and screening for chlamydia in England: 2022 report'. Oct. 2023. Accessed: 23 Sep. 2024. [Online]. Available: https://www.gov.uk/government/statistics/sexually-transmitted-infections-stis-annual-data-tables/sexually-transmitted-infections-and-screening-for-chlamydia-in-england-2024-report.

[2] The National Survey of Sexual Attitudes and Lifestyles (NATSAL). Accessed: 23 Sep. 2024. [Online]. Available: www.natsal.ac.uk.

[3] A. M. Johnson, C. G. Mercer, B. Erens et al., 'Sexual behaviour in Britain: Partnerships, practices, and HIV risk behaviours', *Lancet*, vol. **358**, no. 9296, pp. 1835–1842, 2001.

[4] C. H. Mercer, K. A. Fenton, A. J. Copas et al., 'Increasing prevalence of male homosexual partnerships and practices in Britain 1990–2000: Evidence from national probability surveys', *AIDS*, vol. **18**, no. 10, pp. 1453–1458, 2004.

[5] C. H. Mercer, A. J. Copas, P. Sonnenberg et al., 'Who has sex with whom? Characteristics of heterosexual partnerships reported in a national probability survey and implications for STI risk', *Int J Epidemiol, vol.* **38**, no. 1, pp. 206–214, 2009.

[6] British Association for Sexual Health and HIV. Accessed: 23 Sep. 2024. [Online]. Available: www.bashh.org

[7] British Association for Sexual Health and HIV, 'Mycoplasma genitalium'. 2018. Accessed: 23 Sep. 2024. [Online]. Available: www.bashh.org/resources/19/mycoplasma_genitalium_2018.

[8] British Association for Sexual Health and HIV, 'PID'. 2019. Accessed: 23 Sep. 2024. [Online]. Available: www.bashh.org/resources/6/pid_2019.

[9] CoSRH, 'Intrauterine contraception'. Jul. 2023. Accessed: 23 Sep. 2024. [Online]. Available: https://www.cosrh.org/Common/Uploaded%20files/documents/fsrh-clinical-guideline-intrauterine-contraception-mar-23-amended.pdf.

[10] British Association for Sexual Health and HIV, 'Anogenital herpes'. 2014. Accessed: 23 Sep. 2024. [Online]. Available: www.bashh.org/resources/23/anogenital_herpes_2014.

[11] Herpes Virus Association. Accessed: 23 Sep. 2024. [Online]. Available: https://herpes.org.uk.

[12] NICE, 'NG60. HIV testing: Increasing uptake among people who may have undiagnosed HIV'. Dec. 2016. Accessed: 23 Sep. 2024. [Online]. Available: www.nice.org.uk/guidance/ng60.

[13] S. Ellis, H. Curtis and E. L. Ong, 'HIV diagnoses and missed opportunities: Results of the British HIV Association (BHIVA) National Audit *2010'*, *Clin Med*, vol. **12**, no. 5, pp. 430–434, 2012.

[14] S Madge, P Matthews, S Singh and N Theobald, *HIV in Primary Care*. Lowbury R, editor. 3rd ed. Medfash, 2016.

[15] Association of British Insurers, 'ABI guiding principles for HIV and life insurance'. Jul. 2016. Accessed: 23 Sep. 2024. [Online]. Available: www.abi.org.uk/globalassets/sitecore/files/documents/publications/public/2016/hiv-and-insurance/abi-guiding-principles-for-hiv-and-life-insurance-july-2016.pdf.

[16] Association of British Insurers, 'HIV and life insurance'. Jun. 2016. Accessed: 23 Sep. 2024. [Online]. Available: www.abi.org.uk/globalassets/sitecore/files/documents/publications/public/2016/hiv-and-insurance/hiv-and-insurance-guide.pdf.

[17] A. Palfreeman, A. Sullivan, M. Rayment et al., 'British HIV Association/British Association for Sexual Health and HIV/British Infection Association adult HIV testing guidelines 2020', *HIV Med*, vol. **21** (suppl. 6), pp. 1–26, 2020.

[18] British HIV Association, 'BHIVA/BASHH guidelines on the use of HIV pre-exposure prophylaxis (PrEP)'. 2018. Accessed: 23 Sep. 2024. [Online]. Available: www.bhiva.org/PrEP-guidelines.

[19] N. Phanuphak and R. M. Gulick, 'HIV treatment and prevention 2019: Current standards of care', *Curr Opin HIV AIDS*, vol. **15**, no. 1, pp. 4–12, 2020.

[20] Medicines and Healthcare Products Regulatory Agency, 'Fluoroquinolone antibiotics: Must now only be prescribed when other commonly recommended antibiotics are inappropriate'. Jan. 2024. Accessed: 23 Sep. 2024. [Online]. Available: www.gov.uk/drug-safety-update/fluoroquinolone-antibiotics-must-now-only-be-prescribed-when-other-commonly-recommended-antibiotics-are-inappropriate.

Chapter 7

Cervical Pathology in Primary Care

Halimah Alazzani and Adam N. Rosenthal

Key Points

- Human papilloma virus (HPV) infection is common, affecting most sexually active men and women in the UK. Persistence of infection can cause cervical problems.
- High-risk strains of HPV (HR-HPV), most commonly 16 and 18, cause cervical cancer; HPV immunisation should be encouraged prior to sexual activity.
- Cervical screening is important, including in women who have been immunised against HPV, as immunisation does not prevent infection with all HR-HPV types.
- Cervical screening tests in the UK are now tested for HPV; only those testing positive are examined cytologically. Tests done outside of the screening parameters (e.g. before the age of 25) will be discarded unexamined.
- Since the introduction of primary HPV screening, testing within England has been consolidated into eight labs, all of which refer directly to colposcopy when indicated.
- Cytology reports of suspected glandular neoplasia require fast-track referral; this is done directly from the screening programme but could be needed from primary care, for example a result from abroad.
- An asymptomatic cervical ectropion does not require treatment.
- Cervical screening is a test for asymptomatic women. Women with postcoital bleeding require speculum examination, consideration of sexually transmitted infections testing and possibly referral. Cervical screening can be done if due, but management should not be delayed waiting for the result.
- An abnormal appearance of the cervix requires urgent referral, on the suspected cancer pathway if appropriate, or to colposcopy if cancer is not suspected.
- Women with cervical stenosis or atrophic vaginitis can be treated with topical oestrogens to make cervical screening more comfortable and to reduce inadequate results.
- Women with postmenopausal bleeding require cervical examination, as it can be caused by cervical cancer.

Introduction

The prevalence of cervical cancer has reduced since cervical screening began in 1988 [1]; further reductions are expected due to vaccination against HPV. Many women present to primary care with postcoital bleeding or concerns about cytology results; informed decisions regarding referral and explanation of results ensure that women are managed appropriately, while reducing anxiety.

Understanding of the relevance of HPV infection and its role in the natural history of cervical neoplasia is rapidly developing.

This chapter provides an overview of how cervical anatomy changes over time and under hormonal influence, the cervical screening programme and the impact that HPV testing may have on the future of managing cervical pathology. It is important to understand that a cervical screening test is done on asymptomatic women; those with symptoms need a full clinical assessment, which should not be delayed by waiting for a screening result.

The Cervix

The cervix is a tubular structure in the vagina, at the entrance to the uterus.

The ectocervix is covered in squamous epithelium with characteristic layers maturing from the basement layer up, forming a robust outer coating. The endocervix is lined with mucus-secreting columnar epithelium, with a surface, one cell thick. The two types of epithelium meet at the squamocolumnar junction (SCJ).

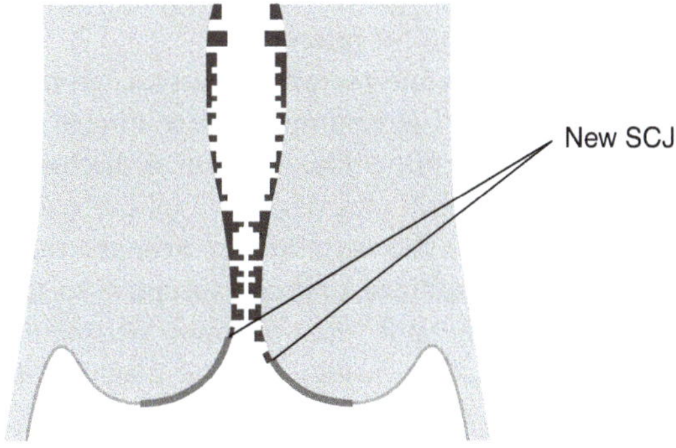

Figure 7.1 The transformation zone.

Prepubertally, the SCJ lies within the endocervical canal. Under the influence of oestrogen at puberty, the cervix everts, leaving the columnar epithelium exposed to the relatively acid vaginal environment, which promotes transformation of the columnar epithelium to squamous epithelium (metaplasia). This results in a new SCJ. The area between the original SCJ and the new SCJ is termed the transformation zone (TZ) (Figure 7.1). Most abnormalities develop in the TZ; this area should be sampled when taking a cervical screening test.

Nabothian follicles are mucus-filled cysts often seen on the cervix (Figure 7.2). They result from mucus-producing glands becoming trapped beneath squamous epithelium as a result of metaplasia. They are a normal finding, always lying within the TZ. Any nabothian follicles should be included in the sampling area when taking a cervical screening test.

Clusters of nabothian follicles can appear alarming to the naked eye. If there is any cause for concern, refer for colposcopic examination, where the characteristic appearances with normal overlying vascular pattern can be visualised and appropriate reassurance given.

Case Scenario 7.1

Ella is a 19-year-old student who is embarrassed to explain her problem when she attends surgery. She has recently started a new relationship and has noticed bleeding after each episode of sex. She wonders if she should have a smear test, even though she isn't 25 yet.

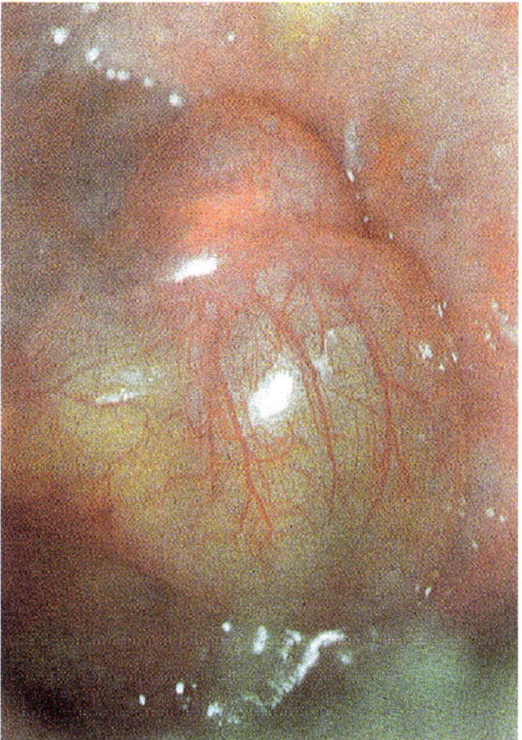

Figure 7.2 Colposcopic appearance of nabothian follicles with characteristic branching pattern of vessels overlying mucus-filled cysts.

Postcoital Bleeding and Intermenstrual Bleeding

Most women presenting with postcoital bleeding (PCB) will not have cancer [2]. Women presenting with PCB need a thorough assessment, including a speculum examination and swabs for infection, but those who are outside of the normal age for cervical screening should not have a screening test taken, as this will be refused by the laboratory. The lower age for cervical screening was moved from 20 to 25 in 2003, because the risk of cervical cancer is very low under the age of 25. Most pre-cancerous changes found in this age group will revert to normal without treatment; screening at this age risks overtreatment, with an increased risk of complications such as bleeding, and future risk of premature delivery [3,4].

Following a speculum examination, woman with a clinical suspicion of cervical cancer should be referred on the suspected cancer pathway [5]. If the cervical screening test is due and the cervix is suspicious, do not take the cervical screening test, as this could disrupt the delicate epithelium, making it harder to diagnose a cancer colposcopically.

If no cause is found with a normal looking cervix, women with persistent PCB or intermenstrual bleeding (IMB) should be referred – referral pathways will vary by area.

NICE does not recommend an ultrasound in primary care for women with IMB but rather that referral is done direct to gynaecology, with hysteroscopy as the first-line investigation; in some areas, however, pathways do not allow gynaecological referral without an initial scan being arranged by the GP [6].

Case Scenario 7.2

Examination of Ella's cervix was normal. Screening for infection demonstrated chlamydia infection, which was treated; she had no further PCB after this. She was advised that she must return for review if her PCB did not settle with treatment of the chlamydia, and this advice was documented in the notes.

Cervical Ectropion

An ectropion (Figure 7.3) describes the appearances when the columnar epithelium extends onto the ectocervix. It can become more pronounced under the influence of oestrogen and is commonly exacerbated by oestrogen-containing contraception [8].

It is a normal finding and requires no treatment, only reassurance, if asymptomatic and found incidentally. Bleeding from an ectropion is common when taking a cervical screening test and is not an indication for referral [8].

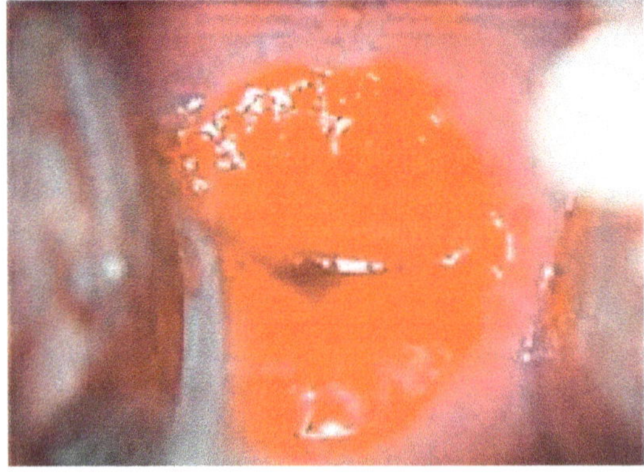

Figure 7.3 Ectropion.

The two commonest symptoms associated with an ectropion are PCB, resulting from trauma to the fragile glandular epithelium, and mucus discharge from the glands within the tissue. If applicable, and if there is diagnostic certainty in primary care, changing the combined oral contraceptive to the progestogen-only pill may resolve symptoms. Referral should be considered if the diagnosis is not certain.

Women with persistent or troublesome PCB and/or discharge who have an ectropion can be referred to gynaecology or colposcopy to be considered for cryocautery, silver nitrate application or diathermy to the cervix [8]. The risk of recurrence should be emphasised, especially in the context of exogenous hormones.

HPV Vaccination

HPV is a key driver of cervical cancer; the NHS has vaccinated against HPV since September 2008. Vaccination was initially for girls only, with a vaccine that covered the two commonest high-risk strains. In 2012, the vaccine type was changed to cover four strains, including two which cause genital warts. The programme was extended to boys in 2019 and in 2023 it was changed to a single dose of a vaccine which covers nine strains of HPV. Those not vaccinated in school can approach their GP for a vaccine up to the age of 25. Men who have sex with men should still have two doses (and can access this via a sexual health clinic up to the age of 45), and those who are immunosuppressed should have a three-dose schedule – this includes those who have HIV and are taking antiretroviral therapy [9].

The Cervical Screening Test

When performing a cervical screening test, the entire cervix must be examined, and the sampling device must be rotated through 360 degrees five times to obtain sufficient material. Only individuals registered as accredited sample-takers should take cervical screening tests. If the cervix cannot be visualised, a bimanual examination will help to identify its position, and changing the speculum size may help. Remember to use a lubricant known to be compatible with liquid-based cytology processing. Refer if you cannot visualise the entire cervix.

Tip: Sometimes, asking the supine patient to 'sit on her fists' or placing her in the left lateral position, with her knees to her chest and the speculum ratchet facing towards the anus, can help, especially if the cervix is very posterior.

Tip: Topical oestrogen therapy is useful where there is difficulty in obtaining an adequate cervical screening test due to the SCJ lying high within the endocervical canal; that is, in postmenopausal women or those using long-term progesterone therapy. The use of oestrogen treatment (or any other hormonal treatment) must be identified on the sample request form to ensure the cytologist understands the relevance of the morphological changes.

Incidental abnormalities may be seen when taking a cervical screening test – these can include cervical polyps, cervical stenosis and congenital abnormalities.

Cervical Polyps

Cervical polyps may arise from the ectocervix, endocervix or be endometrial in origin (Figure 7.4). A submucous fibroid may prolapse through the cervix and present as a polyp. Small polyps may cause IMB, PCB or increased discharge, but the majority are asymptomatic.

Cervical polyps should be removed and sent for histology if they are interfering with the ability to take a cervical screening test (i.e. it is not possible to rotate the sampling device 360 degrees within the external cervical os by a practitioner with appropriate skills), although it is acknowledged that the risk of malignancy is very small [10]. The pathway for this will vary by area – some GPs may be confident removing a polyp in primary care, otherwise this can be arranged by referral to a community clinic run by a GP with an extended role, to colposcopy or to hospital gynaecology.

No further action is required if the polyp was small and asymptomatic, and histology is normal. For a symptomatic polyp, if symptoms persist after removal, further investigations are warranted, for example an ultrasound or referral for hysteroscopy.

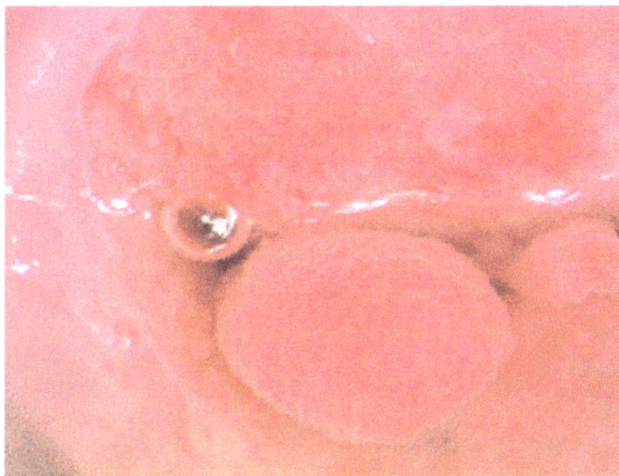

Figure 7.4 Cervical polyp.

Cervical Stenosis

Cervical stenosis may be seen in postmenopausal women or following a large loop excision of the transformation zone (LLETZ) (Figures 7.5 and 7.6). An additional endocervical sample using a small endocervical brush may be needed to get an accurate screening sample. If more than one sample is taken, both samples should be placed in the same pot.

Where cervical stenosis is complete and the women is of screening age, referral to colposcopy or gynaecology (depending on local pathways) should be considered, as an adequate sample is unlikely to be achieved in primary care. Options for women in this situation include cervical dilatation, hysterectomy or withdrawal from the screening programme. Dilatation or hysterectomy is recommended for those with previous high-grade cervical intraepithelial neoplasia (CIN), cervical glandular intraepithelial neoplasia (CGIN) or unexplained high-grade cytology.

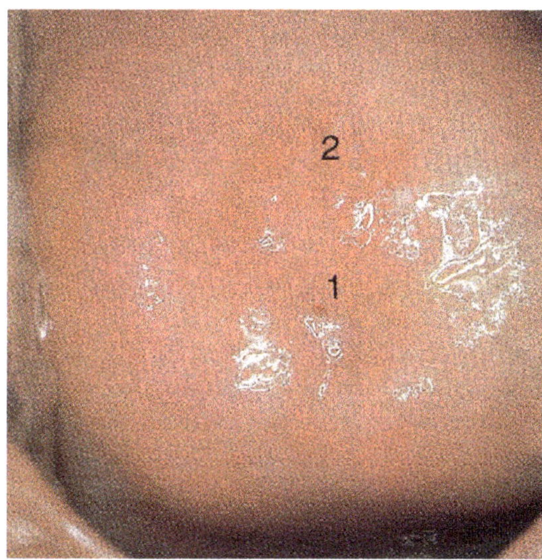

Figure 7.5 Stenosed cervix (1: cervical os; 2: transformation zone).

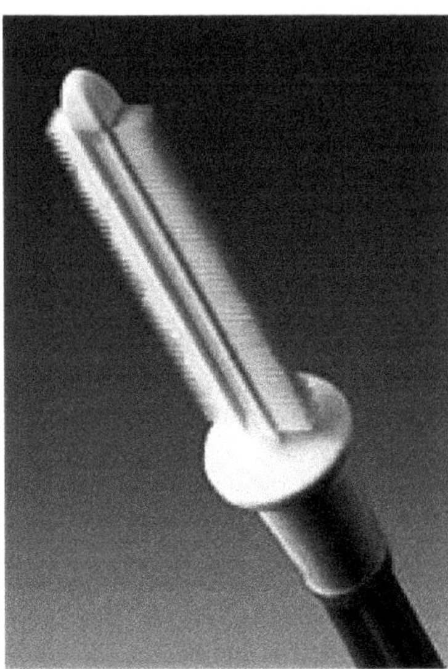

Figure 7.6 Liquid-based cytology (LBC) endocervical sampler for use with a stenosed cervix.

Congenital Anomalies

Embryologically, the cervix, along with the upper vagina, uterus and fallopian tubes, develops from bilateral paramesonephric ducts which fuse during development. Failure of fusion or incomplete fusion leads to anomalies ranging from two distinct cervices to two ossei, with a common endocervical canal. Any such anomaly, or failure to identify a cervix, should trigger investigations into the genital tract anatomy.

If there is more than one cervical os, both must be sampled when taking cytology, with the samples put in separate containers and labelled 'left cervix' and 'right cervix' [11].

The National Cervical Screening Programme

There are approximately 3,200 cases of cervical cancer registered annually in the UK, an incidence of approximately 10/100,000 women. It is the 14th commonest cancer in women in the UK and the 4th commonest worldwide [1,12].

The incidence of cervical cancer in the UK has halved since screening began in 1998; cervical screening is credited with saving 4,500 lives a year in England [11]. The discovery that HPV is the major causative agent for cervical cancer led to changes to the programme, which seem set to further decrease the incidence of cervical cancer in the UK.

Screening intervals vary by country of the UK. As of early 2026, women in England, Scotland and Wales are invited every 5 years from the age of 24.5 to 64. Women in Northern Ireland are invited every 3 years from 24.5 to 49 and then every 5 years until 64. [11,13,14,15].

Tip: Remember this may be the first time a woman has ever had a speculum examination.

The only group of women eligible for more frequent screening are those with HIV, who are invited annually and should ideally also have colposcopy at diagnosis [11]. The forms with which screening tests are sent may have a box to tick indicating that the patient has HIV and needs annual recall. If there is no such box, the practice will need to have their own recall system, to ensure that these women do not slip through the net. Other immunosuppressed women (especially those with solid organ transplants) may be similarly at increased risk but are not currently eligible under the National Cervical Screening Programme (NHSCSP) for more frequent screening. The patient's consultant may wish to discuss this on an individual basis with the local colposcopy team, as only they will be able to take cervical screening tests outside the NHSCSP.

There are no indications for early cervical screening in primary care or for additional routine cervical screening tests, and the cytology laboratories will reject samples taken outside the screening programme. If there is clinical concern, then a referral should be done along the appropriate pathway, or advice should be sought from gynaecology or colposcopy.

Primary HPV Testing

There are more than 150 variants of HPV, which are divided into two groups – high risk (HR) and low risk (LR). Persistent infection with HR-HPV is the main cause of CIN and HPV is found in 99.7% of cases of cervical cancer [16]. In the UK, the two commonest HR types are 16 and 18, but other HR strains are more prevalent in other geographical locations. The LR types 6 and 11 are associated with the development of genital warts.

Testing for HR-HPV increases sensitivity for detection of high-grade lesions. Therefore, following successful pilot studies, the NHSCSP introduced

HR-HPV testing as the primary screening test in England in December 2019, with 'reflex' cytology on samples that test positive for HPV [17]. Primary HR-HPV testing is now used in all four countries of the UK; cervical screening tests are tested for HR-HPV and only samples that test positive for HR-HPV are processed for cytological examination.

If the cytology is normal, these women will be re-screened for HPV in 12 months' time. Women whose samples test negative for HPV at that point will return to routine recall. Women with persistent HR-HPV will need a repeat test in a further 12 months, and if they remain positive for HR-HPV in three consecutive tests, they will be referred for colposcopy assessment [14,15,18,19]. Women who test positive for HR-HPV with any abnormal cytology will be referred for colposcopy assessment.

Figure 7.7 shows the primary care stages of the NHSCSP using HR-HPV as the primary test.

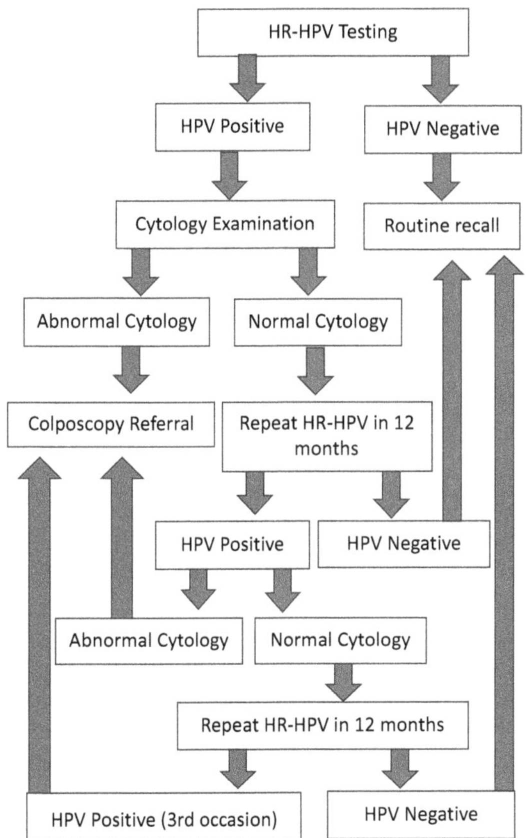

Figure 7.7 Primary stages of the NHSCSP.

Self-Swabbing for HPV

Trials have been carried out whereby women took a self-swab for HPV instead of having a screening test taken by a healthcare professional – if this was negative, they reverted to the normal screening interval [20]. Pilots using this approach for those who are late for their cervical screening are being run in some areas in 2026. It has the potential to reduce costs and to improve screening uptake rates, particularly for women who find screening traumatic, such as those with a history of sexual assault.

A woman having cervical screening must understand how she will receive her result and what will happen if the result is not normal. In England in 2022/2023, 5% of cervical screening tests showed cytological abnormality, with only 1% showing high-grade change [19].

Many women with an abnormal result are concerned that they have cancer and require reassurance. They may also have concerns about being HPV-positive even if the cytology result is negative. Women with such concerns could be signposted to information on the Cancer Research UK website [21] or local information/leaflets; a discussion might include the following information:

- HPV infection is common and transmitted via sexual contact; 80% of the world's population contracts some type of the virus at least once in their lifetime; it should not attract stigma.
- For most women, a normal immune system clears the virus within one to two years with no treatment, but some women have persistent infection for many years. Their previous sample may not have been tested for HPV, if it predated universal HPV screening.
- Women do not have to assume that their current HPV infection has been acquired from a recent sexual encounter of themselves or their partner.
- The term 'high-risk' means the woman has a strain of HPV that has been found in association with cervical cancer and not that she herself is at high risk of developing cancer.
- If the woman smokes, she should try to give up. Smoking is probably associated with a longer persistence of HPV compared with non-smokers; it certainly affects the likelihood of being diagnosed with cervical cancer, and the survival rates for those who are diagnosed [22].

Cervical Screening Tests in Pregnancy [23]

- If a routine cervical screening test is due, this should be deferred until three months after delivery.
- Repeat screening as a follow-up after a low-grade abnormality or treatment should be delayed until three months after delivery.
- Women with an abnormal screening test taken shortly before pregnancy or inadvertently in early pregnancy should have colposcopy in the late first or early second trimester, unless there is a clinical contraindication.

Cervical Screening Tests for Trans Men and Those Who Are Non-binary

Anyone who changes the gender marker on their notes to male may not be recalled under the NHSCSP (exact arrangements vary by country of the UK), but many people in this category will still have their cervix and be at risk of cervical cancer. The Royal College of General Practitioners has called for notes to have two separate markers, one for biological sex and one for gender [24], so that this cohort are not lost to follow-up for cervical screening. This is not currently possible in NHS computer systems and practices must keep a separate record of patients who have a male gender marker but still need screening. They should be recalled manually by the practice when they are due for a screening test and can also be encouraged to keep their own records and contact the practice when screening is due [25].

Withdrawal from Routine Screening [27]

Women may withdraw from the screening programme in writing. There are many reasons why women may choose to withdraw, including the following:

- Women who have never had intimate contact with another person.
- Women who have a terminal illness.
- Women who lack capacity and may find the procedure of taking a cervical screening test distressing. Each woman needs to be considered according to her personal needs; any decision to withdraw should be reconsidered if risk factors and capacity change. Information is available to support professionals, patients and carers in this situation [26].
- Some women choose to withdraw from the screening programme for no clear reason – they must be provided with sufficient information to ensure that this decision is fully informed. A woman who has done this may be reinstated to the programme at her request at any time up to the age of 64.

Ceasing Screening

Screening ceases at the age of 64 unless the woman has not been screened since age 50 or she is due for follow-up after an abnormal cervical screening test. This means that someone who has a normal test after the age of 60 will not be recalled again, as their next test would be after their 65th birthday [28].

Colposcopy

Colposcopy is the examination of the cervix using a magnification system. Colposcopy services in the UK are governed by the British Society for Colposcopy and Cervical Cytology (BSCCP) [23]; practising colposcopists must achieve and retain BSCCP certification.

Indications for Colposcopy [29]

All eight laboratories in England operate direct referral to colposcopy, with no involvement of the GP.

Criteria for referral from the screening programme are as follows:

- HR-HPV detected with any abnormal reflex cytology.
- Persistent HR-HPV detected in three consecutive cervical screening tests 12 months apart.
- Two consecutive HR-HPV tests unavailable or inadequate cytology results.

Colposcopic Examination

The woman lies supine on a colposcopy couch with her legs supported; a speculum examination is performed. The colposcope is a binocular magnifying system that facilitates a clear visual assessment of the cervix. A monitor screen may be available for the woman to also view the findings. Solutions are applied to the cervix to aid diagnosis.

Acetic acid alters the nuclear protein, rendering it opaque. When light from the colposcope meets the cervix, it is reflected back from the opaque nuclear protein, appearing white to the colposcopist. The more dyskaryotic a cell, the larger the nucleus, the more light is reflected and the whiter the area appears.

Cytoplasm is glycogen-rich and stains dark brown with the application of Lugol's iodine. When little glycogen remains, as in a high-grade dyskaryotic cell, there will be little uptake of iodine (Figures 7.8, 7.9, 7.10 and 7.11).

Reports from colposcopy clinics may comment on the presence and density of acetowhite areas and the extent of the cervix staining iodine negative. Other comments include the presence of vascular mosaic and punctation, which refer to abnormal vascular patterns. The more pronounced these features are, the more significant the abnormality.

Results of Cervical Screening and Colposcopy

Dyskaryosis and Cervical Intraepithelial Neoplasia

Dyskaryosis is a cytological abnormality seen in a cervical screening test sample. Dyskaryosis is classified as low-grade (borderline squamous and mild dyskaryosis) or high-grade (moderate and severe dyskaryosis, as well as the rarer 'glandular neoplasia of endocervical type'). Occasionally, cervical screening tests will be reported as showing possible invasion. The higher the level of dyskaryosis, the more of the cell is occupied by the nucleus, referred to as a high nuclear to cytoplasmic ratio.

CIN is a histological diagnosis obtained from a colposcopy sample – it cannot be diagnosed on a cervical screening test. Results of biopsies and treatment specimens will describe any CIN, which can be squamous or glandular. Squamous CIN is categorised according to the depth of involvement of the squamous epithelium. CIN1 is present when the abnormality is confined to the lower third of the epithelium, CIN2, when up to two-thirds are affected, and CIN3 refers to more than two-thirds involvement. Full-thickness involvement CIN3 is sometimes referred to as 'carcinoma in situ' [30]. CGIN is much less common than squamous CIN. It arises in the glandular epithelium of the cervical canal (endocervix). CGIN is a high-grade lesion and is frequently associated with adenocarcinoma.

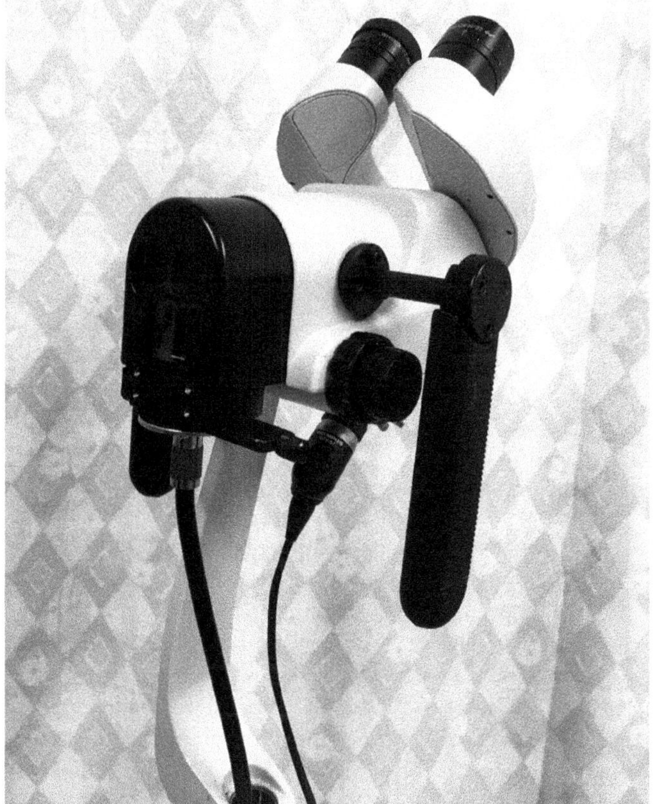

Figure 7.8 Colposcope.

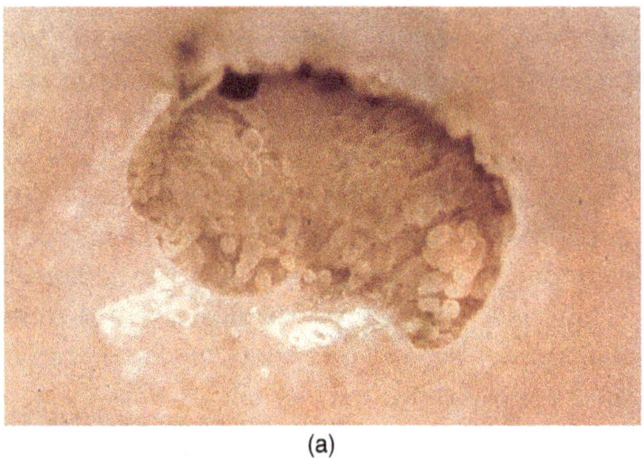

(a)

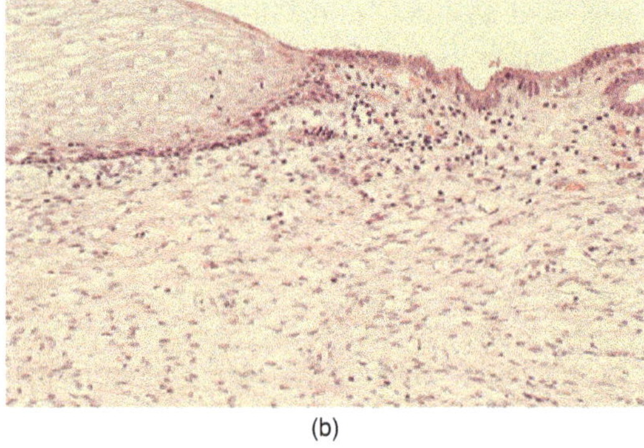

(b)

Figure 7.9 Colposcopy. (a) Colposcopic appearance of the external os showing the SCJ. (b) Histology slide showing SCJ.

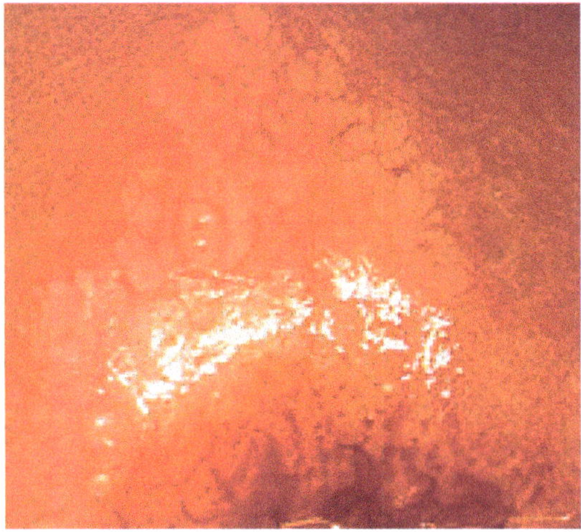

Figure 7.10 Colposcopic image showing mosaicism and punctation.

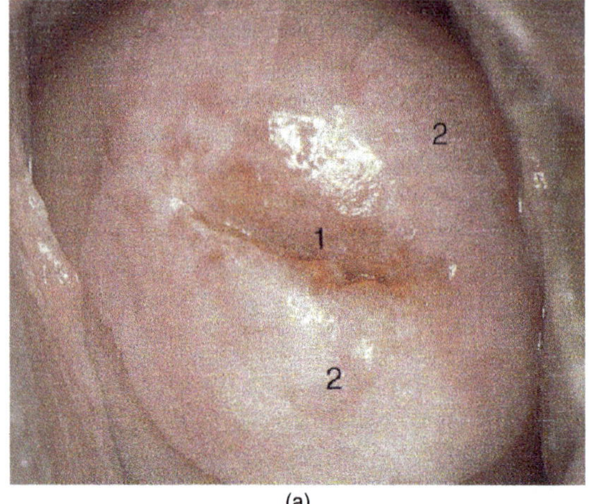

(a)

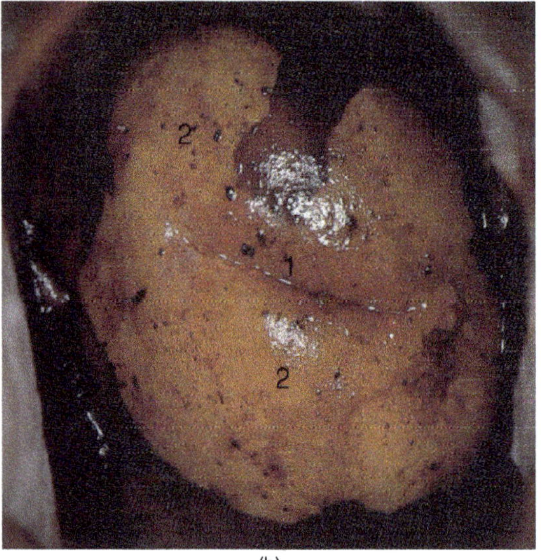

(b)

Figure 7.11 Effect of iodine on abnormal squamous tissue. (a) Before application of Shillers iodine (1: s–c junction; 2: aceto-white staining suggestive of CIN). (b) After application (1: s–c junction; 2: iodine – negative staining suggestive of CIN).

Therefore, cervical screening tests reported as possible glandular neoplasia of endocervical types require an urgent referral to colposcopy. Very rarely, cervical screening tests will be reported as 'glandular neoplasia (non-cervical)'; these are very concerning as they suggest the presence of a non-cervical glandular cancer; for example, endometrial, ovarian or even a non-gynaecological adenocarcinoma. Such cases would be urgently referred by the cytology lab. The grade of cervical screening test does not correlate perfectly with the final histopathological findings; for example, 30% of women referred to colposcopy for persistent low-grade cervical screening tests have high-grade CIN or an underlying cancer [19].

Management of Abnormalities Found at Colposcopy

See and Treat

Many colposcopy clinics offer a 'see and treat' policy for high-grade disease; if the cervical screening test shows high-grade dyskaryosis, and colposcopy shows consistent findings, treatment is offered at the first visit. High-grade dyskaryosis is more likely than low-grade dyskaryosis to progress to cervical cancer if left untreated [31].

Large Loop Excision of the Transformation Zone of the Cervix

The commonest form of treatment is LLETZ (Figure 7.12). The cervix is anaesthetised and a cone-shaped area of cervix is removed using a diathermy wire loop. Further diathermy is then applied to aid haemostasis. There is evidence of a small increase in preterm delivery post-LLETZ [32], so if there is a discrepancy between the cervical screening test result and the colposcopic appearance, a biopsy should be performed at the first visit rather than proceeding immediately to treatment.

To reduce the risk of cervicitis and secondary haemorrhage after LLETZ, it is recommended that a woman abstain from intercourse, using tampons, vigorous exercise and swimming for four weeks; treatment might be delayed if she is due to travel abroad within that time, as there may also be difficulties with travel insurance if complications arise post-treatment. CIN is a slowly progressing condition and such a deferral is unlikely to significantly increase risk, but colposcopic examination should be performed first to exclude malignancy.

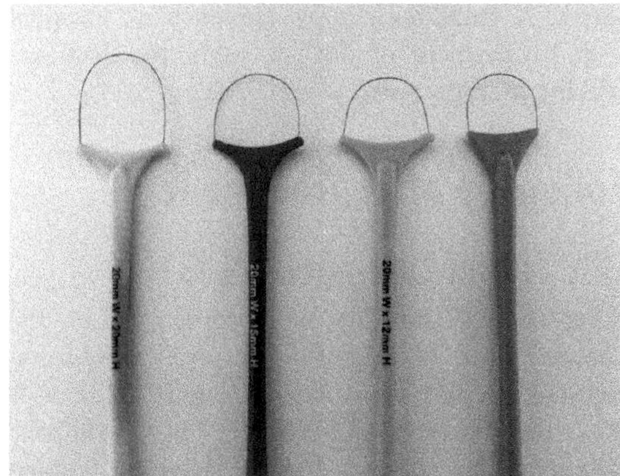

Figure 7.12 Loops used for LLETZ.

Some colposcopists will treat with an intrauterine device (IUD) in situ. There is a lack of evidence to inform best practice in carrying out LLETZ for women with an IUD and so decisions are made on a case-by-case basis. The IUD can be retained, and the threads will likely be cut by the loop. If the IUD is removed, the cervix must have time to heal before reinsertion; this usually takes up to six weeks. Contraception must be considered in the interim, as well as consideration of emergency contraception if needed; that is, if there has been intercourse in the week before the procedure. Resolution of bleeding and discharge after LLETZ procedures is usually an indication that the cervix has healed, but this should be confirmed by speculum examination before any attempt to re-fit an IUD [33].

Criteria for treatment under sedation or general anaesthetic include the following:

- Vaginal access in an awake patient is not sufficient to allow excision with clear margins (e.g. wide lesions/older postmenopausal women).
- The patient declines treatment under local and prefers sedation/general anaesthetic; having this option can prevent women from not attending their colposcopy appointment because of anxiety.
- Some medical conditions, such as poorly controlled epilepsy.

Short-Term Complications of a LLETZ

There is a risk of infection (cervicitis) post-treatment or biopsy, and a woman is informed that if she develops any signs of infection, such as secondary haemorrhage, offensive discharge, temperature or pelvic pain, she should follow the local pathway, which may mean review at the colposcopy clinic or by the GP. Antibiotics should be prescribed, including treatment for anaerobic infection.

It is normal to experience a watery, blood-stained discharge for around four weeks, but if heavy bleeding (worse than her period) occurs, she should contact the unit who treated her, or, if necessary, attend the emergency department. Contact numbers should be provided before leaving the colposcopy clinic.

Long-Term Complications of a LLETZ

LLETZ procedures can increase the risk of premature delivery. The risk is associated with the depth of excision. The risk of preterm labour with a small excision (<10 mm) is comparable to population risk, which is around 7%. However, women with an excision of 10–14 mm have a 9.6% increased risk of preterm labour. This doubles to 18% with deeper excisions of at least 20 mm [34].

Cervical stenosis is rare but can occasionally result in haematometra (collection of blood in the uterus during menstruation) [35].

Cervical dystocia (inability of a scarred cervix to dilate fully in labour) is a rare complication following knife cone biopsy, leading to an increased risk of caesarean section for failure to progress [3].

Other Treatment Methods

Destructive treatments using cold coagulation, cryotherapy or ball diathermy are suitable for treating persistent low-grade disease or ectropion. Some units also use destructive methods to treat high-grade lesions, as these methods carry a lower risk of preterm labour. However, they do not provide histological confirmation of diagnosis, or margin status, and therefore they must only be carried out when specific criteria are met, in accordance with national guidance [31,37].

Knife cone biopsy is sometimes used under general anaesthetic for suspected/proven glandular neoplasia, and high-grade squamous lesions where micro-invasion is a concern. This is because cones usually achieve larger excisions LLETZ and avoid diathermy artefact to the tissue margins, which can make histopathological interpretation harder; this is especially important in cases of micro-invasion or glandular neoplasia.

Laser excision is occasionally used to take a cone or to vaporise vaginal lesions. Hysterectomy is rarely required but may be recommended where there is persistent disease and little remaining intra-vaginal cervix, in women who have completed their families.

Conservative Management [31]

Low-grade disease does not usually require excision; approximately two-thirds of CIN1 will revert to normal spontaneously as the woman becomes immune to HPV [30].

Colposcopic examination with biopsies is, however, required in such cases to make sure the diagnosis of low-grade disease is correct and that a conservative approach is reasonable.

Stopping smoking may increase the likelihood of clearing HPV [22] and hence increase the chances of regression of CIN. If low-grade disease persists for more than 18 months, treatment may be offered as it is then unlikely to regress spontaneously.

Excisional Treatment for Glandular Abnormalities [31]

Women with cervical screening results suggestive of abnormalities in glandular cells should be referred urgently, usually directly from the screening service. These results are more difficult to interpret, the colposcopy is more challenging and there is a significant risk of underlying adenocarcinoma.

The cytology lab will report on the site of origin of the abnormal glandular cells, either cervical or non-cervical. The former are referred urgently to colposcopy, whereas the latter are referred under the fast-track system for suspected cancer.

Generally, where a result is suggestive of cervical glandular neoplasia, excisional treatment will be recommended. Where the result is of borderline changes in glandular cells, management is more variable, and each woman's situation is assessed individually. There is a much higher incidence of high-grade CGIN or cancer with a borderline glandular cervical screening test than with a borderline squamous cervical screening test, and so it is appropriate that more treatments are performed in the former situation, accepting that there will be some negative histology reports from treatment specimens. A multidisciplinary approach is essential with involvement of the patient in the decision-making process.

Follow-Up after Treatment

HPV Test of Cure after CIN [31]

After a LLETZ for CIN, most women will be discharged back to primary care, even if excision margins are not clear of CIN (Figure 7.13). It is likely that diathermy applied after LLETZ will have destroyed any residual disease. However, women aged over 50 with a positive deep (endocervical)

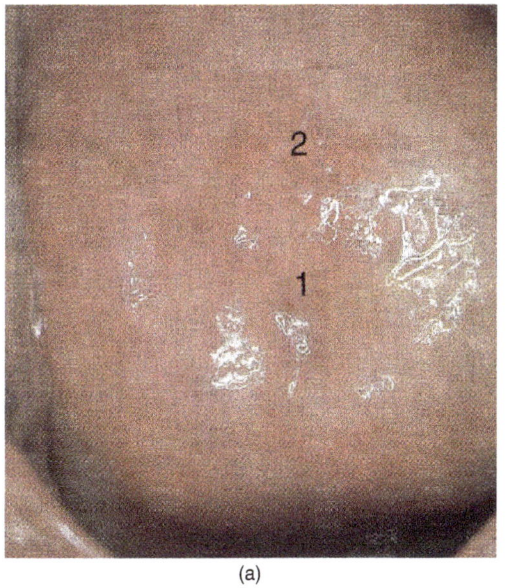

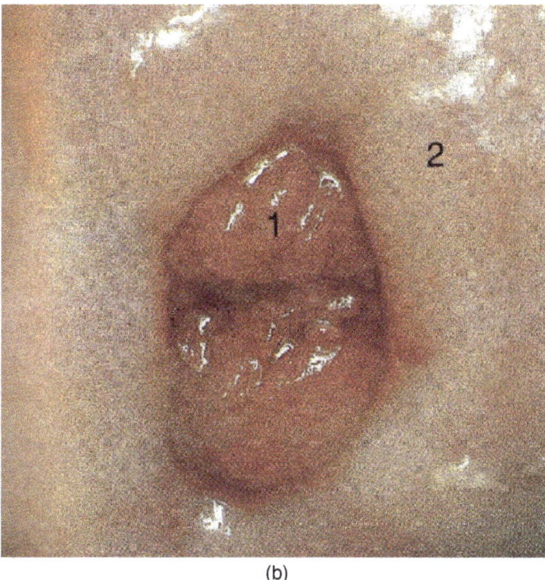

(a) (b)

Figure 7.13 Common appearances post-LLETZ: (a) stenosis (1: cervical os; 2: transformation zone), (b) rosetting (1: columnar epithelium; 2: squamous epithelium).

margin should be offered further excision, as they are at especially high risk of having residual disease.

A cervical screening test should be taken at six months which will be tested for HR-HPV. The results of this cervical screening test could be:

- Negative for HR-HPV; the woman is recalled at three years for a follow-up cervical screening test, regardless of age.
- Positive for HR-HPV reflex cytology testing and referral for colposcopy is done, even if the cytology is negative. Colposcopic findings and biopsy, if indicated, dictate follow-up requirements.

If a woman is aged over 50 at treatment (or lives in a country of the UK where screening is done at five-yearly intervals throughout the lifetime of screening) and her test of cure (TOC) smear is negative, her next cervical screening test should be at three years rather than five. If that cervical screening test is negative, she can revert to routine five-yearly recall.

HPV Test of Cure after CGIN [31]

Following a LLETZ procedure for CGIN where histology indicates complete excision, an HPV TOC is again indicated at six months. If this is negative for HR-HPV, a second TOC is indicated a year later. If both tests are negative, normal recall can resume. Any positive result will lead to continuing follow-up in the colposcopy service.

Incomplete excision of a glandular abnormality generally warrants further excisional treatment, which may require hysterectomy.

Cervical Cancer

It is difficult to comment on the rate of progression of untreated CIN3 to cervical cancer, as further studies in which treatment is not offered would be unethical. Older literature reviews suggest that 12–40% will progress if left untreated [38].

Most cervical cancers arise from squamous cells; about 20% are adenocarcinomas. There are other, rare cervical cancers, such as clear cell, small cell, lymphomas and sarcomas, and mixed squamous and glandular [39]. All cases of cancer will be discussed at a multi-disciplinary team (MDT) meeting.

Cervical cancers are staged from 1 to 4, with subgroups, according to the International Federation of Gynaecology and Obstetrics (FIGO) classification [40]. Stage 1 cancers are confined to the cervix. Stage 1A1 cancers, the earliest stage, where the tumour is less than 3 mm deep, can be adequately treated with LLETZ or cone biopsy. Provided that margins are clear, no further surgical intervention is required [41].

If a woman has a strong desire to retain fertility and the stage of cervical cancer is low (usually less than 1B1) and confined to the cervix, with no pathological lymph nodes on staging it may be possible to offer conisation or radical trachelectomy where the cervix, parametria and upper third of the vagina are removed, as long as clear margins are considered to be achievable [42,43] (Figure 7.14).

There is a higher chance of miscarriage or premature delivery after trachelectomy, even though a cervical cerclage is inserted at the time of the procedure; future deliveries are always by caesarean section [44].

More advanced cancers will be managed in specialist centres with radical surgery, radiotherapy and chemotherapy all playing a part, depending on staging and individual circumstances.

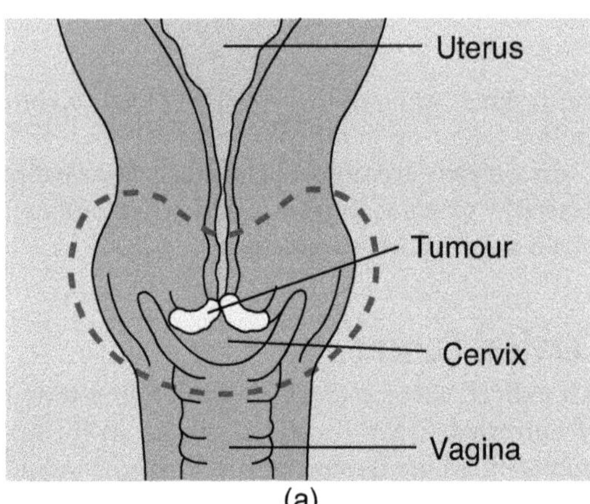

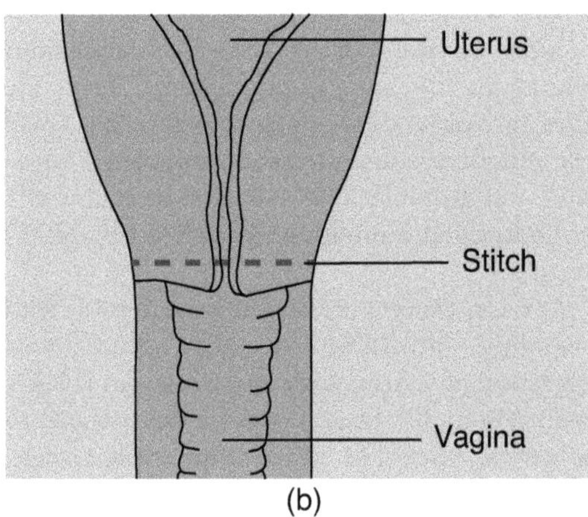

Figure 7.14 Trachelectomy. (a) Pre-op showing area removed. (b) Post-procedure. Source: Images produced by Leeds Teaching Hospitals NHS Trust Medical Illustration Service.

Conclusion

Rates of cervical cancer have reduced in the UK since the introduction of the NHSCSP. Further reductions should be seen as women who are vaccinated against HPV infection reach screening age.

HR-HPV testing is now the primary screening test for the cervical screening programme, with cytology examination used as the reflex triage for colposcopy referral. The use of HR-HPV testing and changes in the screening programme may cause concern to women who do not understand the relevance of their results. It is important for all clinicians in primary care to be aware of changes to the programme so that they can support women appropriately if they have concerns.

References

[1] Cancer Research UK, 'Cervical cancer statistics'. Accessed: 15 May 2024. [Online]. Available: www.cancerresearchuk.org/health-professional/cancer-statistics/statistics-by-cancer-type/cervical-cancer

[2] G. Owens, N. Wood and P. Martin-Hirsch, 'Investigation and management of postcoital bleeding', *TOG*, vol. **24**, no. 1, pp. 24–30, 2021.

[3] UK Health Security Agency. What is the right age for cervical screening? 2014. https://ukhsa.blog.gov.uk/2014/04/28/what-is-the-right-age-for-cervical-screening/

[4] CRUK, 'Routine smear test in women under 25 would cause more harm than good'. Accessed: 15 May 2024. [Online]. Available: https://news.cancerresearchuk.org/2013/11/04/routine-smear-test-in-women-under-25-would-cause-more-harm-than-good.

[5] NICE, 'NG12. Suspected cancer: Recognition and referral'. Oct. 2023. Accessed: 15 May 2024. [Online]. Available: www.nice.org.uk/guidance/ng12.

[6] NICE, 'NG88. Heavy menstrual bleeding: Assessment and management'. May 2021. Accessed: 15 May 2024. [Online]. Available: www.nice.org.uk/guidance/ng88.

[7] P. L. Bright, A. Norris Turner, C. S. Morrison et al., 'Hormonal contraception and area of cervical ectopy: A longitudinal assessment', *Contraception*, vol. **84**, no. 5, pp. 512–519, 2011.

[8] Cambridge University Hospitals NHS Foundation Trust, 'Cervical ectropion'. Accessed: 15 May 2024. [Online]. Available: www.cuh.nhs.uk/patient-information/cervical-ectropion.

[9] UK Health Security Agency, 'HPV vaccination guidance for healthcare practitioners'. June 2023. Accessed: 15 May 2024. [Online]. Available: www.gov.uk/government/publications/hpv-universal-vaccination-guidance-for-health-professionals/hpv-vaccination-guidance-for-healthcare-practitioners.

[10] I. Z. Mackenzie, C. Naish, C. M. P. Rees et al., 'Why remove all cervical polyps and examine them histologically?', *BJOG*, vol. **116**, no. 8, pp. 1127–1129, 2009.

[11] NICE CKS, 'Cervical screening'. Sept. 2022. Accessed: 15 May 2024. [Online]. Available: https://cks.nice.org.uk/topics/cervical-screening/management.

[12] World Health Organization, 'Cervical cancer'. Nov. 2023. Accessed: 15 May 2024. [Online]. Available: www.who.int/news-room/fact-sheets/detail/cervical-cancer.

[13] NHS Inform, 'Cervical screening (smear test)'. Accessed: 15 May 2024. [Online]. Available: www.nhsinform.scot/healthy-living/screening/cervical-screening-smear-test.

[14] Public Health Wales, 'Cervical screening Wales'. Accessed: 15 May 2024. [Online]. Available: https://phw.nhs.wales/services-and-teams/screening/cervical-screening-wales.

[15] nidirect, 'Cervical screening'. Accessed: 15 May 2024. [Online]. Available: www.nidirect.gov.uk/articles/cervical-screening.

[16] K. S. Okunade, 'Human papillomavirus and cervical cancer', *J Obstet Gynaecol*, vol. **40**, no. 5, pp. 602–608, 2020.

[17] Public Health England, 'Significant landmark as primary HPV screening is offered across England'. Jan. 2020. Accessed: 15 May 2024. [Online]. Available: https://phescreening.blog.gov.uk/2020/01/23/significant-landmark-as-primary-hpv-screening-is-offered-across-england.

[18] Public Health England, 'Cervical screening care pathway'. Aug. 2021. Accessed: 15 May 2024. [Online]. Available: www.gov.uk/government/publications/cervical-screening-care-pathway/cervical-screening-care-pathway.

[19] NHS Digital, 'Cervical screening programme, England – 2022–2023'. Nov. 2023. Accessed: 15 May 2024. [Online]. Available: https://digital.nhs.uk/data-and-information/publications/statistical/cervical-screening-annual/england-2022-2023/section-1-call-and-recall.

[20] S. Huntington, K. Puri Sudhir, V. Schneider et al., 'Two self-sampling strategies for HPV primary cervical cancer screening compared with clinician-collected sampling: An economic evaluation', *BMJ Open*, vol. **13**, e068940, 2023.

[21] Jo's Cervical Cancer Trust, 'HPV primary screening'. Dec. 2023. Accessed: 15 May 2024. [Online]. Available: https://www.cancerresearchuk.org/about-cancer/cervical-cancer/getting-diagnosed/screening/results.

[22] M. C. Malevolti, A. Lugo, M. Scala et al., 'Dose-risk relationships between cigarette smoking and cervical cancer: A systematic review and meta-analysis', *European Journal of Cancer Prevention*, vol. **32**, no. 2, pp. 171–183, 2023.

[23] NHSE, 'NHSCSP: Management of cases relating to pregnancy, menopause, contraception and hysterectomy'. Jan. 2023. Accessed: 15 May 2024. [Online]. Available: www.gov.uk/government/publications/cervical-screening-programme-and-colposcopy-management/4-management-of-cases-relating-to-pregnancy-menopause-contraception-and-hysterectomy.

[24] RCGP, 'The role of GPs in transgender care'. Jun. 2019. Accessed: 15 May 2024. [Online]. Available: www.rcgp.org.uk/representing-you/policy-areas/transgender-care.

[25] NHSE, 'NHS population screening: Information for trans and non-binary people'. Jan. 2023. Accessed: 15 May 2024. [Online]. Available: www.gov.uk/government/publications/nhs-population-screening-information-for-transgender-people/nhs-population-screening-information-for-trans-people.

[26] Public Health England, 'Supporting women with learning disabilities to access cervical screening'. Apr. 2019. Accessed: 15 May 2024. [Online]. Available: www.gov.uk/government/publications/cervical-screening-supporting-women-with-learning-disabilities/supporting-women-with-learning-disabilities-to-access-cervical-screening.

[27] Public Health England, 'Ceasing and deferring women from the NHS Cervical Screening Programme'. Sept. 2019. Accessed: 15 May 2024. [Online]. Available: www.gov.uk/government/publications/cervical-screening-removing-women-from-routine-invitations/ceasing-and-deferring-women-from-the-nhs-cervical-screening-programme.

[28] NHS, 'When you'll be invited for cervical screening'. Jun. 2023. Accessed: 15 May 2024. [Online]. Available: www.nhs.uk/conditions/cervical-screening/when-youll-be-invited.

[29] NHSE, 'Cervical screening: Programme and colposcopy management'. Jan. 2023. Accessed: 15 May 2024. [Online]. Available: www.gov.uk/government/publications/cervical-screening-programme-and-colposcopy-management.

[30] V. Mello and R. K. Sundstrom, *Cervical Intraepithelial Neoplasia*. StatPearls Publishing, 2024.

[31] NHSE, 'NHSCSP: Colposcopic diagnosis, treatment and follow up'. Jan. 2023. Accessed: 15 May 2024. [Online]. Available: www.gov.uk/government/publications/cervical-screening-programme-and-colposcopy-management/3-colposcopic-diagnosis-treatment-and-follow-up.

[32] A. Castanon, P. Brocklehurst, H. Evans et al., 'Risk of preterm birth after treatment for cervical intraepithelial neoplasia among women attending colposcopy in England: Retrospective-prospective cohort study', *BMJ*, vol. **345**, e5174, 2012.

[33] CoSRH, 'Intrauterine contraception'. Jul. 2023. Accessed: 15 May 2024. [Online]. Available: https://www.cosrh.org/Common/Uploaded%20files/documents/fsrh-clinical-guideline-intrauterine-contraception-mar-23-amended.pdf.

[34] A. Castanon, R. Landy, P. Brocklehurst et al., 'Risk of preterm delivery with increasing depth of excision for cervical intraepithelial neoplasia in England: Nested case-control study', *BMJ*, vol. **349**, g6223, 2014.

[35] C. S. Sampson and K. Arnold, 'A full uterus: Hematometra from cervical scarring', *Clin Pract Cases Emerg Med*, vol. **4**, no. 1, pp. 88–89, 2020.

[36] J. Y. Han, W. L. Wong and J. K. Y Chan, 'Labor complicated by cervical stenosis following a laser cone biopsy', *J Med Cases*, vol. **12**, no. 1, pp. 13–15, 2021.

[37] P. P. Martin-Hirsch, E. Paraskevaidis, A. Bryant et al., 'Surgery for cervical intraepithelial neoplasia', *Cochrane Database Syst Rev*, vol. **16**, no. 6, CD001318, 2010.

[38] C. Bekos, R. Schwameis, G. Heinze et al., 'Influence of age on histologic outcome of cervical intraepithelial neoplasia during observational management: Results from large cohort, systematic review, meta-analysis', *Sci Rep*, vol. **8**, 6383, 2018.

[39] NICE CKS, 'Cervical cancer and HPV'. Feb. 2022. Accessed: 15 May 2024. [Online]. Available: https://cks.nice.org.uk/topics/cervical-cancer-hpv.

[40] M. Y. Salib, J. H. B. Russell, V. R. Stewart et al., '2018 FIGO staging classification for cervical cancer: Added benefits of imaging', *Radiographics*, vol. **40**, no. 6, pp. 1807–1822, 2020.

[41] CRUK, 'Stage 1 cervical cancer'. Accessed: 15 May 2024. [Online]. Available: www.cancerresearchuk.org/about-cancer/cervical-cancer/stages-types-grades/stage-1.

[42] J. H. Shepherd, C. Spencer, J. Herod et al., 'Radical vaginal trachelectomy as a fertility-sparing procedure in women with early-stage cancer-cumulative pregnancy rate in a series of 123 women', *BJOG*, vol. **113**, no. 6, pp. 719–724, 2006.

[43] T. Chen, J. Li, Y. Zhu et al., 'The oncological and obstetric results of radical trachelectomy as a fertility-sparing therapy in early-stage cervical cancer patients', *BMC Womens Health*, vol. **22**, no. 1, 424, 2022.

[44] A. Tirlapur, F. Willmott, P. Lloyd et al., 'The management of pregnancy after trachelectomy for early cervical cancer', *TOG*, vol. **19**, no. 4, pp. 299–305, 2017.

Chapter 8

Management of Patients with Psychosexual Problems in Primary Care

Leila Frodsham and Angela Wright

Key Points

- Despite our lack of training in psychosexual issues, they are common in primary care. We should consider asking about them as a routine part of our assessment throughout the life course of our patients.
- When assessing the underlying causes of sexual problems, it is important to take a biopsychosocial approach. Sexual issues can have their roots in biological, psychological, relational and cultural factors. Patients may not always be aware of what psychological factors are causing the issue.
- There is a considerable degree of overlap between sexual problems, such as loss of libido, sexual pain conditions, loss of arousal and vaginismus. Psychological problems can lead to physical complications, and vice versa. We need to take an integrated approach to assessment and treatment.
- The Institute of Psychosexual Medicine (IPM) and College of Sexual and Relationship Therapist (COSRT) offer training that can improve confidence in supporting patients with sexual difficulties.

Talking about Sex: Part of Everyone's Job in Primary Care

Sexual Problems Are Common, and Often Cause Distress to Our Patients

Despite our skills and our ideal position to help, research suggests we often feel that giving advice about sex is outside our remit. Beyond a working knowledge of contraception, STIs and erectile dysfunction, other aspects of sex are rarely discussed, if at all. Despite clear evidence of need, training in psychosexual medicine remains poor across all specialities at both undergraduate and postgraduate level.

This lack of training *does not* reflect a lack of need.

Every decade, the National Survey of Sexual Attitudes and Lifestyles (NATSAL) interviews round 10,000 UK citizens, recording their thoughts, attitudes and behaviours about sex. The data gathered allows a unique insight into the sex lives of our patients.

NATSAL 4 (undertaken between 2020 and 2022) has not yet been released. We can, however, look to NATSAL 3 (undertaken in 2010–2012) to provide us with some figures that illustrate just how prevalent psychosexual issues are throughout patients' lives.

- 29% of 16–74-year-olds learned about sex from school, and 33% from friends. Less than 1% learned anything from their doctor.
- 24% used no contraception at first intercourse.

Sexual activity persists with age:

- 26% of 55–64-year-olds' last sex was <7 days ago.
- 10% of 65–74-year-olds' last sex was <7 days ago.

Variety persists with age:

- 8% of 55–64-year-olds' last oral sex was <7 days ago.
- 4% of 65–74-year-olds' last oral sex was <7 days ago.
- 2% of 65–74-year-olds' last anal intercourse was <7 days ago.

Also, 51% of women of all ages (42% of men of all ages) have had *one or more problem with sex for three or more months in the last year.*

Box 8.1 How NATSAL 3 Can Inform Opportunities in Your Own Practice

NATSAL 3 tells us that half of women had one or more problems with sex in the last year. Think about your own practice: are you seeing sexual problems as frequently as this might suggest we should expect to?

Some common opportunities to enquire about this aspect of your patient's life may be:

- at the start of their sexual lives
- contraceptive consultations
- when women consult about gynaecological problems like menorrhagia, endometriosis or PCOS
- after surgery
- during difficulties with conception and assisted conception
- when pregnancy is reported
- when women attend for cervical screenings or swabs
- at the postnatal check
- when prescribing new medications
- during chronic health condition reviews such as diabetes, vascular disease, heart disease, neurological or respiratory disease
- in menopause consultations
- after a cancer diagnosis and treatment (particularly those affecting breasts or sexual organs – especially oestrogen-dependent tumours).

We Need to Take the Lead – Because It Can Feel Difficult to Talk about Sex

Research shows that conversations about sex happen less often than patients would like them to.

For example: during pregnancy and the postnatal period, where sexual problems are commonly expected, one study showed only 31% of pregnant and 15% of postpartum women raised sex with their healthcare practitioner; 76% felt it was the clinician's job to enquire [1,2,3].

When healthcare professionals were asked what holds them back, four themes emerged:

(a) a lack of knowledge about sexual health
(b) attitudes and beliefs that sexual health care is private and not a priority
(c) discomfort discussing sexual health
(d) perceived barriers related to time, responsibility and organisational support.

Point (c) is worth reflecting upon; just like the patients we treat, as health professionals we will differ in our levels of comfort in talking about sex.

It Helps to Consider Sexual Problems through a 'Biopsychosocial Lens'

Sex is affected by what is happening in the body, the mind and the world the patient lives in (Figure 8.1). There can be a complex interplay between each of these areas, with problems originating in one aspect, such as the physical, and the patient then finding this leads to anxiety or a change in sexual confidence, and a partner experiencing their own reaction to the change in how intimacy plays out in the relationship. Often the result is a loss of interest in sex – but the problem may have its roots in something else entirely.

A good example is menopause, with women often presenting with reduced libido and being prescribed testosterone when the actual issue is reduced vulval sensitivity and less satiating orgasms. Very few women will offer information on reduced sexual pleasure and testosterone will not help if the act of sex is not satisfying. In these cases, topical vaginal and vulval oestrogen is preferable to testosterone use, especially noting that 70% of women find most of their sexual pleasure is vulval alone. Menopausal women also often have demanding working lives, teenage children and increasingly dependent parents so the associated anxiety and distraction can reduce mental 'presence' during intimacy.

Ways to Open Up a Conversation about Sex

The PLISSIT model (Figure 8.2) demonstrates that simply opening a conversation about sex and exhibiting an empathetic manner can be enough to help most with a sexual difficulty. It is a counselling framework used to help healthcare providers assess and treat sexual concerns in patients and consists of four stages: permission, limited information, specific suggestion and intensive therapy. The IPM teaches that the patient is the expert and that healthcare professionals are the key or mirror to unlock or reflect what is going on in the subconscious. Most GPs are highly skilled in the nuances of the doctor–patient relationship and can apply the principle

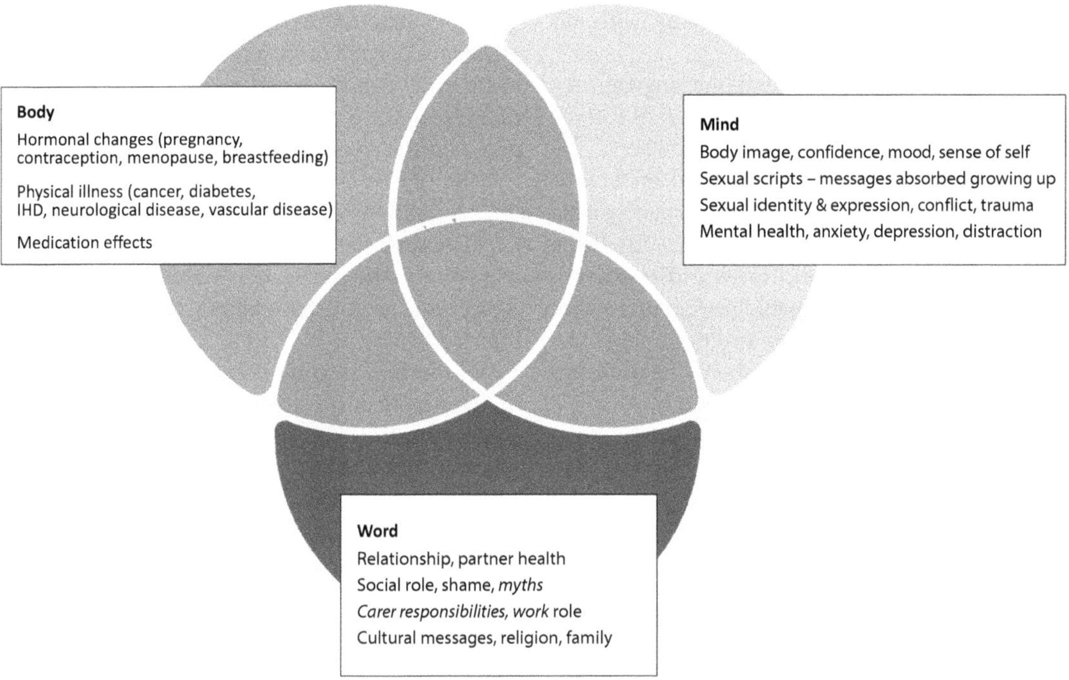

Figure 8.1 A Venn diagram showing the connections between the body, the mind and external factors (the world) and how these can lead to sexual problems.

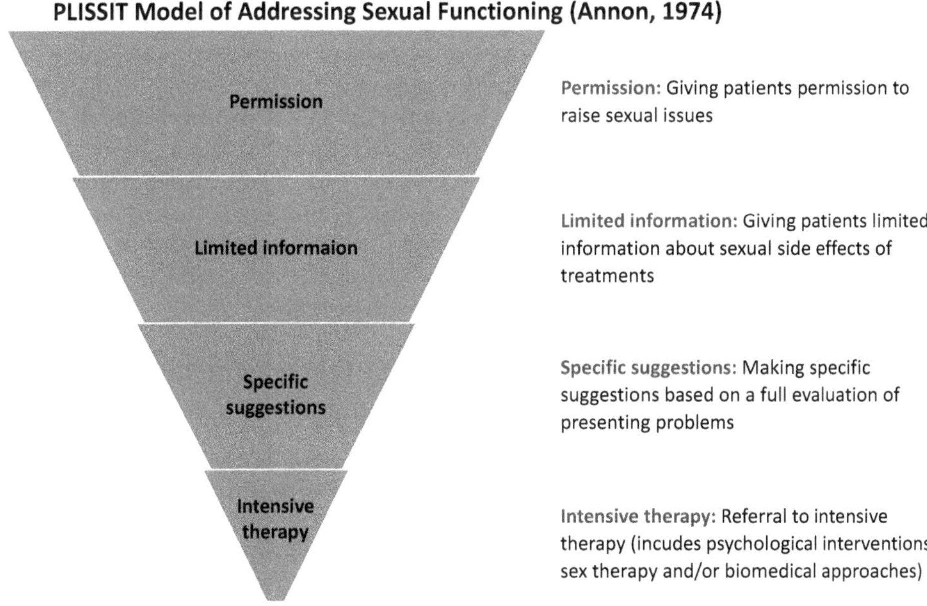

Figure 8.2 The PLISSIT model of addressing sexual functioning. Adapted from J. S. Annon, *The Behavioral Treatment of Sexual Problems: Brief Therapy*. Johns Hopkins University Press, 1974.

to sexual difficulties in the same way as they unpick persistent physical symptoms with no medical explanation.

We may not feel familiar with the language our patients use. Medical training is often very hetero- and mono-normative. Humans, however, are diverse in terms of gender and sexual preference and orientation. Cis- and hetero-normative language may lead to shame and trauma for those with diverse identities. Be curious and respectful: ask your patient how they would prefer you to refer to them and avoid making assumptions about the gender of sexual partners, about relationship structures or about sexual preferences.

Box 8.2 How Your Attitudes and Experiences about Sex Can Inform Your Practice

Think **about your own practice**: what education have you received on sex? Who did you learn from? Were the messages sex-positive or sex-negative? How would you feel talking to your own doctor about sex? Considering how vulnerable this makes your patient feel when you consider your own experiences can make it easier to be open and empathetic.

We may not have received much formal teaching on the subject since school sex education. We may have been raised with strong cultural or religious messages that make us uncomfortable discussing behaviours or attitudes that don't align with our own. We may very reasonably feel we are lacking in the correct skills to tackle these issues or worry that we have no service to refer into.

Primary care is a pressured environment and there is often a fear of 'opening Pandora's box' when we broach difficult conversations. However, we are ideally placed to raise the subject, as we often see patients through large parts of their life course and may have met their partners and know more about the wider context of their stories.

Asking questions about sex does not necessarily have to mean long consultations are needed: in fact, there is ample evidence that even brief intervention can be effective in validating patient's concerns and in improving their sexual wellbeing. They may also reduce consultation time and frequency if the patient is searching for the right clinician to open up to or presenting with other calling cards.

Open questions are best: 'How is sex?'

Many practitioners worry about open-ended questions due to time constraints, but these are more likely to yield useful results, reduce frustration and make both patient and practitioner happier with the consultation.

The IPM uses a ladder to approach consultations called LOFTI, as follows.

Listening: People carefully rehearse what they will say, and the choice of words/delivery are often significant, such as describing their vulva as an infected wound.

Observing: Is your patient tightly buttoned-up/overdressed for the weather? Over 80% of communication is through non-verbal cues. Are they imparting very difficult information with no emotional expression? Do you notice reactions when particular things are said?

Feeling: What are the feelings in the room? Don't be frightened to describe them: 'This all sounds so difficult, I can see why it makes you feel angry'. 'You seem to be describing some really difficult things and I'd expect you to be upset by them'.

Thoughts: What are your impressions of what is going on? 'It seems like things became difficult after you had your baby. I wonder what your delivery was like/how it feels to be a parent?'

Interpretation: You might have a strong feeling of wanting to protect your patient/be maternal/paternal. 'I wonder how things were when you were growing up?'

It is important to acknowledge cultural, sexual and gender differences but also to be aware that some may want to use this as a defence to opening up fully in front of someone who does not fit their background. Don't be frightened to ask your patients what their identity means to them rather than making assumptions.

Approaching the Examination Compassionately

There are simple ways we can ensure our patients always maintain a sense of agency and autonomy over their body.

All healthcare professionals should be aware that patients may have a history of trauma and uncomfortable to declare it. As such, taking a trauma-informed approach to conversations about sex and physical or genital examinations is essential.

The environment for examination needs to feel private and safe. It is important to have somewhere for people to put their bottom clothes. Please tell your patient that they are in control and can stop at any point. You may like to ask them how they would like to alert you to pain or tell you to stop. A common trauma response is to freeze, and patients may struggle to verbalise distress – Broca's area (controlling speech) frequently goes 'offline' when trauma is live – so noticing if this has happened is very important. The process of examination bears some similarities to sex: removing clothes and lying down. People may disclose their feelings about sex more openly during examination. They may also ask questions about their genitalia. There might be a 'phantasy' (a physical fantasy) that might be so strong that it transfers to you, making you also feel anxious about approaching examination. Please don't move too quickly to reassure, even if things look normal. Allow patients to talk about what they are concerned about.

Noticing how a patient behaves during an examination can provide a lot of information and is a key skill in psychosexual assessment. It is important to notice and reflect upon your own feelings, too.

Seek explicit consent: 'It would be helpful to examine you. Is that okay with you? Can I do anything to make this easier for you?'

Make sure you both know what to do to make the examination stop: 'You are in control of this'. 'Is there a way you'd like to tell me if you need to stop?'

Consider reflecting any feelings you notice: 'This must be so difficult for you'. 'I can see that this is making you anxious'.

Box 8.3 A Trauma-Informed Approach to Working with Survivors of Abuse and Trauma

One in Four published a document called 'Survivors' Voices' in 2015, part of a wider 'Survivors' Narratives' project which aimed to improve understanding of the impact of sexual abuse in childhood across professional audiences. It is a document we would urge you to read.

Although research findings in this area vary, it is estimated that between one in four and one in eight men will experience some form of sexual abuse or violence during their lifetime.

The short- and long-term impact of sexual violence and abuse will vary from person to person. It may affect mental, emotional, sexual and physical health and wellbeing.

Trauma is not confined to sexual violence: anything that makes us feel unsafe or helpless may result in trauma. It may be one acute event, or chronic and prolonged. So many forms of trauma exist that as healthcare professionals, we will often be working with people living with trauma. We also may have experienced it ourselves.

Sexual violence or abuse	Community violence (e.g. gender, race, disability, sexuality)
Domestic violence or abuse	Victim or crime
Physical abuse	Life-threatening illness
Emotional abuse	Childbirth
Neglect, deprivation	Traumatic grief
Natural disasters	Witnessing violence
Bullying	Generational trauma
Terrorism Accidents	Secondary trauma

Recovery can take weeks, months or years and does not always occur – meaning that trauma responses may be re-triggered at any point, and someone may need to access further support or counselling in response to life events years after the event. It is common for experiences such as pregnancy, birth or menopause to bring previous trauma to the fore.

Managing Common Sexual Problems in Primary Care

'It Hurts When I Have Sex' – Sexual Pain Disorders

Sex can be painful from the first attempt, but it can also become newly painful at any life stage.

It helps to ask questions to define whether the patient is describing problems with:

- penetration (vaginismus or anismus)
- superficial vulval pain (vulvodynia)
- deeper pain (often caused by inflammation in the pelvis, for example endometriosis, inflammatory bowel disease, irritable bowel syndrome, bladder pain syndrome. It is worth noting that a secondary vaginismus usually occurs with deeper pain).

Remember that penetration is often prioritised by dominant heterosexual scripts – but may not always be important to or wanted by the patient.

Problems with pain may occur with:

- any kind of genital touch (*generalized*)
- a particular type of penetration/touch/partner/situation (*specific*).

It can be very revealing to ask how, or when, perceived problems began.

Causes of Superficial and Deep Dyspareunia

Superficial pain:

- recurrent *Candida*
- herpes simplex virus
- vaginismus (primary or secondary – after *Candida*/endometriosis from reaction to deeper pain)
- vulvar dermatitis (consider common allergens: soaps, shower gels, gel-based sanitary pads and washing powders; consider continence)
- postnatal (including the impact of genitourinary syndrome of menopause (GSM)-like symptoms in breastfeeding women)
- Bartholin's abscess or cyst
- GSM – previously called vulvovaginal atrophy
- genital dermatoses (such as lichen sclerosis)
- low ferritin – 20%.

Less Common Causes

- Iatrogenic (postoperative delivery, perineal trauma, radiotherapy, female genital mutilation).
- Neurologic (neuropathic pain, neurological disease).
- Vaginal structural abnormalities (septum, congenital or iatrogenic skin bridges or scarring).
- Malignancy (vaginal or vulval neoplasia).

Deep Pain

- Endometriosis (deep dyspareunia is a cardinal sign).
- Adnexal or pelvic pathology (cysts, fibroids, pelvic malignancies).
- Pelvic inflammatory disease.
- Iatrogenic (vaginal shortening or narrowing, post-radiotherapy changes, female genital mutilation).
- Chronic pelvic pain.
- Pelvic floor dysfunction (mechanical, anatomical factors, retroversion, prolapse).
- Pelvic congestion (postcoital ache).
- Non-gynaecological (inflammatory bowel disease, irritable bowel disease, urinary tract infections).

When Examining the Patient

Inspect the vulva first: Pay particular attention to vulval dermatoses and perianal skin changes. Vulvitis/vulval eczema can cause microfissures in the posterior fourchette that are not easily seen without stretching the skin slightly.

Proceed gently: All women with sexual pain should have gentle external palpation of the pelvic floor before moving on to digital examination. Unless there is a clear indication for speculum examination, it is preferable to manage the cause of superficial dyspareunia before speculum examination. If not taking a smear, asking the woman to insert instillagel into the vagina before digital examination or speculum examination can really help. It can also help with IUD/IUCD insertions.

General Advice for Managing Painful Sex

The following general advice can be helpful for all women with sexual pain.

1. Wash with an inert oil (e.g. olive/coconut or a plain emollient).
2. Use cotton-only pads or period pants for periods/unbleached tampons. Some women find CBD (cannabidiol) oil tampons can help with endometriosis [4].
3. Avoid biological washing powders.
4. Consider using a low-allergen, unbleached, undyed, unscented toilet paper.
5. Perform pelvic floor massage for a minute twice a day from now on with coconut oil and fingers/thumbs or a bullet vibrator – you might like to apply lidocaine ointment before coconut oil if sore.
6. Refrain from waxing/depilatory creams or shaving your pubic hair and move to clipping to avoid disrupting the microbiome and increasing risk of ingrowing hairs and infections.
7. In women with deep dyspareunia, a depth minimiser like Ohnut can be helpful but only after review by a gynaecologist to exclude treatable causes.

8. Vibratory massage is one of the most effective treatments for sexual pain disorders. One paper demonstrates a 76% reduction in pain [5].
9. Some women like to see a pelvic floor physiotherapist but many also benefit from pelvic floor stretch yoga/Pilates. The Bloume website (www.bloumehealth.com) from the King's College London Psychology Department advises about this (endorsed by the Vulval Pain Society).

Box 8.4 Treating Patients with Genitourinary Syndrome of Menopause

Think about your own practice: are you being proactive about GSM?

The vulva, vagina and bladder are rich in oestrogen and androgen receptors. This means that their structure and function is significantly impacted by hormone loss:

- at perimenopause and menopause
- after surgical, iatrogenic or cancer-induced menopause
- during breastfeeding
- due to anovulatory forms of contraception (progestogen-only pill, implant, injection and the sex hormone-binding globulin-raising impact of combined hormonal contraceptives) which may also result in similar vulvovaginal changes that can impact sexual function.

Atrophic changes to the vagina, vulva and bladder usually respond well to local oestrogens, moisturisers, emollients and massage. Lubricants can also help enormously with all forms of penetrative sex.

GSM can be devastating to sexual function, and also to wider wellbeing. It is preventable with proactive care. Untreated, it can lead to a number of sexual consequences, including:

- loss of arousal and ability to feel pleasure from touch
- loss of volume and sensation in erectile tissue (e.g. clitoris, labia minora)
- difficulty lubricating
- recurrent UTI
- difficulty climaxing
- loss of tissue stretch, leading to painful/difficult penetration
- fissures/bleeding/itch in the vagina and vulva.

Many women will require local oestrogens in addition to systemic hormone replacement therapy to adequately manage symptoms.

Consideration should be given to applying topical oestrogen to the vulva and perineal area, as well as internally. There is increasing evidence to support the use of vaginal and vulval oestrogens in women after hormone receptor positive cancer, for example of the breast.

'Sex Doesn't Feel the Same Anymore' – Arousal Disorders

There are a number of causes of changes in arousal and difficulty in climaxing. Some of these have roots in physical/hormonal changes through the life course:

- the impact of hormonal contraception
- breastfeeding (high prolactin/low oestrogen leading to GSM-like symptoms and prolactin leading to direct suppression of climax)
- post-surgery – direct alteration in anatomy +/– hormone loss
- post-cancer
- impact of medication (selective serotonin reuptake inhibitors (SSRIs), antihypertensives, hormone blockers, antipsychotics, antihistamines)
- degenerative neurological conditions such as multiple sclerosis
- the impact of poorly controlled diabetes.

Medication changes can be impactful – a trial of mirtazapine in place of SSRI, for example, or considering a Mirena in place of a low-dose combined hormonal contraceptive pill.

Anxiety – Distraction/Dissociation

The brain is often considered our biggest sexual organ, and it certainly acts as a powerful volume switch for arousal. Anticipation can dial up sensation and arousal, but distraction and dissociation are often part of a low arousal picture. Trauma is a common source of dissociation and may relate to sexual abuse or violence, medical care including cancer treatment and childbirth or other triggers. Many women will benefit from the use of mindfulness and psychological support.

Persistent Genital Arousal Disorder

Persistent genital arousal disorder (PGAD) is a poorly recognised and distressing condition affecting around 0.6–2.7% of women [6]. It is characterised by highly distressing persistent genital sensations, sensitivity and arousal in the absence of sexual desire. It often co-exists alongside other sexual dysfunctions and sufferers are more likely to have a Tarlov cyst and may also be more likely to be diagnosed with restless legs.

Climax can temporarily relieve symptoms, but they often return within hours. Psychological distress is often very high. Treatment usually includes pelvic floor physiotherapy, pelvic floor massage and psychological therapies, as well as the use of medications such as antidepressants and nerve pain agents. There is no published evidence to support treatments but anecdotally women seem to improve with a combination of topical vaginal oestrogens in the peri/menopausal group (which is when this appears more prevalent) and pelvic floor massage. More published data is urgently required.

SSRIs and Sexual Dysfunction

SSRIs are commonly prescribed in primary care. They have a direct effect on inhibition of climax and can, in a dose-dependent manner, lead to anorgasmia. They also decrease genital blood flow and subjective measures of sensation.

There are increasing reports of persistent changes in sexual function despite stopping medication. It is important prescribers are aware of this issue and include discussion of sexual function changes when counselling patients about these drugs.

Use of Toys/Erotica to Intensify Arousal

Sexual arousal is the result of the balance of inhibitory and excitatory factors. Where arousal is diminished, it can help to consider intensifying sensation or sexual novelty/psychological turn-on.

There are a number of non-salacious websites that may be suitable for discussion with patients who ask for further information (see Helpful Resources at the end of this chapter).

'I Don't Feel Like Sex' – Dealing with Low Libido

Libido is a complex biopsychosocial phenomenon. It is impacted by a number of issues, including:

- our physical health (including illness, medication, mobility and pain)
- our sex hormones
- our psychological wellbeing
- our lived experiences (including trauma)
- our sexual scripts and sexual identity
- our relationships
- our partner's health
- how distracted we are by our various roles and responsibilities.

If a Patient Is Experiencing Low Desire, Ask 'Why Now?'

What was her level of desire previously? Ask whether it is impacting any relationship she is in. Is the loss of desire generalised or specific to a partner or situation?

Remember loss of libido is often the logical end point of another problem with sex that might need addressing, such as loss of arousal, pain during or after sex, dryness or anorgasmia. This may be the primary issue rather than libido.

There is no 'normal' level of libido. Human sexual interest can range from identifying as asexual through to a very high interest in sex. Distress about loss of interest is required by both the *Diagnostic and Statistical Manual of Mental Disorders* (DSM) and International Classification of Diseases (ICD) to diagnose a 'problem' with desire.

Explaining Desire to Patients

Our cultural and societal references tend to propagate the idea that sexual desire is always a spontaneous phenomenon. Research suggests this is not always the case.

We may experience sexual desire: *spontaneously* (like hunger) or *responsively*, in reaction to a cue (similar to noticing the smell of baking bread and *then* wanting to eat).

Spontaneous desire is common early in relationships. Research suggests many women in long-term relationships may experience more responsive desire.

Previous positive outcomes (e.g. pleasure, orgasm, emotional connection to a partner, relationship security, a good night's sleep) make us more likely to respond with interest to a sexual cue. However, negative outcomes (e.g. pain, UTI or shame felt by not lubricating when touched) can result in barriers to responding to, or being receptive to, a sexual cue.

Role of Testosterone and Other Hormones

Much of the narrative around women and libido tends to centre on the role of testosterone, especially at menopause. Although it can play an important part in sexual thoughts, fantasy and interest, it is better thought of as just one jigsaw piece in the more complex picture that is human sexual interest and function.

Testosterone and its precursors are made by the ovaries and the adrenals. About 50% of the total circulating level is made through peripheral conversion from these precursors. Women whose ovaries are removed or damaged (i.e. after cancer treatment) have lower circulating testosterone levels.

Both androgens and oestrogens also help maintain the genital tissues and structures and are involved in vaginal lubrication.

There is a weak association between testosterone and desire, orgasm and self-image in premenopausal women. It is also associated with desire, arousal and masturbation frequency in midlife women.

The loss of testosterone due to surgical menopause does increase the prevalence of hypoactive sexual desire disorder (HSDD). Studies do not suggest there is a clear level of circulating androgens that signals HSDD.

When Should We Use Testosterone in Primary Care?

The main indication for testosterone in primary care is for postmenopausal women with low desire. The British Menopause Society Consensus suggests clinicians use a biopsychosocial assessment first, to make sure that we properly consider addressing any other physical, psychological and relational factors contributing to the loss of sexual interest [7].

If you suspect that changes in hormone levels may be affecting desire, start by offering local oestrogen (vaginal and vulval) and systemic hormone replacement therapy (improving oestrogen levels locally, and systemically, is usually the most impactful measure).

If this is not helpful, then a three- to six-month trial of testosterone supplementation may be of benefit [7,8,9].

Other Factors That Influence Sexual Function

The Impact of Other Medications or Health Conditions

The physical aspect of sexual function is often impacted by co-existing medical issues. Anything that changes the neurovascular or endocrine picture in the body has the potential to affect sexual interest or response. This includes surgery and serious illness such as cancer and neurological conditions.

Many commonly prescribed medications will also impact and teaching on this can be poor: watch out for these common culprits:

- SSRIs and SNRIs (post-SSRI syndrome is rare but can leave patients with long-lasting genital numbness and pleasureless orgasm; shorter-term commoner impacts include loss of genital sensation, delayed or absent climax and loss of libido)
- antihypertensives (betablockers and ACE inhibitors in particular)
- antihistamines and antimuscarinics (can be drying)
- hormonal medications (hormone blockers can lead to GSM and diminished desire and arousal; combined oral contraceptives can reduce circulating androgens and diminish libido and contribute to vulvovaginal dryness or pain)
- antipsychotics.

Partner Issues

Sexual expression can have solo and partnered components [10]. It is important to remember sex may still be very important to those without a current partner.

Research shows that partner health is one of the biggest factors impacting female sexual satisfactions scores. Remember to ask patients about their partner/s when talking about sex. This can also be a valuable early warning system about other preventable health issues in the partner (e.g. in the case of erectile dysfunction, the loss of men's morning erections can herald the development of angina within two to five years).

Helpful Resources

Books

- *Mind the Gap* – Karen Gurney
- *Better Sex through Mindfulness* – Lori Brotto
- *The Body Keeps the Score* – Bessel Van Der Kolk
- *Sexology* – Silva Neves

Websites

- www.postbabyhankypanky.com
- www.OMG-Yes.com

Useful Resources for Vaginismus

- www.bloumehealth.com
- https://weareferly.com
- www.thevaginismusnetwork.com
- https://theflowerempowered.com
- www.tightlywoundfilm.com
- www.vaginamuseum.co.uk

Podcasts

- Vaginismus: 'My body won't let me have sex': www.bbc.co.uk/news/av/world-europe-49695670
- The problem with sex – Science Weekly podcast: www.theguardian.com/science/audio/2019/may/10/the-problem-with-sex-science-weekly-podcast
- The diagnosis and treatment of dyspareunia, *BMJ*: www.listennotes.com/podcasts/the-bmj-podcast/the-diagnosis-and-treatment-l2K0GQn1XhR

Review Articles on Sexual Problems

- F. Cowan and L. Frodsham, 'Management of common disorders in psychosexual medicine', *The Obstetrician & Gynaecologist*, vol. **17**, pp. 47–53, 2015.
- G. Mumford, 'How to look after your vulva'. *The Guardian*, 8 Dec. 2019. Accessed: Dec. 2024. [Online]. Available: www.theguardian.com/lifeandstyle/2019/dec/08/how-to-look-after-your-vulva.
- H. Horton, 'Pain and vaginismus: The condition that destroys lives'. *The Guardian*, 31 Aug. 2020. Accessed: Dec. 2024. [Online]. Available: www.theguardian.com/lifeandstyle/2020/aug/31/pain-vaginismus-destroys-lives-misunderstood-common-conditions-surgery-treatment.

References

[1] Barrett G, Pendry E, Peacock J, Victor C, Thakar R, Manyonda I. Women's sexual health after childbirth: a longitudinal study of prevalence and associated factors. *Br J Obstet Gynaecol*, vol. **107**, no. 2, pp. 186–195, 2000.

[2] M. Serati, S. Salvatore, G. Siesto et al., 'Female sexual function during pregnancy and after childbirth', *J Sex Med*, vol. **7**, pp. 2782–2790, 2010.

[3] E Bartellas, J. M. Crane, M. Daley, K. A. Bennett and D. Hutchens, 'Sexuality and sexual activity in pregnancy', *Br J Obstet Gynaecol*, vol. **107**, no. 8, pp. 964–968, 2000.

[4] P. Wang, J. Chen, X. Zhou, C. Xiong, Y. Wang and Z. Huang, 'Efficacy and usability of a cannabidiol-infused tampon for the relief of primary dysmenorrhea', *J Cannabis Res*, vol. **5**, no. 1, 45, 2023.

[5] Y. Reisman, R. C. Rosen, S. Althof et al., 'The use of vibratory stimulation for the treatment of sexual dysfunction: A review of current evidence', *Int J Impot Res*, vol. **32**, no. 6, pp. 611–617, 2020.

[6] R. A. Jackowich, L. Pink, A. Gordon and C. F. Pukall, 'Prevalence, characteristics, and correlates of persistent genital arousal disorder in women', *J Sex Med*, vol. **17**, no. 1, pp. 69–82, 2020.

[7] British Menopause Society, 'Testosterone replacement in menopause: A British Menopause Society factsheet'. Dec. 2022. Accessed: Dec. 2024. [Online]. Available: https://thebms.org.uk/wp-content/uploads/2022/12/08-BMS-TfC-Testosterone-replacement-in-menopause-DEC2022-A.pdf.

[8] Primary Care Women's Health Forum, 'Top tips on testosterone use for women'. Accessed: Dec. 2024. [Online]. Available: https://pcwhf.co.uk/resources/top-tips-on-testosterone-use-for-women-2/#.

[9] S. J. Parish, J. A. Simon, S. R. Davis et al., 'International Society for the Study of Women's Sexual Health clinical practice guideline for the use of systemic testosterone for hypoactive sexual desire disorder in women', *J Sex Med*, vol. **18**, no. 5, pp. 849–867, 2021. https://doi.org/10.1016/j.jsxm.2020.10.009. PMID: 33814355.

[10] D. Lovell, N. Hayfield and Z. Thomas, '"No one has ever asked me and I'm grateful that you have": Men's experiences of their partner's female sexual pain'. *Sex Relatsh* Ther, vol. **40**, pp. 1–24, 2023. https://doi.org/10.1080/14681994.2023.2293766.

Infertility Management in Primary Care

Stephanie Cook and Clare Searle

Key Points

- Fertility problems are common and affect up to one in seven couples.
- Fertility consultations are often emotional and require time and sensitivity to fully explore the relevant factors and concerns.
- Likely barriers to success should be addressed early to optimise outcomes, including lifestyle issues for both partners.
- Couples facing fertility problems should be seen together; both partners are affected by decisions surrounding investigation and treatment.
- Basic investigations are necessary from both partners prior to referral.
- Understanding of local referral pathways and criteria is important.
- Women with a past gynaecological history of note or aged over 35 should be referred into a specialist fertility clinic after six months of trying to conceive naturally.
- Single women (or same-sex couples) should be fully informed of their available options.

Introduction

Reproductive medicine has developed rapidly over recent years; a complex array of possibilities and alternative options for parenting now exists. In today's world, having a family is possible for most, though in some cases parents have to accept that their babies may not be entirely their own biological material.

In general, fertility is much more complicated than it has ever been, and this is particularly true in primary care, where the assessment and investigations begin. These consultations require a truly holistic and patient approach.

Principles of Care

Infertility is broadly defined as a failure to conceive fter one year of regular unprotected penetrative sexual intercourse. Couples in whom there are reasons for sub-fertility, or where the woman is over the age of 35 years, should be identified as high risk and referred on at six months. The cause of infertility can be due to female or male factor causes or both; it is important to keep an open mind. Ideally, regular intercourse should occur two to three times per week, throughout the month, and not just around the time of ovulation [1].

The Broader Issue

NICE estimates that on average, one in seven couples in the UK will have difficulty conceiving. Although some couples may struggle with fertility, more than 80 out of 100 couples will become pregnant within one year of trying (if the woman is aged under 40) and this rises to 90% in the second year [2].

Fertility consultations may involve a heterosexual couple struggling to conceive, a same-sex couple or a woman wishing to conceive without a partner.

Female Infertility

The causes of female infertility may be broadly divided into three groups: failed ovarian function, anatomical abnormalities and environmental factors.

Failed Ovarian Function

Failure to ovulate is thought to account for around 25% of presentations and is usually related to abnormal hormone function.

Hormonal Dysfunction

This is the most common cause for anovulation. The process of successful ovulation depends upon a complex balance of hormones and their interactions. There are three main causes of ovulatory dysfunction:

- *Hypogonadotropic hypogonadism.* The hypothalamus is the part of the brain which sends signals to the pituitary gland, which then sends hormonal stimuli to the ovaries in the form of follicle-stimulating hormone (FSH) and luteinising hormone (LH), to initiate egg maturation. If the hypothalamus fails to trigger and control this process, immature eggs will result. This is the cause of ovarian failure in 20% of cases. The most common presentation of this is in women with a low body mass index (BMI) and/or high exercise regimens. One cause of this phenomenon is excessive exercise combined with inadequate energy intake. In 2014, the term 'RED-S' was introduced by the International Olympic Committee. RED-S (Relative Energy Deficiency in Sport) is caused by low energy availability and can lead to an anovulatory state. In recent years the scientific community has begun to recognise this syndrome, and to raise awareness of the consequences of low energy availability, a state when the body doesn't have enough calories to support all of its functions [3].
- *Pituitary gland dysfunction.* The pituitary produces and secretes FSH and LH. The ovaries will be unable to ovulate properly if too much or too little of these hormones are produced. Common causes include physical injury, tumours and chemical imbalances, such as Sheehan's syndrome.
- *Ovarian dysfunction.* In approximately 50% of cases, the ovaries do not produce normal follicles in which the eggs can mature. Ovulation is rare if the eggs are immature, and the chances of fertilisation then reduce significantly. Polycystic ovary syndrome (PCOS) is the most common disorder responsible for this problem. Symptoms include amenorrhoea, hirsutism, anovulation and infertility. The syndrome is characterized by a reduced production of FSH, and normal or increased levels of LH, oestrogen and testosterone. This abnormal ratio of gonadotrophins causes partial development of ovarian follicles; follicular cysts therefore develop which are detectable on ultrasound. Please refer to Chapter 14.

Scarred Ovaries

Physical damage to the ovaries may result in failed ovulation. For example, infection or extensive or multiple surgeries for ovarian cysts may damage or scar the capsule of the ovary, so follicles cannot mature properly and ovulation does not occur.

Premature Ovarian Insufficiency and 'Age-Related Infertility'

Human biology dictates that a woman's store of eggs is fixed from birth. From puberty onward that store depletes each month, programmed to be exhausted at menopause, when reproductive life comes to an end. Most studies show this decline starts at around age 35 with the perimenopause beginning around age 45 and menopause at age 51. In premature ovarian insufficiency this decline is quicker, and loss of ovarian function occurs under the age of 40. Women are now living longer, and the average age of childbirth is slowly rising [4] (see Figure 9.1). Premature ovarian insufficiency is a growing concern for women who are going through fertility investigations at an older age.

There has been increasing media interest in the subject of women choosing to have their eggs frozen. The technique of vitrification, with rapid freezing of cells preventing the formation of ice crystals known to damage the genetic structure of the egg, was initially used to preserve fertility ahead of cancer treatments [5] but it is increasingly being used in the private sector to buy time as the biological clock continues to tick. Recent research suggests that pregnancy and live birth rate ('post thaw') show promising outcomes, especially if eggs are frozen at a younger age and if 15 eggs or more were frozen per patient [5]. Although social egg freezing is becoming increasingly popular, the actual use of frozen eggs rate remains low to date [5].

Anatomical Issues

- *Uterine leiomyomas.* Fibroids are very common, typically affecting women aged 30–45. They may be asymptomatic, may cause heavy menstrual bleeding, or may cause symptoms via pressure on other organs such as the bladder. Depending on their position, they can interfere with embryo implantation, while large fibroids may distort the shape of the abdomen or narrow the uterine cavity, leading

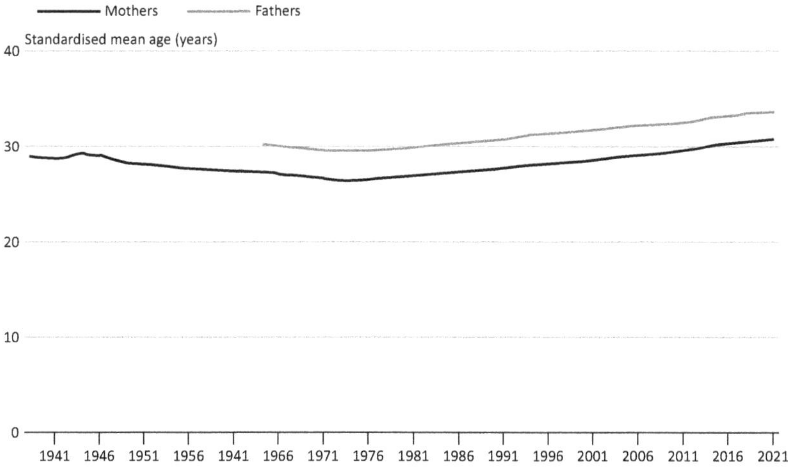

Figure 9.1 Average age of parents remains at record highs. Standardised mean age of mothers and fathers, England and Wales, 1938–2021. Source: www.ons.gov.uk. (n.d.). *Birth Characteristics in England and Wales – Office for National Statistics*. [Online]. Contains public sector information licensed under the Open Government Licence v3.0. Available: www.ons.gov.uk/peoplepopulationandcommunity/birthsdeathsandmarriages/livebirths/bulletins/birthcharacteristicsinenglandandwales/2021#age-of-parents.

to increased risk of miscarriage or preterm delivery.

- *Poorly functioning fallopian tubes.* Tubal disease affects approximately 20% [2] of infertile couples and varies from mild adhesions to complete tubal blockage. Treatment for tubal disease can be surgical. With advances in microsurgery and lasers, success rates (defined as the number of women who become pregnant within one year of surgery) are as high as 30% overall; however, in many cases recognising this as 'absolute infertility' and moving to in vitro fertilisation (IVF) early is recommended. The main causes of tubal damage include the following:
  - *Infection.* This is caused by bacteria and viruses, usually transmitted sexually. Infection commonly causes inflammation and tubal scarring. Sometimes a hydrosalpinx can be seen on ultrasound – this is where the fallopian tube is occluded at both ends and fluid collects in the tube.
  - *Abdominal diseases.* The most common of these are appendicitis and colitis, causing peritoneal inflammation leading to fallopian tube scarring and blockage.
  - *Previous surgery.* Pelvic or abdominal surgery can leave adhesions that damage fallopian tubes.
  - *Ectopic pregnancy.* Pregnancies that occur within the fallopian tube often cause irreversible tubal damage.
  - *Congenital defects.* Rarely, women may be born with genetic defects leading to tubal or uterine abnormalities, such as septate uterus.

Endometriosis

Endometriosis has long been implicated in sub-fertility [6]. The fecundity of healthy couples is approximately 15–20% per month and is directly affected by maternal age, whereas the fecundity of women with endometriosis drops to 2–10% per month [1].

Endometriotic spots occur not only in the uterus (adenomyosis) but also elsewhere in the abdomen, commonly affecting the fallopian tubes, ovaries, pouch of Douglas and pelvic peritoneum. A positive diagnosis has traditionally only been made by diagnostic laparoscopy, but MRI now plays more of a role in the diagnostic process.

The management of endometriosis-related infertility requires a multidisciplinary approach, with input from a fertility specialist. Surgical treatments should be discussed and offered to patients with endometriosis-related sub-fertility, as they may improve the chances of natural conception [6].

Environmental Factors

Environmental factors affecting male and female infertility include air pollution, chemotherapy, radiotherapy and lifestyle factors (such as smoking and obesity). For example, obesity affects both female and male infertility in a variety of ways, from hormonal dysfunction and a negative effect on oocyte quality to an adverse impact on DNA and gene expression. Rising levels of obesity, and its associated morbidity, are a key global concern. As well as the negative impact on fertility, obesity is associated with increased risk of pregnancy and birth complications for both mother and infant. It is essential that lifestyle factors are raised early on in the fertility journey (ideally long before patients begin the referral process, such as at contraceptive reviews and routine health checks) [7].

Male Infertility

Problems with production and maturation of sperm are the commonest causes of male infertility [8]. Sperm may be immature, abnormally shaped or unable to move properly. Sperm may also be normal but produced in abnormally low numbers (oligospermia) or seemingly not at all (azoospermia).

Causes include the following:

- *Infection or inflammation*, such as sexually transmitted infections (STIs), prostatitis or mumps.
- *Endocrine or hormonal disorders*, such as Kallmann syndrome (an absence of or decrease in the function of the male testes).
- *Immunological disorders*; some men produce antibodies to their own sperm.
- *Environmental and lifestyle factors.*
- *Genetic diseases*, which are directly or indirectly associated with sperm abnormalities.
- *Anatomical abnormalities.* Obstructions of the genital tract can cause infertility by partially or totally blocking seminal fluid flow. This is commonly due to infection and inflammation, previous surgery or the presence of varicose veins in the scrotum (scrotal varicoceles).
- *Immotile cilia syndrome.* Here, the sperm count is normal, but the spermatozoa are non-motile, for example Kartagener's syndrome.
- *Mitochondrial deletions.* Mitochondria are structures in the cell responsible for energy production. There is a set of genes in the mitochondria separate from the normal chromosome set contained in the nucleus. Recently, it has been discovered that these genes, when altered or deleted, can affect a person's health and/or fertility.
- *Liver disease, renal disease or treatment for seizure disorders.*
- *Other factors.* Other factors may arise from the defective delivery of sperm into the female genital tract. This could be caused by impotence or premature ejaculation.

Changing Family Demographics

According to figures from the Human Fertilisation and Embryo Authority (HFEA), increasing numbers of single patients and patients in female same-sex relationships are using IVF and donor insemination to get pregnant [9]. NICE has produced clear guidelines on available NHS-funded fertility options for same-sex couples [1].

Initial Assessment

The first consultation is important, as time is paramount for a successful outcome. Women often present alone for the first consultation, and this allows exploration of any guilt or stigma attached to sub-fertility, and sensitivity when discussing histories of previous pregnancies, pelvic infection and sexual abuse. This can evoke significant negative emotions for women and may not have been shared with their current partner. It may be appropriate to encourage future transparency with their partner, who is usually the major support system for the woman. Psychological support and counselling may also be helpful. However, the primary aim should not be lost or overshadowed by the psychological element, as this will often be resolved by achieving a live birth. Both partners should be encouraged to attend future appointments.

Infertility History

General

For both parties, the basic history should include the following:

- age
- smoking status
- alcohol consumption
- BMI
- history of STIs
- frequency of unprotected vaginal sexual intercourse
- history of surgery to abdomen or genital organs

- previous history of major medical or surgical illness
- consanguinity.

Female

- Nature of relationship; heterosexual, same-sex, single parent.
- Length of time trying to conceive.
- Parity.
- Smear results.
- Menstrual history; age started, duration, regularity of cycle, contraception.
- Sexual history; pain during intercourse.
- Intermenstrual or postcoital bleeding.
- Genetic abnormalities.
- Psychosexual difficulties.

Male

- Any previous fathered pregnancies.
- Problems with erection and/or ejaculation.
- Previous history of trauma, torsion or operation to testes.
- Use of steroids, for example for muscle building.

A questionnaire may be useful to avoid omissions and save time.

Examination

Examination may be helpful to exclude any major findings and identify higher-risk patients for early onward referral. This would include patients with a fibroid mass, evidence of hirsutism and clinical signs of PCOS, and patients where the pelvis feels fixed or there is nodularity suggestive of endometriosis.

A male genital examination might reveal small or undescended testes, hernia or hydrocele, all potential causes of abnormal sperm.

Advice

General

All patients should be given the following advice.

- Lifestyle factors such as weight, smoking and alcohol intake play a major role in fertility and should be optimised to give the best chance of pregnancy. A BMI between 20 and 29 is ideal for both men and women. Smoking cessation is essential.
- Vaginal sexual intercourse two to three days every week is advisable.
- Female fertility and (to a lesser extent) male fertility declines with age.
- Stress can reduce libido and frequency of intercourse, which can contribute to the fertility problems.
- Contacting a fertility support group or having counselling may be helpful.

Local guidelines differ, but ideally patients must have stopped smoking for at least six months and have a BMI of less than 30 to qualify for NHS treatment. If couples are made aware of the guidelines early on, it gives them an opportunity to achieve the target BMI before investigation or treatment starts. It will also help with spontaneous conception.

Advice for Specific Risk Factors

- *Tight underwear.* There is an association between elevated scrotal temperature and reduced semen quality, but it is uncertain whether wearing loose-fitting underwear improves fertility.
- *Occupation.* An enquiry about occupation should be made as some occupations involve exposure to hazards that can reduce male/female fertility; appropriate advice should be offered.
- *Drug use.* Advice should be provided regarding prescription, over-the-counter or recreational drugs which may interfere with male and female fertility.
- *Folic acid.* Women should take folic acid (recommended dose: 0.4 mg/day) before conception and up to 12 weeks' gestation to reduce the risk of having a baby with neural tube defects. A higher dose of 5 mg/day is recommended by NICE for the following groups [10]:
  - As of 2026, NICE no longer recommend a higher dose for women with a BMI >30, but RCOG guidance does still advise this.
  - Women with a child with a neural tube defect.
  - Women who are taking anti-epileptic medication.
  - Women with diabetes, coeliac disease, sickle-cell disease or thalassaemia.
- *Complementary therapy.* The effectiveness of complementary therapies for fertility problems has not been properly evaluated; further research is needed before such interventions

can be recommended. Women wishing to know more about this could be directed to the HFEA website [11].

Investigations

Initial investigations are done in primary care, while further investigation and management requires referral.

Primary Care Investigations [1]

- Local referral criteria should be checked as to the exact tests required before referral.
- Female tests to consider at the point of referral include the following:
  - FSH and LH – between days 2 and 4 of the cycle
  - Day 21 progesterone (if irregular cycle, can be repeated a week later)
  - FBC, TFTs, oestradiol, prolactin, testosterone and sex-hormone binding globulin
  - Rubella and chlamydia screening
  - Transvaginal ultrasound scan (TVUS) is optional at this stage. A more detailed scan will be repeated within the infertility service.
  - Anti-Müllerian hormone, which some GPs may have access to in primary care – as of early 2026 this access is not universal.
- Male tests:
  - Semen analysis – if the first result is abnormal, repeat the test no sooner than three months later (or as soon as possible if there is azoospermia or severe oligospermia)
  - If the repeat semen analysis is abnormal, then FSH, LH, prolactin, testosterone, TSH tests and genetics tests such as karyotyping, CFTR mutation and Y-chromosome microdeletion should be performed. These may be requested by the specialist fertility team.

Baseline tests for both halves of the couple are imperative as more intrusive investigations should only be proceeded with if the couple are both actively engaged.

Investigations Usually Conducted within an Infertility Service

- *Ovarian reserve testing.* The day 2–4 FSH is a useful predictor of ovarian reserve and is crucial in guiding the choice of IVF protocol. Additionally, two other tests of ovarian reserve are supported by NICE:
  - Total antral follicle count, ≤4 for a low response and >16 for a high response (this is assessed as part of a baseline 3D transvaginal ultrasound scan – see below).
  - Anti-Müllerian hormone (AMH), ≤5.4 pmol/L for a low response and ≥25.0 pmol/L for a high response [12].
- *Ultrasound scanning.* A 3D TVUS assesses antral follicle reserve and helps to identify anatomical causes of infertility, such as a bicornuate uterus or intramural fibroids.
- *Hystero-salpingogram (HSG).* An HSG is the simplest test to check tubal patency. Radio-opaque dye is inserted through the cervical os, visualising an outline of the uterus and tubes. HSG can identify adhesions, polyps and fibroids, as well as congenital abnormalities. The dye may show up tubal blockages.
- *Hysterosalpingo contrast sonography (HyCoSy).* This uses an ultrasound scan and contrast medium to get a more detailed image of the uterus, ovaries and tubes. It is used to check for polycystic ovaries, fibroids, polyps and other problems in the pelvis, as well as tubal patency. It has become increasingly popular in recent years and has the advantage over HSG of not involving ionising radiation.
- Magnetic resonance hysterosalpingography (MR-HSG). An MR-HSG is a relatively new and less invasive test than HSG or HyCoSy. Studies show similar diagnostic performance to HyCoSy [13].
- *Laparoscopy.* This is more invasive, but it is often considered the 'gold standard'. It is usually performed if a woman has a history of pelvic surgery (such as an appendectomy), pelvic pain or other symptoms, or if an HSG (or HyCoSy) has highlighted a possible problem. Laparoscopy has the advantage of being able to examine the outside of the tubes and uterus to check for adhesions and endometriosis. A dye is usually passed through the inside of the tubes to check they are patent. An exploratory laparoscopy allows treatment of conditions such as endometriosis or adhesions at the same time. A hysteroscopy may be performed at the same time as laparoscopy to assess the uterine cavity.

These tests will support the decision-making for NHS IVF referral.

NICE [1] recommends that women with no known comorbidities (such as pelvic inflammatory disease, previous ectopic pregnancy or endometriosis) should be offered HSG or, where appropriate expertise is available, HyCoSy, to screen for tubal occlusion. This is a reliable test for ruling out tubal occlusion and is less invasive. It makes more efficient use of resources than laparoscopy. A systemic review and meta-analysis showed a 92% sensitivity for diagnosing tubal occlusion and 95% specificity in HSG and similar results for HyCoSy [14].

Management Strategies

Female Factor Infertility

- *Ovulation disorders: polycystic ovaries.* Ovarian stimulation treatments include clomifene citrate, metformin or a combination of these. If there is resistance to clomifene, laparoscopic ovarian drilling, combined treatments of clomifene and metformin or gonadotropins should be considered.
- *Tubal and uterine disorders.* For women with mild tubal disease, tubal surgery may be more effective than no treatment. Women with hydrosalpinx should be offered salpingectomy, preferably by laparoscopy, before IVF. Women with amenorrhoea and intrauterine adhesions should be offered hysteroscopic adhesiolysis to restore menstruation and improve their chance of pregnancy.
- *Managing endometriosis.* There is no proven association between the extent of the disease and symptom severity. Women with mild, moderate or severe disease should be offered laparoscopic surgical ablation or resection of endometriosis plus adhesiolysis to improve fertility. Women with ovarian endometriomas should also be offered laparoscopic cystectomy.

Male Factor Infertility

Dependent on the cause and severity, the following may be considered.

- Assisted reproductive technologies:
  - *Artificial insemination.* This procedure places large numbers of healthy sperm either at the entrance of the cervix or into the partner's uterus.
  - *IVF, GIFT and other techniques.* In vitro fertilisation and gamete intrafallopian transfers have been used to treat male infertility. As is the case with artificial insemination, IVF and similar techniques offer the opportunity to prepare sperm in vitro, so that oocytes are exposed to an optimal concentration of high-quality, motile sperm.
  - *Microsurgical fertilisation* (microinjection techniques, such as intracytoplasmic sperm injection). This treatment is used to facilitate sperm penetration by injection of a single sperm into the oocyte.
- *Drug therapy.* A small percentage of infertile men have a hormonal disorder that can be treated with hormone therapy.
- *Surgery.* This is designed to overcome anatomical barriers that impede sperm production and maturation or ejaculation. Procedures to remove varicose veins in the scrotum (varicocele) can occasionally improve the quality of sperm.

Unexplained Infertility

A great deal of research has gone into the medical management of unexplained infertility, and it is clear that there is much overtreatment. This observation has been supported by a number of publications, including a 2015 meta-analysis from the Netherlands in which the authors point out that treatment often seemed to delay the much-wanted successful outcome [15]. It is important to recognise the huge psychological impact on couples going through fertility investigations and treatment and to bear in mind that where no cause is found, there is an excellent chance of having a pregnancy naturally.

Perhaps the message should be – 'Just think of the number of women who became pregnant spontaneously after several treatment cycles failed'. NICE states that women with unexplained fertility should not be treated with ovarian stimulation drugs but should be encouraged to have regular unprotected sex for a total of two years (this includes up to one year before investigations) before IVF will be considered.

Prediction of IVF Success

The key to cost-effective management is the identification of those most likely to achieve a live birth through IVF, which has led to the introduction of access criteria.

NICE guidelines [1] suggest that women aged 40 or under who have never had IVF should be offered three full cycles of IVF if they have evidence of a good ovarian reserve, with one cycle being offered to those who are aged 40–42.

Because of current financial pressures, there is, however, widespread variation on the adoption of the NICE guideline, for example exclusion of those with an existing child, leading to a concern about a 'postcode lottery' in care.

Post-Treatment Outcomes

Fertility care doesn't end with a positive pregnancy test. Many couples will have increased risks relating either to their fertility problem or to maternal age alone. In addition to this, despite the HFEA aim to reduce twin pregnancy rates down to 10% for IVF patients, the rates can still be considerably higher and vary between centres. Twin pregnancies are by definition a high-risk pregnancy and NICE supports single embryo transfer in those with higher chances of successful treatment.

NICE advises that patients are told that the absolute risks of long-term adverse outcomes in children born as a result of IVF are low.

Conclusion

Many women are unaware of the decline in fertility after the age of 30, as well as the negative impact of obesity and smoking on fertility outcomes. Contraception consultations present an opportunity to raise these issues, as well as to provide education about the increasing risks of pregnancy, including miscarriage, with age.

Investigations in primary care should be undertaken promptly to prevent delay in referral; recognizing 'at-risk groups' early on allows referral without delay.

The first consultation is essential to managing expectations. The patient should have a clear idea of the process and timescales involved. As a GP, it is critical to know the local criteria for NHS-funded treatment, allowing the patient a head-start on stopping smoking and reducing their weight where relevant. Empathy and transparency of the clinician as well as local support groups and fertility forums may be invaluable in supporting patients along their journey.

References

[1] NICE, 'CG156. Fertility problems: Assessment and treatment'. Sept. 2017. Accessed: 9 Sep. 2024. [Online]. Available: www.nice.org.uk/guidance/CG156.

[2] NICE CKS, 'Infertility'. Jul. 2023. Accessed: 9 Sep. 2024. [Online]. Available: https://cks.nice.org.uk/topics/infertility.

[3] M. Mountjoy, J. K. Sundgot-Borgen, L. M. Burke et al., 'IOC consensus statement on relative energy deficiency in sport (RED-S): 2018 update', *Br J Sports Med*, vol. **52**, no. 11, pp. 687–697, 2018.

[4] Office for National Statistics, 'Births in England and Wales: Summary tables'. Feb. 2024. Accessed: 9 Sep. 2024. [Online]. Available: www.ons.gov.uk/peoplepopulationandcommunity/birthsdeathsandmarriages/livebirths/datasets/birthsummarytables.

[5] P. Kakkar, J. Geary, T. Stockburger et al., 'Outcomes of social egg freezing: A cohort study and a comprehensive literature review', *J Clin Med*, vol. **12**, no. 13, 4182, 2023.

[6] C. Bulletti, M. E. Coccia, S. Battistoni et al., 'Endometriosis and infertility', *J Assist Reprod Genet*, vol. **27**, no. 8, pp. 441–447, 2010.

[7] A. Sahu, S. Pajai, A. Sahu et al., 'The impact of obesity on reproductive health and pregnancy outcomes', *Cureus*, vol. **15**, no. 11, e48882, 2023.

[8] S. Minhas, C. Bettocchi, L. Boeri et al. (EAU Working Group on Male Sexual and Reproductive Health), 'European Association of Urology guidelines on male sexual and reproductive health: 2021 *update* on male infertility', *Eur Urol*, vol. **80**, no. 5, pp. 603–620, 2021.

[9] HFEA, 'Key facts and statistics'. Accessed: 9 Sep. 2024. [Online]. Available: www.hfea.gov.uk/about-us/media-centre/key-facts-and-statistics.

[10] NICE CKS, 'Antenatal care – uncomplicated pregnancy'. Feb. 2023. Accessed: 9 Sep. 2024. [Online]. Available: https://cks.nice.org.uk/topics/antenatal-care-uncomplicated-pregnancy.

[11] HFEA, 'Complementary and alternative therapies'. Accessed: 9 Sep. 2024. [Online]. Available: www.hfea.gov.uk/treatments/complementary-and-alternative-therapies.

[12] A. La Marca, G. Sighinolfi, D. Radi et al., 'Anti-Müllerian hormone (AMH) as a predictive marker

in assisted reproductive technology (ART)', *Hum Reprod Update*, vol. **16**, no. 2, pp. 113–130, 2010.

[13] L.-S. Chen, Z.-Q. Zhu, L. Jing et al., 'Hysterosalpingo-contrast-sonography vs. magnetic resonance-hysterosalpingography for diagnosing fallopian tubal patency: A systematic review and meta-analysis', *European Journal of Radiology,* vol. **125**, 108891, 2020.

[14] S. Maheux-Lacroix, A. Boutin, L. Moore et al., 'Hysterosalpingosonography for diagnosing tubal occlusion in subfertile women: A systematic review with meta-analysis', *Syst Rev*, vol. **2**, 50, 2013.

[15] F. Kersten, R. P. Hermens, D. D. Braat et al., 'Overtreatment in couples with unexplained infertility', *Hum Reprod*, vol. **30**, no. 1, pp. 71–80, 2015.

Chapter 10

Ectopic Pregnancy from a Primary Care Perspective

Jacqui Tuckey and Chantal Simonis

Key Points

- Always include ectopic pregnancy in your differential diagnosis for women of reproductive age with abdominal pain.
- Pain and bleeding in early pregnancy is an ectopic pregnancy until proven otherwise.
- Not all women with ectopic pregnancy have typical symptoms.
- Most women with ectopic pregnancy do not have any known risk factors.
- Women with a history of ectopic pregnancy should be offered access to early ultrasound scanning in any subsequent pregnancy to determine location.
- No method of contraception is contraindicated in a woman solely because she has had an ectopic pregnancy.
- The psychological sequelae of ectopic pregnancy are often overlooked.

Case Scenario 10.1: Laura

Laura is a 37-year-old patient presenting to a tertiary fertility clinic with a four-year history of secondary sub-fertility. She had a right salpingectomy for ectopic pregnancy in a previous relationship. Diagnostic laparoscopy in 2014 had shown an absent right fallopian tube, a normal, patent left tube and the presence of mild endometriosis. Her partner had a normal semen analysis and two conceptions with a previous partner (resulting in a termination of pregnancy and an ectopic).

The couple underwent an IVF cycle resulting in the transfer of two embryos. Two weeks later a urinary pregnancy test was positive. Laura attended at seven weeks' gestation for an early pregnancy scan. On questioning, she commented that she had noticed a small amount of brown vaginal loss the week before. This had settled and she had not had any pain.

Transvaginal pelvic ultrasound scan showed an empty uterus with a thickened endometrium. A left adnexal mass could be seen and there was a small amount of blood in the pouch of Douglas. Laura was transferred straight to the gynaecology ward and underwent emergency laparoscopy. This confirmed the diagnosis of left ampullary ectopic pregnancy and she underwent laparoscopic salpingectomy.

Introduction

An ectopic pregnancy is one which implants outside of the endometrial cavity. Without timely diagnosis and treatment, it may be a life-threatening condition [1]. Most ectopic pregnancies are tubal (98%), with the remainder occurring in the abdomen, ovary or cervix. Of tubal pregnancies, 80% occur in the ampulla [2].

Prevalence

There are approximately 120,000 ectopic pregnancies in the UK each year with a prevalence of 11:1,000 pregnancies [3]. The incidence is increasing worldwide, mainly due to the increased incidence of pelvic inflammatory disease, in many cases caused by *Chlamydia trachomatis*. Ectopic pregnancy is more common following IVF, with an incidence of 4% [4]. This is mainly due to the proportion of women undergoing assisted conception who have underlying tubal pathology.

Heterotopic pregnancy, with the presence of a simultaneous intra- and extra-uterine pregnancy, occurs in 1:4,000 pregnancies. It is more common after IVF because of the increase in multiple pregnancies [4]. It is of vital importance, therefore, that a healthcare professional carrying out pelvic ultrasound scan for pregnancy is informed if the patient has had IVF and how many embryos have been replaced. Any practitioner must be adequately trained and must fully assess the pelvis, even if an intrauterine pregnancy is seen, so that this rare type of pregnancy is not missed.

Risk Factors

The main risk factor for ectopic pregnancy is tubal damage from previous ectopic pregnancy, pelvic inflammatory disease, endometriosis or tubal surgery. Faulty implantation of developing embryos occurs because of a defect in the anatomy or function of the damaged fallopian tube. The incidence of tubal damage increases with successive episodes of PID (13% after a single episode, 35% after two and 75% after three episodes) [5]. Overall, a patient with a history of ectopic pregnancy has a 10–25% chance of a further ectopic pregnancy [5].

Much has been written about the risk of ectopic pregnancy with IUD use for contraception. A meta-analysis of case-control studies published in the 1990s reported no increased risk of ectopic pregnancy associated with copper IUD use [6]. NICE guidance on long-acting reversible contraception (LARC) states that the risk of ectopic pregnancy associated with the use of copper IUDs is lower than using no contraception [7]. The UK medical eligibility criteria (UKMEC) for contraceptive use considers past ectopic pregnancy to be a condition for which there is no restriction for the use of IUDs [8]. The absolute risk of ectopic pregnancy is not increased by the use of intrauterine contraception because the method is highly effective. However, if a woman becomes pregnant using an IUD, it is likely to be ectopic and so this must be excluded. The bottom line is that IUDs are better at preventing pregnancies in the uterus than the tube. CoSRH guidance on intrauterine contraception states that women should be advised that the overall risk of ectopic pregnancy is very low, approximately 1 in 1,000 at five years of use [9]. Regardless, women choosing intrauterine methods of contraception should be informed about symptoms of ectopic pregnancy.

Complications

Ectopic pregnancy presents a major health problem for women of reproductive age. Failure to make a prompt diagnosis can result in tubal rupture, which in turn can lead to haemorrhage, shock, disseminated intravascular coagulation (DIC) and ultimately death. Details of these fatal cases are included in the MBRRACE-UK (Mothers and Babies: Reducing Risks through Audits and Confidential Enquiries) report which includes the national Confidential Enquiry into Maternal Deaths (CEMD), reported yearly [10].

A significant consequence of ectopic pregnancy is tubal sub-fertility. Approximately 40% of women with a history of ectopic pregnancy will face difficulties in conceiving an intrauterine pregnancy spontaneously and 25% of couples having assisted conception treatment will have a diagnosis of tubal sub-fertility [2].

When to Suspect an Ectopic Pregnancy

In a recent MBRRACE-UK report (November 2022), a chapter was dedicated solely to maternal deaths from early pregnancy disorders [10]. The UK death rate from ectopic pregnancy increased from five in the previous report to eight. Importantly, a disproportionate number of vulnerable and young women died from ectopic pregnancy in 2018–2020. Knight et al. observed multiple structural and other biases in UK maternity care [10] which are being addressed by NHS England in their Three-Year Delivery Plan for Maternity and Neonatal Services, 2023 [11].

One of the concerns of the CEMD was the difficulty in diagnosing the condition. In our case study, Laura was a fertility patient with a history of previous ectopic pregnancy. She had minimal symptoms, yet the pregnancy was easily detected on ultrasound scan – this is not a common scenario. About one-third of women will have no known risk factors and atypical presentation is common [12,13].

Ectopic pregnancy should be suspected in women with vaginal bleeding or abdominal pain, especially if they are known to be pregnant, have missed or have irregular periods. A review of studies reported in NICE guidelines found that 93% of women with ectopic pregnancy present with abdominal or pelvic pain, 73% with amenorrhoea and 64% with vaginal bleeding [12]. Many women have poor recall for their menstrual history; it is crucial to remember that what is described as a period may not be. Less common symptoms include gastrointestinal symptoms, dizziness, fainting and shoulder tip pain.

The report of the Confidential Enquiry states that GPs should ask all women of reproductive age who have abdominal pain with diarrhoea and/or vomiting about the risk of pregnancy. If there is any possibility, a urinary pregnancy test (UPT) should be carried out in the surgery. NICE recommend that all healthcare professionals caring for women of reproductive age should have access to pregnancy tests. The Confidential Enquiry report goes further in suggesting that GPs should consider carrying a pregnancy test in their emergency bag. Fainting and dizziness are uncommon with gastroenteritis but may occur with a bleeding ectopic pregnancy.

How to Manage a Suspected Ectopic Pregnancy

Management depends primarily on how stable the patient is. Women with bleeding or other symptoms of an early pregnancy complication should have their pulse and blood pressure assessed. Those women who are not haemodynamically stable should be transferred to hospital by ambulance with intravenous fluids, if available. Women who are haemodynamically stable should have a UPT to confirm pregnancy and an abdominal examination should be carried out. If abdominal tenderness is elicited, an ectopic pregnancy should be strongly suspected, and immediate admission arranged to an early pregnancy assessment unit (EPAU) or out-of-hours gynaecology service. If abdominal pain and tenderness is absent, a pelvic examination should be carried out to check for pelvic or cervical motion tenderness, and if present urgent admission arranged as above. It is recommended by the NICE Guideline Development Group (GDG) that palpating for adnexal masses when performing pelvic examination for women with pain should be avoided because of the risk of tubal rupture [12].

As an aside, women of reproductive age who present to the emergency department should have a UPT and Focussed Assessment with Sonography in Trauma (FAST) scan before thrombolysis is considered for a diagnosis of possible pulmonary embolism [10]. In the 2022 MBRRACE report, three women died from ruptured ectopic pregnancies after receiving thrombolysis. A FAST scan had not been performed in any of these women, despite symptoms suggestive of ectopic pregnancy.

Laura was asymptomatic and haemodynamically stable. She did, however, have clear ultrasound findings consistent with an ectopic pregnancy. Had she presented to her GP with this scenario, a same-day referral to an EPAU would have been the appropriate course of action.

Early Pregnancy Assessment Unit

Assessment and ultrasound scanning facilities should ideally be available seven days a week for the management of women with complications of early pregnancy. They should offer a dedicated service provided by healthcare professionals competent to diagnose and care for women with pain and bleeding in early pregnancy. These units should have the facility to accept self-referrals from women with previous ectopic pregnancy and recurrent miscarriage. In the primary care setting, expectant management may be used for women less than six weeks' gestation with light bleeding, but no pain. Women need to be given clear advice on symptoms to be aware of and how to access emergency care. It is vital that GPs know their own local facilities and referral pathways.

The recommendations for women less than six weeks' gestation are based on evidence reviewed by NICE [12]. It demonstrates that ultrasound scanning does not always confirm a diagnosis at less than six weeks and that many women have spotting in early pregnancy that resolves without needing investigation. Additionally, the expert reviewers were of the opinion that a negative UPT virtually rules out an ectopic. Remember, there are always exceptions, and it is crucial to be guided by the patient's signs and symptoms. It is not possible to be certain of gestation due to irregular menses or a patient's inaccurate recall of their menstrual cycle.

Support and Information Giving

Early pregnancy complications can cause significant distress to women and their partners. They should always be treated with dignity and respect, even when the pregnancy is unplanned. Past history will contribute to how a patient manages the situation in which she finds herself. Women will react differently to early pregnancy complications and need to be provided with information and support in a sensitive way. If you make a referral, it is important to explain what she can expect to happen next and why.

Diagnosis in Secondary Care

Women who are haemodynamically unstable will be admitted for urgent surgical management. For stable women in whom an ectopic pregnancy is suspected, a transvaginal ultrasound will be carried out to determine if the pregnancy is intrauterine, definite or probable ectopic, a molar pregnancy or a pregnancy of unknown location. If the diagnosis is uncertain, serial human chorionic gonadotrophin (hCG) levels, repeat transvaginal scans or laparoscopy may be used [12,13]. It is important that the woman understands that it can sometimes require repeated investigations to make a diagnosis – this clearly may add to her distress.

Treatment Options

The treatment options for a haemodynamically stable woman may be expectant, medical or surgical. The choice depends on clinical stability, site of implantation, risk of rupture, serum hCG, level of pain and acceptability of the method of treatment to the woman. A small proportion of women with an ectopic pregnancy with very minimal or no symptoms can simply be watched. Intervention may be required if symptoms develop or worsen, or if hCG levels are not steadily falling.

NICE recommends medical management with methotrexate as a first-line treatment, provided the woman can return for follow-up [12]. They must have no significant pain, an unruptured ectopic pregnancy with an adnexal mass less than 35 mm and no visible heartbeat, hCG level 1,500–5,000 IU/L and no intrauterine pregnancy on scan.

Methotrexate is a folic acid antagonist which can be given intramuscularly (IM) or injected into the ectopic pregnancy. Direct injection into the ectopic requires laparoscopy and success rates are lower than with systemic methotrexate. The currently used regimen is IM methotrexate 50 mg/mg. Serum hCG levels are checked on days 4 and 7 with repeat transvaginal pelvic ultrasound. A second dose of methotrexate should be considered if hCG levels do not fall by at least 15% [13]. Serum hCG levels are continued weekly until a negative result is obtained. Approximately 14% of women will require a repeat dose and less than 10% will require subsequent surgical intervention. Three in four women will experience pain and a proportion of women will require hospital admission for observation. Conjunctivitis, stomatitis and gastrointestinal upset may occur secondary to methotrexate use.

Surgery may involve removal of the tube (salpingectomy) or tubal incision and removal of the pregnancy (salpingotomy). Following salpingotomy, serial hCG levels will be required to ensure that no persistent trophoblasts remain. Salpingectomy is the treatment of choice as a damaged or diseased tube is associated with a high risk of recurrence. Salpingotomy should only be offered, as an alternative, to those with contralateral tubal damage; however, up to one out of five of these women will require further treatment, either medical or surgical [12]. Laparoscopy is preferable to laparotomy, but evidence suggests no benefit in terms of future fertility. Women who are rhesus negative and undergo surgical management should be offered anti-D prophylaxis [12,13].

In view of her previous history of ectopic pregnancy, it was appropriate that Laura was advised to have a salpingectomy. She had four years of secondary sub-fertility following her first ectopic and therefore medical management or conservative surgery would not have been a prudent choice for a clearly damaged tube.

Fertility after Ectopic Pregnancy

A woman who has an ectopic pregnancy will want to know what her chances are of having a successful pregnancy in the future. Figures vary, but the Ectopic Pregnancy Trust advises that chance of future intrauterine pregnancy is 65% at one year and 85% at two years [14].

Controversy exists on the impact of different treatment options on future fertility. An observational population-based study including 1,064 women with ectopic pregnancy between 1992 and 2008 concluded a two-year cumulative rate of intrauterine pregnancy to be 67% after salpingectomy, 76% after salpingotomy and 76% after medical treatment [15]. It must not be forgotten that other factors have an impact on pregnancy rates, with a significantly lower rate for women >35 years. The two-year cumulative risk of recurrence was 18.5% after surgical treatment and 25.5% after methotrexate.

A multicentre RCT looking at 446 women with a healthy contralateral tube concluded that there is no significant difference in fertility rates after salpingotomy or salpingectomy [16].

Laura's only option for fertility was further assisted conception; fortunately, she had some frozen embryos stored. Despite the absence of both fallopian tubes, she will still have a very small risk of cornual ectopic pregnancy. Surgical removal of the tubes will always be as complete as possible, but a cornual stump may remain. Laura will need to have an early ultrasound scan at approximately six weeks' gestation in any future pregnancy to confirm location.

Follow-Up

The psychological cost of ectopic pregnancy is frequently overlooked and is often not considered in the same way as other pregnancy loss [4]. In fact, women often have the same grief reaction as those who experience miscarriage but may also have the additional stress of future fertility concerns.

Follow-up is an important part of the process. Sadly, this is not always offered in the hospital setting and may fall to the GP thus it is important to be well informed. It is vital to ensure that any arrangements that have already been made for antenatal care are cancelled and this requires vigilance. There is nothing more distressing to a woman who has experienced an early pregnancy loss than receiving, for example an appointment for a nuchal scan.

Laura had not yet arranged antenatal care, although her GP was of course advised of her ectopic pregnancy. Laura and her partner were offered counselling within the sub-fertility clinic setting. It is a requirement of the Human Fertilisation and Embryology Authority (HFEA) that clinics offering assisted conception offer access to specialist counselling if required.

The woman needs to be given the opportunity to discuss any questions she may have about her treatment, future fertility and risk of recurrence. Subsequent pregnancies should be reported promptly so that early location scanning can be arranged. Psychological wellbeing needs to be assessed. Grief, anxiety and depression are common after early pregnancy loss and may be as intense as that following any other form of bereavement. Distress is commonly at its worst after four to six weeks and may last for many months. Referral for counselling, preferably with a counsellor experienced in dealing with pregnancy loss, may be appropriate. The Ectopic Pregnancy Trust (www.ectopic.org.uk) is a charity supporting patients who have experienced ectopic pregnancy and healthcare professionals looking after them. The Miscarriage Association (www.miscarriageassociation.org.uk) offers similar support.

Don't forget that, like any other conception, an ectopic pregnancy may have been unplanned and unwanted and contraceptive advice may be required. The issues around IUD use have been discussed above, but the recommendations from CoSRH are that no form of contraception is contraindicated after ectopic pregnancy. Women need reliable, effective contraception; a method with a low failure rate will have a low risk of ectopic. Even women who wish a further pregnancy may require short-term reliable contraception until they have recovered both emotionally and physically and are ready to try again. Women who are treated with methotrexate should be advised to avoid pregnancy for three months as there is a possible teratogenic risk – this needs to be clearly stated when they choose this treatment method.

As she no longer had either fallopian tube, Laura could not conceive spontaneously and therefore did not require contraceptive advice.

Conclusion

Ectopic pregnancy is a common complication of early pregnancy, and the incidence has risen worldwide due to the increase in pelvic infection, mainly as a result of rising chlamydia rates. It can result in significant morbidity, affecting both physical and mental health. Future fertility may be affected and there is a risk of recurrence, which may vary depending on method of treatment undertaken. Tubal infertility accounts for the diagnosis in about one-quarter of couples attending fertility services.

Ectopic pregnancy can be difficult to diagnose and this was one concern raised by the CEMD. Deaths from early pregnancy complications are low, but ectopic pregnancy remains the most common cause. The 2022 report concluded that almost all women who died could have had better care. Any maternal death is a tragedy; we will only avoid deaths from ectopic pregnancy by vigilance and raising awareness among both health professionals and the public. The adage that a woman of reproductive age with abdominal pain has an ectopic pregnancy until proven otherwise is one that is well worth remembering.

References

[1] C. M. Farquhar, 'Ectopic pregnancy', *Lancet*, vol. **366**, no. 9485, pp. 583–591, 2005.

[2] K. T. Barnhart, 'Clinical practice: Ectopic pregnancy', *NEJM*, vol. **361**, no. 4, pp. 379–387, 2009.

[3] Health Services Safety Investigation Body, *The Diagnosis of Ectopic Pregnancy*. Healthcare Safety Investigation Branch, 2020. Accessed 29 Feb. 2024. [Online]. Available: www.hsib.org.uk.

[4] J. L. Tay, J. Moore and J. J. Walker, 'Ectopic pregnancy', *BMJ*, vol. **320**, no. 7239, pp. 916–919, 2000.

[5] V. P. Sepilian, 'Ectopic pregnancy'. *Medscape*, 2041923, 2022.

[6] X. Xiong, P. Buekens and E. Wollast, 'IUD use and the risk of ectopic pregnancy: A meta-analysis of case-control studies', *Contraception*, vol. **52**, pp. 23–34, 1995.

[7] National Institute for Health and Clinical Excellence Clinical Guideline [CG30], 'Long-acting reversible contraception: The effective and appropriate use of long-acting reversible contraception'. 2005 (updated 2019). Accessed 29 Feb. 2024. [Online]. Available: www.nice.org.uk.

[8] CoSRH, 'UK medical eligibility criteria for contraceptive use UKMEC April 2016 (amended September 2019)'. Accessed 29 Feb. 2024. [Online]. Available: www.fsrh.org.

[9] CoSRH, 'Clinical guideline: Intrauterine contraception'. Mar. 2023 (amended July 2023). Accessed 29 Feb. 2024. [Online]. Available: www.fsrh.org.

[10] M. Knight, K. Bunch, R. Patel R et al., on behalf of MBRRACE-UK, 'Saving lives, improving mothers' care core report – Lessons learned to inform maternity care from the UK and Ireland Confidential Enquiries into Maternal Deaths and Morbidity 2018–20'. National Perinatal Epidemiology Unit, University of Oxford, 2022.

[11] NHS England, 'Three year delivery plan for maternity and neonatal services'. Mar. 2023. Accessed 29 Feb. 2024. [Online]. Available: www.england.nhs.uk.

[12] National Institute for Health and Clinical Excellence, 'National Guideline (NG 126): Ectopic pregnancy and miscarriage: Diagnosis and early management'. 17 Apr. 2019 (updated 23 Aug. 2023). Accessed 29 Feb. 2024. [Online]. Available: www.nice.org.uk.

[13] C. J. Elson, R. Salim, N. Potdar et al., on behalf of the Royal College of Obstetricians and Gynaecologists, 'Diagnosis and management of ectopic pregnancy', *BJOG*, vol. **123**, e15–e55, 2016.

[14] The Ectopic Pregnancy Trust, 'Trying to conceive again'. 2021. Accessed 29 Feb. 2024. [Online]. Available: www.ectopic.org.uk.

[15] M. De Bennetot, B. Rabischong, B. Aublet-Cuvelier et al., 'Fertility after tubal ectopic pregnancy: Results of a population-based study', *Fertil Steril*, vol. **98**, no. 5, pp. 1271–1276, 2012.

[16] F. Mol, N. M. van Mello, A. Strandell et al., 'European Surgery in Ectopic Pregnancy (ESEP) study group, Salpingectomy vs salpingotomy in women with tubal pregnancy (ESEP study): An open-label, multicenter randomized controlled trial', *Lancet*, vol. **383**, pp. 1483–1489, 2014.

Management of Miscarriage in Primary Care

Dominique Warren

Key Points

- Miscarriage is defined as the spontaneous loss of a pregnancy before 24 weeks' gestation.
  - Early miscarriage is before 12 weeks.
  - Late miscarriage is 12–24 weeks.
- Miscarriage occurs in up to 25% of pregnancies and 50% of cases of miscarriage are due to chromosomal abnormalities.
- Recurrent miscarriage is defined as three or more consecutive miscarriages.
- The most common signs associated with threatened miscarriage are pain and bleeding. It is important to exclude an ectopic pregnancy in women who have bleeding and pain in early pregnancy.
- An ectopic pregnancy may also present with pain, no bleeding and atypical gastrointestinal symptoms.
- Primary care clinicians must have a low threshold for performing a pregnancy test in sexually active women presenting with pelvic pain.
- Clinicians should be aware that women with a history of bleeding and previous miscarriage can be offered vaginal progestogen after an intrauterine pregnancy is confirmed by scan.
- Miscarriage can have a long-lasting, psychological effect on a woman and her partner, and ongoing emotional support may be needed following the loss and in future pregnancies.
- The management of missed miscarriage includes the following choices: expectant, medical and surgical. It is important that the woman is involved in making the choice.

Definition

A miscarriage is defined as the spontaneous loss of a pregnancy before viability, which is defined as before 24 weeks' gestation [1]. Most of these losses will be defined as an early miscarriage occurring before 12 weeks and they account for 98%. Late miscarriages are defined as occurring between 12 and 24 weeks' gestation [15].

Miscarriage Matters

Miscarriage is common, affecting one in five women nationally, and accounts for an estimated 50,000 admissions [6] to secondary care hospitals for both elective and emergency management. There is also a burden on the primary care sector for both the initial consultation and after-care counselling. The psychological impact on the patient and her family is significant and can be long-lasting, as shown by recent studies [6,4]. Nine months after a pregnancy loss, 18% women are diagnosed with post-traumatic stress, 17% for moderate to severe anxiety and 6% for moderate to severe depression [11].

For this reason, a general practitioner should be versed in the understanding of miscarriage management and its after-care.

Risk Factors and Causes

In most early miscarriages, no cause will be found, although it is thought that chromosomal abnormalities account for many of these cases [3]. There is better understanding of the causes of second-trimester losses but often after investigation reasons can still be vague and multifactorial.

The lack of direct causes can add to the parents' distress as they look for a reason or something to change to prevent a recurrence.

Causes of miscarriage include:

- genetically balanced parental translocation
- abnormal fetal development
- uterine abnormality

- cervical insufficiency (second-trimester miscarriage)
- placental failure
- multiple pregnancies
- immunological issues
- infections
- endocrine, such as luteal phase deficiency or polycystic ovarian syndrome.

Risk factors include:

- age
- high body mass index (BMI) (>30 kg/m^2) is associated with reduced fertility and increased risk of miscarriage
- low BMI (<18 kg/m^2)
- the longer the length of time it takes for the woman to conceive, the higher the chance of miscarriage
- a new partner
- paternal age over 45 years
- smoking
- underlying health conditions such as autoimmune disorders
- multiple pregnancies
- previous miscarriages.

In most cases, the cause of early miscarriage is not directly identified, though certain risk factors are strongly associated with it. Advanced maternal age, defined as 35 or older, is linked to increased fetal chromosomal abnormalities and a decline in oocyte quality, leading to higher rates of abnormal embryos. Miscarriage rates are lowest (12%) in women aged 20–29, rising with age to 65% for those 45 and older. Paternal age over 40 also increases miscarriage risk.

Both being underweight (BMI under 18.5) and obesity (BMI over 30) are associated with higher miscarriage rates. Women with a BMI under 18.5 are 1.6 times more likely to miscarry, while those with a BMI over 30 are 1.9 times more likely.

Black women are at greater risk of miscarriage, with recent studies showing a 40% miscarriage rate in this group. The reason for this is not yet understood but may be related to the increased incidence of medical conditions, for example fibroids, diabetes and hypertension, and also to inequities in healthcare.

Maternal conditions, including autoimmune disorders such as antiphospholipid antibodies and thyroid issues as subtle as subclinical thyroid diagnoses, also increase the risk.

Additionally, the risk of miscarriage increases with the number of prior miscarriages. A systematic review has reported the miscarriage rates to be 11.3%, 17.0%, 28.0%, 39.6%, 47.2% and 63.9% for women with no, one, two or three, four, five and six previous miscarriages, respectively [10]. A lengthier time conceiving has also been linked to higher risk.

Types (Classification)

Miscarriage is defined as below, with management varying for each type [3,6]:

- *Threatened miscarriage*: usually mild symptoms of bleeding with little or no pain. The cervical os is closed.
- *Inevitable miscarriage*: usually presents with heavy bleeding with clots and pain. The cervical os is open. The pregnancy will not continue and will proceed to incomplete or complete miscarriage.
- *Incomplete miscarriage*: this occurs when the products of conception are partially expelled. Many incomplete miscarriages can be unrecognised missed miscarriages.
- *Missed miscarriage*: the fetus is not viable but retained. The uterus is small for dates.
  A pregnancy test can remain positive for several days after the fetus has died. It usually presents with a history of threatened miscarriage and persistent, brown discharge. Early pregnancy symptoms may have decreased or gone.
- *Recurrent miscarriage*: when a woman suffers three or more consecutive miscarriages.

Differential Diagnosis

Bleeding in early pregnancy is common and occurs in approximately one-third of pregnancies [3]. It is important to determine the cause of bleeding, as there are several issues which may be totally unrelated to the pregnancy and potentially serious. In every case the woman needs to understand if her pregnancy is viable.

The main causes of bleeding in early pregnancy:

- normal viable pregnancy
  - implantation bleeding
  - subchorionic hematoma
  - cervical polyps

- cervical ectropion
- cervical malignancy
- ectopic pregnancy
- molar pregnancy.

Abdominal pain can occur in early pregnancy and is more concerning. This must be investigated to exclude the following:

- normal viable pregnancy
- pain associated with corpus luteum
- ectopic pregnancy
- torsion or rupture of ovarian cysts
- urinary tract infection
- appendicitis
- fibroid torsion.

Case Scenario 11.1

Chioma is a 32-year-old primary school teacher who attends evening surgery in tears. She and Adam, her partner, have been trying to conceive for 18 months and she is now 7 weeks pregnant. Chioma experienced a previous first-trimester miscarriage earlier this year which was managed at home after confirmation by scan.

In this pregnancy, Chioma started bleeding at work today and has requested an emergency appointment. She tells you that her bleeding has been light and painless.

It is important that Chioma was seen as an emergency appointment because of her symptoms and her anxiety surrounding pregnancy. The degree of pain and amount of bleeding experienced will give some indication as to the urgency of her management.

A threatened miscarriage is the most common complication of early pregnancy, occurring in approximately 20% of pregnant women before 20 weeks of gestation. Although many women who have had a threatened miscarriage go on to have a successful pregnancy, there is a 2.6-times increase in the risk of miscarriage in the pregnancy and 17% of women will go on to have further complications later in the pregnancy.

A woman who presents with bleeding and associated pain, or pain alone, in early pregnancy should have an ectopic pregnancy excluded as a matter of urgency. Ectopic pregnancies affect 11 in every 1,000 pregnancies and are associated with significant morbidity and a maternal mortality rate of 0.2%. Ectopic pregnancy can present with a variety of symptoms (see Box 11.1).

There are also many women who have no symptoms or signs during their early pregnancy but will be diagnosed with a missed miscarriage at their first antenatal scan.

It is necessary for primary care services to have access to in-house pregnancy testing for women who present with pelvic pain ± vaginal bleeding who may have not considered pregnancy before their consultation.

Who to Refer to Early Pregnancy Services?

It is important for the primary care team to understand the referral route and triage system into the local early pregnancy assessment unit (EPAU) to avoid delay in managing cases of early pregnancy pain and bleeding.

Box 11.1 Symptoms and signs of ectopic pregnancy

Common symptoms:

- abdominal or pelvic pain
- amenorrhoea or missed period
- vaginal bleeding with or without clots.

Other reported symptoms:

- gastrointestinal symptoms
- breast tenderness
- dizziness, fainting or syncope
- shoulder tip pain
- urinary symptoms
- passage of tissue
- rectal pressure or pain on defecation.

Most common signs:

- vaginal examination – adnexal tenderness
- abdominal examination – tenderness.

Other reported signs:

- cervical motion tenderness
- rebound tenderness or peritoneal signs
- pallor
- abdominal distension
- enlarged uterus
- tachycardia (more than 100 beats per minute) or hypotension (less than 100/60 mmHg)
- shock or collapse.

Typically, EPAUs will accept women with bleeding and/or pain or other early pregnancy complications for those with:

- a pregnancy of six weeks' gestation or more
- a pregnancy of uncertain gestation
- a previous ectopic pregnancy.

The National Institute for Health and Care Excellence (NICE) has advised expectant management for women with a pregnancy of less than six weeks' gestation who are bleeding, but not in pain. The rationale is that ultrasound scan at this gestation can be unreliable and lead to multiple inconclusive scans, creating more anxiety.

The expectant management options advised in primary care settings are:

- repeating a urine pregnancy test after 7–10 days and review if it is positive
- a negative pregnancy test means that the pregnancy has miscarried
- for the woman to return if her symptoms continue or worsen
- women who return with worsening symptoms and signs should then be referred.

There should be a low threshold for urgent referral for women with a positive pregnancy test and signs and symptoms associated with ectopic pregnancy. NICE guidance and MBRACE 2024 (Mothers and Babies: Reducing Risks through Audits and Confidential Enquiries across the UK) advise that atypical presentation of ectopic pregnancy can include gastrointestinal symptoms and that about a third of women with an ectopic pregnancy will have no known risk factors. Many EPAUs will review patients with a lower gestation, especially with risk factors for ectopic pregnancy.

Example of EPAU Triage System

Urgency of review will be dependent on symptoms and medical history (Table 11.1).

A transvaginal ultrasound scan is the gold-standard examination in early pregnancy, and the woman should be advised of this before attending to minimise any distress it could engender [1,3]. Reassurance should be given that the scan will have no detrimental effect on the pregnancy itself. Transabdominal scan will be used in conjunction with a transvaginal scan if there is concomitant pathology leading to difficulty in visualization or if the uterus is enlarged and rising out of the pelvis, for example with fibroids. Transabdominal scans can be undertaken if a transvaginal scan is deemed intolerable to the patient, but women should be advised that it can often give a limited view and inaccuracy in early gestation pregnancies.

Table 11.1 Example of EPAU triage system

Urgent – refer to A&E immediately
• Haemodynamically unstable
• Significant abdominal pain
• Heavy bleeding
Review within 24 hours
• Pain with or without bleeding
Review within 48 hours
• Light bleeding with no pain

Case Scenario 11.2

Chioma is referred to the local EPAU and an appointment is made for the following morning. She is given safety-net advice in case she develops heavier bleeding or significant pain overnight.

Emotional Support and Information Giving

Healthcare professionals will need to offer emotional support to the patient and her partner.

Each woman's reaction to complications or the loss of a pregnancy will vary and support should be individualized and managed sensitively [7]. Healthcare professionals helping to manage these patients should consider attending communication courses to ensure language is appropriate.

The primary care team should be meticulous in identifying women where there is a language barrier. Women should be offered an interpreter at every consultation and family members should not be used to translate. This is paramount to ensure that all are given equal access to care.

Social deprivation has been identified as a risk factor for poor outcomes in maternity and early pregnancy. Primary care teams are well placed to identify those where there is more need for accessibility and flexibility due to social concerns and this should be highlighted when referring to EPAU.

Women and their partners should be kept fully informed about the possible causes, anticipated course and investigations they will receive together with timings. Evidence-based information should be provided in a variety of formats and include the following.

- When and how to seek help if existing symptoms worsen or new symptoms develop, including a 24-hour contact telephone number.
- What to expect during the time waiting for an ultrasound scan.
- What to expect during care, such as the potential length and extent of pain and/or bleeding, and the possible side effects.
- Information about postoperative care (for women undergoing surgery).
- What to expect during the recovery period – for example, when it is possible to resume sexual activity and/or try to conceive again, and what to do if she becomes pregnant again.
- Information about the likely impact of treatment on future fertility.
- Where to access support and counselling services, including leaflets, web addresses and helpline numbers for support organisations.

These consultations require sufficient time to discuss issues with additional appointments if required. A follow-up appointment should also be offered to all women following pregnancy loss.

Case Scenario 11.3

Chioma is seen in the EPAU on the following day and has a transvaginal ultrasound scan. The scan confirms a viable six-week pregnancy. She, however, is still experiencing bleeding. She is offered vaginal 400 mg micronised progestogen to be administered twice a day as support for her pregnancy. She is offered a follow-up scan in two weeks.

All women with ongoing bleeding and a normal scan can be offered vaginal micronised progesterone 400 mg twice daily. This has been shown to increase the livebirth rate from 57% to 72% [12].

Case Scenario 11.4

Chioma is seen in the EPAU a few days later complaining of increased bleeding and has a transvaginal ultrasound scan (Box 11.2). The scan confirms a non-viable pregnancy. Condolences and support are offered. She is given the option of expectant, medical or surgical treatments and she opts for expectant management.

Management of Miscarriage

The three management options for miscarriage are:

- expectant
- medical
- surgical (local or general anaesthetic).

Expectant Management

A woman with a confirmed diagnosis of miscarriage can be offered expectant management for up to 14 days initially, assuming there are no other clinical or social concerns, such as infection or increased bleeding risk, or language barriers indicating difficulty in healthcare access.

Women should be informed about the risk of infection (1 in 100), the risk of haemorrhage warranting blood transfusion (2 in 100) and emergency surgery. In some women, bleeding and pain will not occur at all, which may indicate that the process of miscarriage has not started. In some women, bleeding will persist or increase, which may suggest incomplete miscarriage. In both scenarios, a repeat scan should be offered, and all treatment options (continued expectant, medical or surgical management) should be discussed, allowing her to make an informed choice. If she opts for continued expectant management, a further review should be arranged 14 days after the first follow-up appointment.

Women undergoing expectant management of miscarriage are offered verbal and written information about what to expect throughout the process, advice on pain relief and where and when to get help in an emergency. They are advised to remain in contact during this time with EPAU to discuss their progress. Once expectant management is completed, a woman is advised to undertake a urine pregnancy test after three weeks and to contact the healthcare professional if it is positive.

Medical Management

National guidance has advanced to include the administration of an antiprogestogen to improve outcomes for those undergoing medical management for a missed miscarriage. Most EPAUs will offer:

- 200 mg oral mifepristone and

Box 11.2 NICE Criteria for Diagnosing and Managing Miscarriage Based on Transvaginal Ultrasound [6]

If no visible fetal heart is seen, measure crown rump length (CRL), or if no fetal pole, mean gestational sac (MGS) diameter:

CRL	<7 mm	Rescan in 7 days
	>7mm	Seek second opinion on viability of pregnancy and/or rescan in 7 days
MGS	<25 mm	Rescan in 7 days
	>25 mm	Seek second opinion on viability of pregnancy and/or rescan in 7 days

- 48 hours later, 800 µg misoprostol (vaginal, oral or sublingual) unless the gestational sac has already been passed.

This regime has been shown to have an 83% success rate of complete resolution of miscarriage without the need for surgical intervention.

Vaginal misoprostol can also be offered for incomplete miscarriage at doses of 600 mcg or 800 mcg administered vaginally, orally or sublingually.

All women receiving medical management of miscarriage are offered pain relief and anti-emetics as needed. They need to know what to expect throughout the process, including the length and extent of bleeding and the potential side effects of treatment, including pain, diarrhoea and vomiting. The woman should also be advised to undertake a urine pregnancy test after three weeks following her medical management and to contact a healthcare professional if it is positive. The risk of infection and haemorrhage is the same as for expectant management.

Surgical Management

The options for surgical management include:

- manual vacuum aspiration
- surgical management under general anaesthesia.

Manual Vacuum Aspiration

Manual vacuum aspiration (MVA) is undertaken under local anaesthetic in an outpatient or clinic setting. A local anaesthetic is injected into the cervix and the cervix is then gradually dilated (if required). A narrow suction tube is inserted into the uterus to remove the pregnancy tissue by aspiration. The procedure duration is expected to be between 10 and 20 minutes.

Surgical Management of Miscarriage

Surgical management of miscarriage (SMM) is carried out in theatre under general anaesthetic. All women undergoing SMM are provided with oral and written information about the treatment and what to expect during and after the procedure. The risks associated with surgical management are:

- infection (2–3 in 100)
- perforation of uterus (1 in 200), plus possible damage to other organs and blood vessels
- haemorrhage (less than 1 in 200)
- the need for a repeat procedure for evacuation of retained products
- general anaesthetic reaction (1 in 10,000) and death (1 in 100,000) or local anaesthetic reaction (in case of MVA)
- hysterectomy (1 in 30,000) if there is uncontrolled bleeding or severe damage to the uterus.

Case Scenario 11.5

Chioma miscarries at home and after a few days her bleeding settles. She returns to the surgery to ask for a sick note as she feels unable to return to her busy job working with young children. She is tearful and anxious about the same problem happening if she was to become pregnant again.

She is signposted to the Miscarriage Association website, local support services and offered a further appointment after a week for a further consultation. Adam has been very supportive, but he has had to return to work as a self-employed joiner.

Post-Miscarriage Care

Women should be informed about how to access support and counselling services, including leaflets, web addresses and helpline numbers for support organisations. Tommy's, the Pregnancy and Baby Charity, has an accessible helpline available to women to contact for support with details on their website [11]. The Royal College of Obstetricians and Gynaecologists (RCOG) and the Miscarriage Association have useful patient information leaflets that can be accessed through their websites [9].

Women who do not wish to become pregnant should be advised to commence contraception immediately after the miscarriage. Further information on the use of contraception can be obtained from the Faculty of Sexual and Reproductive Healthcare or Family Planning Association websites [3,7].

Anti-D rhesus prophylaxis should be given at a dose of 250 IU (50 mg) to all rhesus-negative women who have a surgical procedure to manage an ectopic pregnancy or a miscarriage.

Anti-D rhesus prophylaxis is not given to women in the following cases:

- medical management for an ectopic pregnancy or miscarriage
- threatened miscarriage or complete miscarriage
- pregnancy of unknown location.

Recurrent Miscarriage

Recurrent miscarriage is defined as:

- three or more first-trimester miscarriages [10].

Clinicians are advised to consider referral to a dedicated recurrent miscarriage clinic earlier if they are concerned that there may be a cause for recurrent losses. The risk of recurrent miscarriage is higher if a woman:

- is over the age of 35 and her partner is over the age of 40
- is overweight
- has had previous miscarriages (with an incremental risk of miscarriage reaching 30–40% after three losses).

The known causes of recurrent miscarriage are:

- anti-phospholipid syndrome (APLS)
- blood-clotting disorders (factor V Leiden, factor II (prothrombin), gene mutation and protein S deficiency)
- chromosomal abnormalities
- cervical insufficiency
- other causes that may play a part but there is not enough evidence: uterine anomalies (bicornuate or septate uterus), polycystic ovarian syndrome (PCOS), infections (toxoplasmosis, rubella) and immune problems (raised levels of uterine NK cells).

All women who have had recurrent miscarriage should be offered a referral to the gynaecology department for investigations. The recommended tests include:

- assessment for antiphospholipid antibodies (lupus anticoagulant and anticardiolipin). Two blood tests done 6–12 weeks apart
- thyroid function tests and assessment for thyroid peroxidase (TPO) antibodies
- 3D pelvic ultrasound to detect uterine abnormalities
- investigations for fetal genetic abnormalities: cytogenetics (if fetal tissue is available)
- investigations for genetic abnormalities in both partners, if an abnormality is found after examination of fetal tissue or if no tissue is available
- thrombophilia screen (if history of late miscarriages).

Women with recurrent miscarriage should be advised to a maintain healthy lifestyle including smoking cessation, reducing alcohol consumption, maintaining a BMI between 19 and 25 kg/m^2 and limiting caffeine to less than 200 mg/day.

They should be advised that it may not be possible to determine the cause for recurrent miscarriages, but women in whom no cause is found may be reassured that the prognosis for a future successful pregnancy is 75%.

Primary care may have to initiate treatment with aspirin and heparin for women diagnosed with antiphospholipid syndrome, as it should be offered from a positive test until 34 weeks of gestation. This would have been advised by a specialist clinic and following a discussion of the risks and benefits.

In women with infertility and miscarriage it has been shown that uterine anomalies are prevalent in 24.5% of cases versus 5.5% of women in the general population. If the ultrasound shows any abnormality, then hysteroscopy or laparoscopy may be offered to confirm the diagnosis and managed by specialist gynaecologists.

Psychological Effects

It is clear from research that healthcare professionals can make a huge difference to a woman's experience of early pregnancy complications and loss. The healthcare professional is unable to do much in terms of changing the outcome of the pregnancy, but being an empathetic ear, listening to the woman and really understanding the significant loss for her and her partner can make a big difference [1].

The language used when describing miscarriage can have a negative effect on the woman and/or her partner. The RCOG recommends that more patient-focused terminology should be adopted.

It is very common for women and their partners to blame themselves after a pregnancy loss, and the first thing a healthcare professional needs to do is to reassure them both that this is not the case [5]. This is often worse if the couple have been trying to conceive for a long time or experienced previous loss, so being aware of the history is vitally important.

Sometimes, women and their partners feel they must just get on with their lives and that the pregnancy loss should be dismissed as it occurred early. Women should be encouraged that every miscarriage matters, and they should be given the opportunity to talk about the loss. Bereavement reactions, including sadness, anger and guilt, should be expected. This emotional process is often made more difficult with early miscarriage because there is not a recognisable fetus to bury and mourn [4]. EPAUs will offer choice to the woman of how she would want the pregnancy tissue to be managed with hospital management versus patient-planned ceremony and burial.

The recent "Independent Pregnancy Loss Review" has lobbied for a baby loss certificate to be available to help patients register their loss and backdate any previous pregnancy losses. This can be accessed on the www.gov.uk website and is voluntary. It is designed to give patients who require it official validation of their loss and to show that the government acknowledges that a life has been lost [14].

Within the first six months following miscarriage, 30–50% of women will have symptoms of depression; the woman needs to be reassured that this is common and likely to improve with time, but that it should be addressed and managed accordingly [1,14].

There can be lots of stresses on a relationship and often the partner who is trying to support the woman feels like he is unable to grieve himself and, as with other problems around perinatal mental health, his needs are often ignored. As a healthcare professional, it is important to also consider the partner in cases of miscarriage.

Some women appear to cope well initially after the miscarriage but require support later. It is important to discuss this with the woman and consider offering a delayed appointment.

Case Scenario 11.6

Chioma returned to clinic after a week to request a renewal of her sick note for a further week. She found the online information supportive and had spoken to friends, who she found out had also had miscarriages. She found this support helpful and it enabled her to be honest about how she was feeling and seek psychological support with the aim to return to work. She has applied for a government baby loss certificate to identify her now two pregnancy losses. Chioma is advised that she can consider trying to conceive again once she is ready. If she were to have a repeat loss, then her case would be reviewed and referred a specialist clinic. She can be can be reassured that the prognosis for a successful future pregnancy with supportive care alone is in the region of 75% [10].

Conclusion

Miscarriage is a common complication of early pregnancy that requires sensitive management. Timely referrals, individualised care and holistic support are essential to optimise outcomes. Counselling and reassurance about future pregnancies are crucial. Women and their partners should be directed to reputable support organizations for additional help and guidance.

Further information is available from the Miscarriage Association: www.miscarriageassociation.org.uk.

References

[1] BMJ Best Practice, 'Miscarriage: Symptoms, diagnosis and treatment'. Accessed: 11 Nov. 2025. [Online]. Available: https://bestpractice.bmj.com/topics/en-gb/666?locale=en_GB.

[2] B. G. Darney, M. R. Weaver, N. Stevens, J. Kimball and S. W. Prager, 'The Family Medicine Residency Training Initiative in miscarriage management: Impact on practice in Washington state', *Fam Med*, vol. **45**, no. 2, pp. 102–107, 2013.

[3] L. W. Prine and H. MacNaughten, 'Office management of early pregnancy loss', *Am Fam Physician*, vol. **84**, no. 1, pp. 75–82, 2011.

[4] L. F. Smith, J. Frost, R. Levitas, H. Bradley and J. Garcia, 'Women's experience of three early miscarriage management options: A qualitative study', *Br J Gen Pract*, vol. **56**, no. 524, pp. 198–205, 2006.

[5] L. F. Smith, P. D. Ewings and C. Quinlan, 'Incidence of pregnancy after expectant, medical or surgical management of spontaneous first trimester miscarriage: Long-term follow-up of miscarriage treatment (MIST) randomised controlled trial', *BMJ*, vol. **339**, 3827, 2009.

[6] NICE, 'Ectopic pregnancy and miscarriage: Diagnosis and initial management in early pregnancy of ectopic pregnancy and miscarriage'. NICE guidelines [NG126]. Apr. 2019 [updated Aug. 2023].

[7] M. J. Cameron and G. C. Penney. 'Terminology in early pregnancy loss: What women hear and what clinicians write', *J Fam Plann Reprod Health Care*, vol. **31**, no. 4, pp. 313–314, 2005.

[8] K. Levine and S. T. Cameron, 'Women's preferences for method of abortion and management of miscarriage', *J Fam Plann Reprod Health Care*, vol. **35**, no. 4, pp. 233–235, 2009.

[9] C. Jansson and A. Adolfsson, 'A Swedish study of midwives' and nurses' experiences when women are diagnosed with a missed miscarriage during a routine ultrasound scan', *Sex Reprod Healthc*, vol. **1**, no. 2, pp. 67–72, 2010.

[10] L. Regan, R. Rai, S. Saravelos et al. 'Recurrent Miscarriage Green-Top Guideline No. 17'. RCOG Green-Top Guidelines, 2023.

[11] Tommy's, 'Baby loss information and support'. Accessed: 11 Nov. 2025. [Online]. Available: www.tommys.org.

[12] A. Coomarasamy, A. J. Deval, V. Cheed et al., 'Randomized trial of progesterone in women with bleeding in early pregnancy', *N Engl J Med*, vol. **380**, pp. 1815–1824, 2019.

[13] 'Saying goodbye'. Accessed: 11 Nov. 2025. [Online]. Available: www.sayinggoodbye.org.

[14] 'The independent pregnancy loss review: Care and support when baby loss occurs before 24 weeks gestation'. Jul. 2023.

[15] 'ESHRE Guideline on the management of recurrent pregnancy loss'. European Society of Human Reproduction and Embryology, 2023.

Chapter 12

Pregnancy-Related Issues Relevant for Primary Care

Jenny Blackman and Alexandra Bain

Key Points

- Preconceptual counselling is essential for women with complex medical needs.
- Optimize medical conditions before pregnancy and provide appropriate contraception until this is achieved.
- Check medication for women of reproductive age and wherever possible use agents with a known low-risk profile for pregnancy.
- It is important to be able to explain common pregnancy symptoms from a physiological point of view.
- Liaise between specialties and refer women with pre-existing conditions to joint medical/obstetric clinics. Regional maternal medicine networks are valuable for multi-disciplinary team (MDT) discussion and advice.
- Use the Royal College of Obstetricians and Gynaecologists (RCOG) Green-Top Guidelines for pregnancy-related queries such as chickenpox exposure, genital herpes and intrahepatic cholestasis of pregnancy.
- MBRRACE-UK (Mothers and Babies: Reducing Risk through Audits and Confidential Enquiries across the UK) report summaries will provide the latest recommendations.
- The recommended vaccination schedules in pregnancy should be known.
- Use the postnatal follow-up visit to give specific lifestyle guidance and advice regarding future pregnancies, such as for women with gestational diabetes or hypertension in pregnancy.

Introduction

This chapter focuses on common pregnancy-related symptoms and key issues relevant to primary care in the preconceptual, antepartum and postnatal periods. Intrapartum events and obstetric emergencies are not covered here.

Using cases to illustrate clinical scenarios related to the pregnant patient, this chapter aims to give stepwise and logical approaches to common problems with discussion around the subject after each one.

Type 1 Diabetes

Case Scenario 12.1

A 22-year-old patient comes to see you. She has had type 1 diabetes since the age of 15. Last month she had a first-trimester miscarriage. She thinks she might have thrush again and is requesting treatment.

She has been taking long- and short-acting insulin but struggles with her blood sugar control at times because of a stressful job and shift work. She has a body mass index (BMI) of 29. There is no other relevant past history, and she does not smoke. She is in a stable long-term relationship with a supportive partner.

The patient's presenting complaint should be investigated with a vaginal swab for *Candida* and treatment as necessary. The consultation should also be used to explore whether her recent pregnancy was planned or unplanned.

If she is hoping to conceive again, control of diabetes should be reviewed, and the opportunity taken to address aspects from a preconceptual point of view.

Discussion regarding a suitable contraceptive may be appropriate if she is not planning another pregnancy or until control of diabetes is optimal.

Pre-conceptionally, she should be aiming for the same capillary plasma target ranges as all people with type 1 diabetes: fasting glucose 5–7 mmol/L on waking and 4–7 mmol/L before meals. The Diabetes in Pregnancy Pathway updated by the National Institute for Health and Care Excellence (NICE) in

2020 emphasizes the importance of preconceptual care for women with pre-existing type 1 diabetes, aiming for a pre-pregnancy HbA1c of 48 mmol/mol and strongly advising against pregnancy if the HbA1c is greater than 86 mmol/mol [1].

Women with diabetes who have a BMI greater than 27 should be given advice on weight management in line with NICE guidance on obesity.

Careful counselling about the risks of pregnancy with diabetes includes consideration of effects of the pregnancy on disease and effects of the diabetes on the pregnancy for both the mother and fetus. This counselling is particularly important as the risks are reduced with tighter diabetic control. Maternal diabetes is associated with an increased risk of miscarriage, congenital abnormalities, pre-eclampsia, infections, sudden intrauterine fetal demise, macrosomia and intrauterine growth restriction. There is an increased chance of caesarean delivery and intrapartum problems such as shoulder dystocia.

Folic acid at the higher dose of 5 mg daily is recommended from three months prior to conception in all women with diabetes.

A dose of 150 mg daily aspirin is recommended from 12 to 36 weeks' gestation to reduce the risk of pre-eclampsia (see Case Scenario 8 for more details about use of aspirin in pregnancy).

Women with type 1 diabetes who are planning to become pregnant should be offered ketone testing strips and meter; they are advised to test for ketonaemia if they become hypoglycaemic or unwell. They should also be advised that nausea and vomiting, often associated with early pregnancy, may affect blood glucose control.

Women with diabetes should be informed of the increased risk of hypoglycaemia and impaired awareness of these episodes in pregnancy.

There is an increased progression of nephropathy and retinopathy in pregnancy. Retinal screening and renal function should be performed pre-conceptually if not done within the past six months.

Early referral to a joint obstetric and endocrine clinic is advised, preferably pre-conceptually.

Nausea and Vomiting in Early Pregnancy

Case Scenario 12.2

A 29-year-old Asian lady presents with persistent vomiting. She has been unable to tolerate food and can only sip water. She has an appointment to see the midwife for a booking visit next week and thinks she is seven weeks pregnant. You saw this lady frequently in the first trimester of her previous pregnancy with severe nausea and vomiting requiring admission to hospital on two occasions.

Nausea and vomiting in the first trimester of pregnancy is extremely common, but hyperemesis gravidarum occurs in less than 2% of pregnancies. Hyperemesis gravidarum describes prolonged, persistent nausea and vomiting unrelated to other causes, weight loss (usually at least 5% of pre-pregnancy body weight), dehydration and electrolyte imbalance. It is a diagnosis of exclusion.

As there is not one confirmatory test, it is essential to exclude other causes of nausea and vomiting by means of history, examination and urine testing. The most common of these is a urinary tract infection. Rarer causes include Addison's disease, peptic ulcer disease, pancreatitis and thyrotoxicosis. Physical examination will establish the degree of dehydration. Postural hypotension and tachycardia are important signs. A previous history of hyperemesis makes the diagnosis more likely. It is important to remember the presence or absence of ketouria in pregnancy is not an indicator of dehydration [4].

Any patient with vomiting not successfully controlled in primary care should be considered for ambulatory day care for intravenous fluids. Women with recurrent hyperemesis despite intravenous fluids will need to be managed as an inpatient. Complications of hyperemesis include Mallory–Weiss tears, Wernicke's encephalopathy due to thiamine deficiency, hyponatraemia, thrombosis, depression and psychological effects. An ultrasound should be performed to date the pregnancy and exclude multiple and molar pregnancy [2].

Common recommendations include taking small and frequent meals, avoiding spicy or fatty foods and avoiding sensory stimuli that may act as triggers. However, there are few studies evaluating this advice [3]. Acupressure and electrical stimulation wrist bands as interventions have mixed evidence. Acupuncture may have some benefit.

There is good evidence for the safety and effectiveness of an H1 receptor antagonist antihistamines (such as cyclizine or promethazine), phenothiazines and Xonvea. Xonvea is a slow-release combination of doxylamine and pyridoxine and the only licensed treatment of nausea and vomiting of pregnancy in the UK. Many women require a combination of two or more antiemetics [4].

Second-line options include dopamine antagonists such as metoclopramide and ondansetron. There is evidence that ondansetron is safe and its use should not be discouraged if first-line antiemetics are ineffective. Women can be reassured regarding a very small increase in the absolute risk of orofacial clefting with ondansetron use in the first trimester, which should be balanced with the risks of poorly managed hyperemesis gravidarum [4].

Epilepsy

Case Scenario 12.3

A 19-year-old woman with epilepsy comes for review. She has not had a seizure for the past eight months. She has been taking lamotrigine for several years. She is unsure of the date of her last menstrual period, but thinks it was more than five weeks ago and has a positive pregnancy test. She is unsure how she feels about pregnancy as she often rows with her partner and he is unemployed at present.

Epilepsy is a high-risk condition in pregnancy. However, the majority of these pregnancies proceed without difficulties. Women who have been free from seizures for many years are unlikely to experience seizures in pregnancy providing their medication is continued. The greatest risk of seizures is at the time of labour and the immediate postnatal period. Sudden unexplained death in epilepsy (SUDEP) remains the predominant cause of death for women with epilepsy in pregnancy. Seventeen of the women featured in MBRRACE-UK's Saving Lives, Improving Mothers' Care 2023 report died from causes related to epilepsy, and 14 of these deaths were due to SUDEP. Red flags for SUDEP include night-time seizures, uncontrolled seizures and poor compliance with medication [5].

The risks of uncontrolled convulsive seizures largely outweigh the potential teratogenic risk of medication and women with epilepsy are advised to continue their medication during pregnancy. Sodium valproate is contraindicated in women of childbearing potential unless a Pregnancy Prevention Programme (sometimes called PREVENT) is in place, which involves ensuring annual review by a specialist and a highly effective contraceptive. Most studies show a two- to threefold increase in major fetal malformations (neural tube defects, orofacial clefts and heart defects) for women on anti-epileptic medication, compared with the general population. Phenytoin, primidone, phenobarbitone, carbamazepine and sodium valproate all cross the placenta and are teratogenic. The risk of fetal malformation increases with use of multiple agents [2].

Abrupt withdrawal or changes in medications are not recommended, even in women presenting with an unplanned pregnancy taking high-risk medication. Changes should be in consultation with a specialist team and allow the woman to make informed choice about the balance of risks.

Most women with epilepsy of childbearing age are currently prescribed lamotrigine. The dose may need to be increased two- to threefold during pregnancy.

Preconceptual counselling and discussion in early pregnancy for women with epilepsy are often overlooked, but should be robustly delivered in all care settings and on an opportunistic basis. Early referral for joint care with the obstetrician and neurologist is indicated. All women should be prescribed 5 mg folic acid daily, if possible for three months prior to conception.

Group B Streptococcus

Case Scenario 12.4

You are looking at some results on behalf of a colleague. A pregnant woman was recently seen with vulval irritation and vaginal discharge in the second trimester of pregnancy. A vaginal swab showed *Candida* and Group B streptococcus.

This lady only needs treatment for *Candida*. The community midwife needs to be aware of the result showing Group B streptococcus, as this patient should be counselled and offered intravenous antibiotics in labour.

Group B streptococcus does not usually cause severe infections in well adult women (unlike Group A streptococcus, which can cause a rapid and severe sepsis in pregnancy and the puerperium). However, Group B streptococcus is recognised as the most frequent cause of significant infection in the neonate in the first week of life.

The UK National Screening Committee does not recommend routine screening for Group B streptococcus as there is insufficient evidence that the benefits outweigh the risks and it has not been shown to be cost effective [6]. Therefore, vaginal swabs should not be taken during pregnancy without clear clinical indication.

If, however, a swab is indicated by vaginal discharge or pre-labour spontaneous rupture of the membranes and Group B streptococcus is identified, intrapartum intravenous antibiotics are offered to women.

If a woman has a urine infection with Group B streptococcus, a course of antenatal antibiotics is given at the time of detection and intravenous antibiotics are recommended during labour.

Intrapartum antibiotics are offered in labour to women who have had a previous newborn with Group B streptococcal infection.

Chickenpox Exposure

Case Scenario 12.5

You have been asked to phone a lady back who rang the receptionist in a panic this morning. She is 27 weeks pregnant and this is her first pregnancy. She is booked with the midwife, is low-risk, has no relevant past history and has been well in her pregnancy. The day before yesterday she went to her nephew's birthday party and her sister phoned to say that he is now covered in what appears to be chickenpox.

You need to establish the risk for this exposure by asking if she has had chickenpox before or has scars from past chickenpox. If she has previously been infected, she can be reassured.

Next you need to establish if significant exposure has occurred. This is defined as face-to-face contact or being in the same room as an infected individual for more than 15 minutes [7].

More than 90% of women born in the UK are immune to varicella zoster. However, if there is no definite history of infection, maternal blood can be tested (usually by adding the test onto the booking bloods) to see if she is seropositive. If this is the case, she can be reassured.

Contracting varicella zoster is not known to increase the risk of miscarriage but carries a small risk of fetal varicella syndrome under 28 weeks' gestation. In the last four weeks of pregnancy there is a significant risk of varicella infection in the newborn.

Varicella immunoglobulin (VZIG) can be given to non-immune women up to 10 days after exposure. This is not only for fetal effects of varicella zoster infection but also because chickenpox during pregnancy has greater risks to the pregnant women than in the non-pregnant state, including pneumonia, hepatitis and encephalitis.

If chickenpox develops, then treatment is with aciclovir. If a woman develops respiratory symptoms or any other deterioration in her condition, she should be referred immediately to hospital.

Seronegative women could be offered immunization outside of pregnancy.

Vaccinations in Pregnancy, Normal Pregnancy Physiology and Management of Anaemia

Case Scenario 12.6

You see a 34-year-old lady who is currently 29 weeks into her fifth pregnancy. She asks you whether she should have the flu vaccine. She saw on the news that it is not a very effective injection this season, but her midwife has suggested she has it. She also mentions how tired she is and says she feels short of breath climbing the stairs at home.

Influenza vaccination (inactivated vaccine) is recommended for all pregnant women. There are several benefits to receiving the vaccine, including protection for both mothers and their babies and avoiding the complications that arise from the flu. Covid-19 vaccination is considered safe in pregnancy and women should be recommended to stay up to date with Covid-19 vaccinations as per national guidance.

Pertussis vaccine is also recommended in pregnancy and is safe for both mother and baby. Vaccination is offered from 16 to 32 weeks but can be given up to term. This vaccination programme was initiated in 2012 in response to a pertussis outbreak and since then there has been a decrease in the number of whooping cough cases in babies under six months of age.

The following vaccinations are contraindicated in pregnancy: BCG, measles, mumps, rubella, varicella, vaccinia (smallpox) and human papillomavirus (HPV) [9]. Women who are found in pregnancy to be non-immune to rubella should be offered rubella immunisation (MMR vaccine) after delivery which is considered safe if breastfeeding.

Physiological changes in normal pregnancy mean that most women are aware of feeling shorter of breath. This is partly due to the effects of progesterone on ventilation.

A full blood count to screen for antenatal anaemia is routinely taken at booking and the 28-week midwife visit. Physiological changes lead to a normal dilutional anaemia. However, pregnancy also causes a significant increase in iron and folate requirements. The definition of normal haemoglobin levels in pregnancy are >110 g/dL in the first trimester and >105 g/dL in the second and third trimesters.

Dietary advice and a trial of oral iron is the first-line management of anaemia in pregnancy, providing haemoglobinopathy has been excluded. Serum ferritin is the most useful parameter for assessing iron deficiency; levels below 15 μ/L are diagnostic of iron deficiency and below 30 μ/L should prompt treatment. An increase in haemoglobin must be demonstrated after two weeks, otherwise further tests are required [8].

Referral and consideration of parenteral iron should be initiated from the second trimester onwards for all women with confirmed iron deficiency who fail to respond to or are intolerant of oral iron.

Iron deficiency is associated with preterm delivery, low birth weight, placental abruption and increased peripartum blood loss.

Itching in Pregnancy

Case Scenario 12.7

A lady comes to see you at 34 weeks' gestation in her second pregnancy. She is very distressed by severe itching.

Itching in pregnancy is a common symptom, causing significant distress and loss of sleep for some women.

Intrahepatic cholestasis of pregnancy (ICP) is a diagnosis to consider (previously termed obstetric cholestasis). It can cause widespread itching, but often affects the palms of the hands and soles of the feet. If this lady had ICP in a previous pregnancy, then this makes the diagnosis more likely as it has a high recurrence rate. A rash is not a feature of ICP. Bile acids are raised and both liver function and the itching resolve after birth. Note, serum alkaline phosphatase (ALP) is increased in normal pregnancy as it is made by the placenta so does not indicate disease.

Other causes of itching and liver dysfunction such as drugs, hepatitis, autoimmune conditions and gall stones need to be excluded.

Other pregnancy-specific conditions to be considered in any woman with abnormal liver function are pre-eclampsia and acute fatty liver of pregnancy.

Women with ICP should be referred to an obstetric team and will have regular liver function tests and consideration of timing of delivery. Over the years, ICP has caused anxiety and iatrogenic prematurity because of the association with stillbirth. The risk of stillbirth in women with ICP and a singleton pregnancy is known to be increased when the concentration of bile acids is >100 μmol/L. Once the woman has had her baby, symptoms and liver function should return to normal. Checking liver function tests and bile acids can be deferred until the postnatal check. She can be reassured about the lack of long-term sequelae for herself and her baby [10].

Postnatal Hypertension

Case Scenario 12.8

You are asked to see 33-year-old lady 10 days postnatally. Unfortunately, there is very little information on the discharge summary about her antenatal and intrapartum care, but she tells you that she had to be induced at 37 weeks' gestation because her blood pressure was very high, she had a headache and her blood tests were abnormal. She laboured quickly and had a normal vaginal birth. She has recovered quickly and feels well now. Her midwife has now handed over care to the health visitor but asks if her labetalol can be 'weaned off'.

Ideally this lady should have been discharged with a clear plan regarding the postnatal period, but often this is not the case. The dangers of hypertension during the postnatal period are of eclampsia and stroke.

All women should be aware of associated symptoms such as headache, nausea, vomiting, visual disturbance and epigastric pain. The blood pressure should be checked by the community midwife on alternate days for two weeks after discharge for women with hypertension during pregnancy and/or labour. Any woman after childbirth with a diastolic blood pressure greater than 90 with symptoms, or sustained over 4 hours, or a systolic blood pressure greater than 150 should be reviewed and have bloods taken, including a full blood count and renal and liver function.

Most women with antenatal hypertension will need antihypertensives for at least two weeks following delivery. Blood pressure medication can be reduced when the blood pressure is consistently 130–140/80–90 mmHg [11].

If medication is still required at six weeks post-delivery, then investigation for other causes is warranted as 13% of women thought to have gestational hypertension or pre-eclampsia have underlying disease. Urine should be checked at the six-week postnatal check, and if proteinuria still exists, then renal function should be reviewed and further investigated.

Severe early onset (requiring delivery before 34 weeks) pre-eclampsia has a recurrence rate of 40% in future pregnancies, although the onset of disease usually occurs two to three weeks later and is less severe. Mild pre-eclampsia at term has a recurrence risk of 10% [12].

Screening for pre-eclampsia would happen automatically in a future pregnancy as blood pressure, symptoms and urine testing are addressed routinely at each point of contact with the community midwife for every woman.

In this lady's next pregnancy she should take low-dose aspirin 150 mg daily from 12 to 36 weeks of gestation. In addition to women with previous pregnancy-related hypertension, other women who should receive low-dose aspirin include those with pre-existing hypertension, diabetes, chronic kidney disease and those with a history of autoimmune disorders such as SLE or antiphospholipid syndrome and women with more than one of the following risk factors – primigravida, maternal age above 40 years, pregnancy interval of greater than 10 years, BMI above 35, family history of pre-eclampsia and multiple pregnancy. Evidence shows a 17% reduction in the risk of developing pre-eclampsia if low-dose aspirin is taken by these women [13].

Gestational Diabetes

Case Scenario 12.9

A 36-year-old lady had her second baby 6 weeks ago. She had a glucose tolerance test at 28 weeks because her BMI is 44. Following this, she was diagnosed with gestational diabetes mellitus (GDM) and was taught how to monitor her blood sugars. Her GDM was managed with diet and she had extra growth scans. She was induced at 38 weeks and had an emergency caesarean delivery for fetal distress. She was not given any further advice apart from that she did not need to monitor her blood sugars after delivery.

A fasting glucose test should be offered 6–13 weeks postnatally to exclude diabetes. If this is below 6.0 mmol/L, she will need an annual HbA1c test to check her blood glucose level is normal and she should be told she has a moderate risk of developing type 2 diabetes in the future, with appropriate advice and guidance (NICE – 'Preventing type 2 diabetes'). A referral into the NHS Diabetes Prevention Programme should be offered.

She has a significant risk of developing gestational diabetes in future pregnancies and should be offered early testing in the first trimester. She should be given lifestyle advice and encouragement to normalize her BMI.

Women with a fasting glucose of 6.0–6.9 mmol/L should be told that they have a high risk of developing type 2 diabetes. Women with a fasting level greater than 7.0 mmol/L are highly likely to have type 2 diabetes and therefore need confirmatory tests [1].

All women who have had a previous caesarean delivery are considered high risk for future pregnancies and are usually seen by an obstetrician at 20 weeks' gestation for discussion about mode of delivery. There is a 72–75% chance of a successful vaginal birth in the woman's next pregnancy and the scar rupture rate is approximately 0.5%. All women who have had a previous caesarean who are planning a vaginal birth are advised to labour with fetal monitoring and intravenous access in a hospital delivery suite [14].

Hypothyroidism

Case Scenario 12.10

A 39-year-old woman who has recently moved from Poland has joined your practice. She is nine weeks into her second pregnancy. She tells you she has been on 'levothyroxine for years' and asks for a repeat prescription and the details of how to book with a midwife.

Hypothyroidism affects around 1% of pregnancies. Pregnancy itself is thought to have no effect on hypothyroidism. Maternal and fetal outcomes are good for those women on sufficient thyroxine replacement. In around 25% of women the dose of levothyroxine will need to be increased in pregnancy [2].

If hypothyroidism remains untreated in pregnancy, it can be associated with an increase in miscarriage, anaemia, pre-eclampsia and low birth weight. There is also a link with neurodevelopmental delay in the child [2].

Thyroid function should be checked in all hypothyroid women pre-conceptionally. For those women on adequate replacement, thyroid function should be checked once in each trimester. Following a thyroxine dose adjustment, thyroid function should be checked after four to six weeks. Postnatally, women should switch back to their pre-pregnancy dose of thyroxine.

Those patients who have previously had Grave's disease, had radioiodine treatment or had a thyroidectomy should be referred to the maternal medicine team. These women may have the presence of thyroid-stimulating hormone receptor antibodies. There can be transplacental passage of these antibodies which can lead to fetal/neonatal thyrotoxicosis [2].

References

[1] National Institute for Health and Care Excellence (NICE), 'Diabetes in pregnancy: Management from preconception to the postnatal period'. Clinical Guideline NG3. National Institute for Health and Care Excellence, February 2020.

[2] C. Nelson-Piercy, *Handbook of Obstetric Medicine*, 6th edn. CRC Press, 2021.

[3] R. C. Boelig, V. Berghella, A. J. Kelly, S. J. Barton and S. J. Edwards, 'Interventions for treating hyperemesis gravidarum', *Cochrane Database Syst Rev*, vol. **6**, CD010607, 2013.

[4] Royal College of Obstetricians and Gynaecologists, 'The management of nausea and vomiting in pregnancy and hyperemesis gravidarum'. Green-Top Guideline No. 69. RCOG, 2024.

[5] MBRRACE-UK, 'Saving Lives, Improving Mothers' Care: Lessons learned to inform maternity care from the UK and Ireland confidential enquiries into maternal deaths and morbidity 2019–21'. Oct. 2023.

[6] Royal College of Obstetricians and Gynaecologists, 'Prevention of early onset neonatal Group B streptococcal disease, early onset'. Green-Top Guideline No. 36. RCOG, 2017.

[7] Royal College of Obstetricians and Gynaecologists, 'Chickenpox in pregnancy'. Green-Top Guideline No. 13. RCOG, 2015.

[8] British Society for Haematology, 'UK guidelines on the management of iron deficiency in pregnancy'. British Committee for Standards in Haematology, 2011.

[9] P. S. Arunakumari, S. Kalburgi and A. Sahare, 'Vaccination in pregnancy', *Obstetr Gynaecol*, vol. **17**, no. 4, pp. 257–263, 2015.

[10] Royal College of Obstetricians and Gynaecologists, 'Intrahepatic cholestasis of pregnancy'. Green-Top Guideline No. 43. RCOG, 2022.

[11] National Institute for Health and Care Excellence (NICE), 'Hypertension in pregnancy: Diagnosis and management'. Clinical Guideline CG107. National Institute for Health and Care Excellence, 2023.

[12] M. Smith, J. Waugh and C. Nelson-Piercy, 'Management of postpartum hypertension', *Obstetr Gynaecol*, vol. **15**, no. 1, pp. 45–50, 2013.

[13] F. Mone and F. M. McAuliffe, 'Low-dose aspirin and calcium supplementation for the prevention of pre-eclampsia', *Obstetr Gynaecol*, vol. **16**, no. 4, pp. 245–250, 2014.

[14] Royal College of Obstetricians and Gynaecologists, 'Birth after previous caesarean birth'. Green-Top Guideline No. 45. RCOG, 2015.

Chapter

13

Postnatal Care in Primary Care

Carrie Ladd

Key Points

- Women need adequate contraception from three weeks postnatal; breastfeeding alone has a relatively high failure rate.
- If a woman is concerned that she has a perinatal mental health problem, do not dismiss her or normalise her symptoms.
- Venous thromboembolism can occur even if a woman has been adequately anticoagulated.
- Infection can be serious in the postnatal period: there are red flags for admission.
- Prescribing in pregnancy and breastfeeding needs careful consideration of risks and benefits. If necessary, take advice before stopping or starting medication.

At the GP six- to eight-week maternal postnatal consultation:

- Use a template.
- Ask about mental health first, before discussing physical health.
- Discuss physical health issues relevant to the pregnancy and the birth. The postnatal discharge letter should offer advice about future health screening requirements, such as annual HbA1c following gestational diabetes mellitus (GDM).
- Ask about bowel and bladder function to identify any issues with pelvic floor muscles.
- Think about preconception care for the next pregnancy.
- Offer advice about issues, such as weight, exercise, smoking and alcohol.

This chapter will discuss the postnatal period as relevant to GPs. It considers the mental and physical health of the mother in the time after discharge from hospital. The postnatal period begins immediately after the birth of a child and extends for about eight weeks [1]. This is approximately the time that it takes for a woman's body to return to the non-pregnant state. For postnatal mental illness (PMI), the period extends to 12 months after childbirth [2].

Normal Physiological Changes in the Postnatal Period

The Uterus

The pregnant-term uterus weighs about 1,000 g; by six weeks after birth it weighs 50–100 g. The endometrial lining rapidly regenerates and by the 16th day it is restored throughout the uterus, except at the placental site. The size of the placental bed decreases by half immediately after birth because of uterine contractions. Vaginal discharge (lochia) comes from the placental bed, decreases rapidly after initial uterine contraction and has usually stopped by five weeks postnatal [3].

Vagina

The vagina shrinks rapidly in size, but never back to its prepregnant size. By three weeks, the rugae start to reappear in women who are not breastfeeding. In breastfeeding mothers, who have persistently decreased oestrogen levels, the vaginal epithelium remains atrophic for a variable period and women may experience dyspareunia.

Perineum

Swelling and engorgement of the vulva rapidly resolves within one to two weeks. Most of the muscle tone is regained by six weeks, but it may not return to normal, depending on the extent of injury during birth.

Abdominal Wall

The abdominal wall remains soft and poorly toned for many weeks.

Ovaries

Resumption of normal ovarian function is variable, with a mean time to first menses of seven to nine weeks in formula-feeding mothers. However, ovulation can occur as early as 28 days after birth, therefore contraception is needed from 21 days.

In breastfeeding women, resumption of menses also varies, depending on how much and how often the baby is breastfed and whether supplementary formula is used. Anovulation in lactating women is caused by elevated prolactin levels. If a woman is less than six months postnatal, amenorrhoeic and fully breastfeeding (including at night), the lactational amenorrhoeic method (LAM) is over 98% effective in preventing pregnancy [4]. This is, however, a much higher failure rate than some other methods, particularly long-acting contraception such as the implant [5], and so women who could rely on LAM may also choose to use another method of contraception. The risk of pregnancy for women using LAM is increased if breastfeeding decreases (particularly stopping night feeds), when menstruation recurs, or if the woman is more than six months postnatal.

Breasts

Lactation can be experienced after a miscarriage or termination at 16 weeks gestation or more. If not breastfeeding, the prolactin level returns to normal within two to three weeks. Colostrum is already present in the breasts at birth; suckling by the newborn triggers its release during the first two to four days. For most women having their first baby the milk will 'come in' at three to four days, but this may be sooner after subsequent births.

Transition to Motherhood

Becoming a mother is a major life transition and women usually spend time considering and imagining the kind of mother they will be when their baby is born; the reality may be different. If a woman is more able to adjust her expectations of herself and the relationship with her baby, she may cope better.

Timing of Routine Postnatal Care

This is covered by National Institute for Health and Care Excellence (NICE) postnatal care guidelines and quality standards [1,6]. The care that women can expect to receive is illustrated in Figure 13.1. In the immediate period after birth, the midwifery team are responsible for postnatal care, but this transfers to the GP at around 7–14 days. Although many women appear to recover well after pregnancy, incontinence, perineal pain, anxiety and depression are common and can persist for months or years.

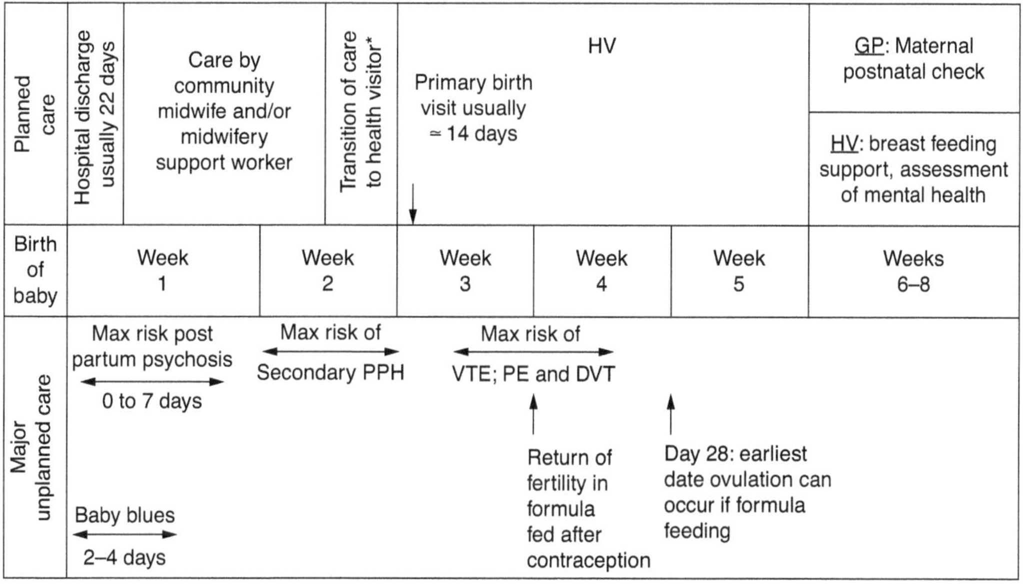

Figure 13.1 Planned and major unplanned postnatal care by primary healthcare professionals.

About a quarter of women now have a caesarean section and maternal factors such as obesity, older age and conditions such as diabetes or hypertension increase the risk of intervention and hence the complexity of postnatal care.

The GP Six- to Eight-Week Maternal Postnatal Consultation

Since April 2020 there has been a contractual requirement for every woman who gives birth to be offered a GP appointment six to eight weeks postnatally for a maternal postnatal consultation; 90% of women report having received it four to eight weeks after birth. There has been a lack of evidence for the purpose and content of this check with varying consistency and standards of appointment offered. In 2023, Healthwatch [7] analysed experiences shared by 2,693 new mothers since April 2020; 10% had not received the six- to eight-week check. Of those who had, only 22% were satisfied with the time taken and 30% said that mental health was not mentioned; 15% of checks were carried out on the phone. This study should be interpreted in the context of many of these checks taking place during the Covid-19 pandemic, but the findings echo those of a 2014 survey [8], which also found dissatisfaction with time taken and the lack of focus on mental health.

A 2023 guidance document published by NHS England illustrates what the GP six- to eight-week check should include [9]. Key features include perinatal mental health, physical health, pelvic health, family planning and health promotion. There are varying ways that practices can offer this check; it may be helpful to consider the following and develop a template to ensure consistency.

Organisation of the Appointment

- Who will do it? The usual GP, a GP of the woman's choice or a GP with a special interest?
- Will women be invited for the check and, if so, by whom and how will they do this?
- Will it happen on the same day as the baby check?
- How much time is needed?

Conducting the Consultation

As per NICE guidance, the maternal postnatal consultation should be conducted by a GP and cover the following areas.

- Perinatal mental health – transition to motherhood, any mental health issues.
- Physical health – recovery from the birth; ask about common morbidities and identify longer-term health risks which need follow-up, such as annual HbA1c checks for those who have had GDM.
- Pelvic health – ask direct questions regarding bowel and bladder function to enable identification of problems with pelvic health promptly; refer onward appropriately, for example to pelvic floor physiotherapy.
- Family planning and health promotion – including contraception, smoking cessation advice, lifestyle advice and future family planning support.
- Explore any other concerns that the woman has.

Review the maternity discharge letter; it will contain important information about the delivery and any immediate concerns such as pre-eclampsia.

Case Scenario 13.1: A Complex Pregnancy with Multimorbidity

Jane is aged 38, had her first child six weeks ago and attends for her postnatal check. She has obesity (body mass index (BMI) 35) and developed GDM and pre-eclampsia during pregnancy. Her pregnancy was managed by the joint obstetric–diabetic clinic and she had a normal delivery at 39 weeks. There were no other problems during the pregnancy. She was managed by diet alone and her blood sugar and blood pressure were normal on discharge from hospital, with no proteinuria.

- Her discharge letter should contain information and recommendations for her care.
- She has made the transition to motherhood well and has no mental health problems.
- She has recovered well with no persistent morbidities.
- She has risk factors for her next pregnancy and her future health – obesity, past GDM and pre-eclampsia.
- Her choice of contraception needs to balance her preferences against any risks identified, using the UK medical eligibility criteria (UKMEC) [10].

Issues Raised from Jane's Case Study

Obesity

Supporting Jane in the postnatal period to change her eating habits and physical activity levels may improve the future health and risk of her whole family, and the outcomes of future pregnancies.

At her six-week check she should be weighed and her BMI calculated. She should be offered a referral for advice on healthy eating and exercise [9].

Gestational Diabetes Mellitus

Women diagnosed with GDM have a sevenfold increased risk of type 2 diabetes. Jane has a higher-than-population risk of developing GDM in subsequent pregnancies but could reduce her risk if she lost weight.

In addition to addressing her obesity with lifestyle advice, and possibly referral (depending on local pathways), Jane should have either a fasting plasma glucose at 6–13 weeks postnatally or an HbA1c after 13 weeks (unreliable before then) [11]. This might be normal, show non-diabetic hyperglycaemia (NDH, previously known as prediabetes) or show that she has developed diabetes, in which case it should be repeated to confirm the diagnosis.

If the test is normal or shows NDH, she needs an annual HbA1c, and is also eligible for the NHS England diabetes prevention programme (DPP; similar programmes exist in the devolved nations). If she has developed diabetes, she should be managed in the usual way that the practice manages patients with diabetes. More information about the management of those at high risk of diabetes can be found in the NICE guidance on prevention of diabetes in those at high risk [12].

Pre-eclampsia

Jane has a risk of recurrence of subsequent pregnancy hypertensive disorders and pre-eclampsia (Box 13.1) [13]. Jane should be advised to contact her GP before she starts trying for another baby, and advice may be needed from the obstetric preconception clinic. Aspirin is advised from 12 weeks gestation if there are no contraindications to reduce the risk of developing pre-eclampsia; this use of aspirin is unlicensed and so it should be prescribed rather than advising over-the-counter purchase [13].

She also has an increased lifetime risk of hypertension and cardiovascular disease. Unfortunately, pregnancy hypertension is not included as a risk factor in the QRisk3 tool [14] so it is difficult to accurately predict her risk.

Contraception in the Postnatal Period

Women should be advised that they can ovulate as early as three weeks postnatally and therefore should be using an adequate form of contraception as soon as they resume having sex after birth. Factors to be taken into consideration include the woman's preference, breastfeeding status, any medical complications during pregnancy or birth (e.g. high blood pressure) and a woman's medical history before the last pregnancy. More information can be found in the UKMEC [10] and other guidance on the CoSRH website: www.cosrh.org.

Postnatal Mental Health Problems

These conditions are common and affect about 20% of postnatal women. Treatment is clear, evidence based and effective [15,16] and the

Box 13.1 Risks for Future Pregnancies of Hypertension in Pregnancy [13]

Women who have had gestational hypertension should be told that their risk of developing:

- gestational hypertension in a future pregnancy is 11–15%
- pre-eclampsia in a future pregnancy is approximately 7%.

Women who have had pre-eclampsia should be told that their risk of developing:

- gestational hypertension in a future pregnancy is approximately 6–12%
- pre-eclampsia in a future pregnancy is approximately 33% if they gave birth between 28 and 34 weeks and 23% if they gave birth at 34–37 weeks. The risk is likely to be higher for those who gave birth before 28 weeks, but exact data is not available.

Table 13.1 Rates of perinatal psychiatric disorder per thousand maternities [19]

Postnatal psychosis	2/1,000
Chronic serious mental illness	2/1,000
Severe depressive illness	30/1,000
Mild to moderate depressive illness and anxiety states	100–150/ 1,000
Post-traumatic stress disorder	30/1,000
Adjustment disorders and distress	150–300/ 1,000

JCC-MH: Guidance for commissioners of perinatal mental health services. RCPsych 2021.

Royal College of General Practitioners (RCGP) has produced a tool to aid with practical implications of the NICE guidance [17]. Not all PMI is depression; Table 13.1 shows the rates of different disorders. PMI ranges from mild to moderate illness that can be managed in primary care (90% of all PMI) to severe illness that needs to be managed by specialist perinatal psychiatrists.

Baby blues is not PMI; it affects most women within a few days of birth. This can include feeling upset, with mood swings, and wanting to cry for no particular reason. These feelings disappear after a few days and never last longer than two weeks.

Mild to moderate PMIs are important because of the devastating effects and distress they can have on women who are not identified early and treated adequately. They can compromise the healthy emotional, cognitive and physical development of the child, with long-term consequences [18,19]. Effects on the child vary – for example, maternal anxiety doubles the risk of mental health problems in the child from 5% to 10% but the effect is not inevitable. If the duration of illness is short, and there is no social adversity, the risks to the child are generally low [20]. PMIs can also have lasting effects on partner and family relationships. There is emerging evidence that 10% of fathers may suffer perinatal depression, or a range of anxiety symptoms [21,22].

Women who have experienced postnatal depression are at risk of suffering further episodes of illness following subsequent deliveries and unrelated to childbirth. After one postnatal episode the risk of recurrence is at least 25% [23].

There are barriers to the identification of PMI; as many as half of mothers meeting diagnostic thresholds for perinatal depression and anxiety may be unidentified [24], despite frequent routine contact with a range of primary care services. NICE recommends that women should be asked at each postnatal contact about their emotional health and encouraged to discuss how they are feeling (Figure 13.2) [1].

A 2015 report [25] has shown that the greatest barrier to providing better support to women is the low level of identification of need. Barriers to identification were identified, including the following.

Barriers to Identification for Women

- Poor awareness of perinatal mental illness among women, their partners and families.
- Stigma and fear among women that their baby might be taken away.
- Feeling dismissed or overly reassured when discussing their problems with GPs.

Barriers to Identification for GPs

- Time pressures on GPs consultations.
- Insufficient training and confidence among GPs in managing PMI.
- A lack of contact between GPs and women during pregnancy and inconsistent team-working between GP practices and midwives and health visitors.
- A lack of focus on mother and baby wellbeing after the initial six- to eight-week check.
- A lack of specialist resources and long waiting times when a referral is made.

Red Flags for GPs [9,17]

- Recent significant change in mental state or emergence of new symptoms.
- New thoughts or acts of violent self-harm.
- New and persistent expressions of incompetency as a mother or estrangement from the baby.

Consider asking about intrusive or distressing thoughts or images if there are concerns about mental health – these may not always be volunteered, even if present.

At a woman's first contact with services in pregnancy and the postnatal period, ask about:

- any past or present severe mental illness
- past or present treatment by a specialist mental health service, including inpatient care for any severe perinatal mental illness in a first-degree relative (mother, sister or daughter).
- refer to a secondary mental health service (preferably a specialist perinatal mental health service) for assessment and treatment, all women who:
  - have or are suspected to have severe mental illness
  - have any history of severe mental illness (during pregnancy or the postnatal period or at any other time).

At a woman's first contact with primary care or her booking visit, and during the early postnatal period, consider asking the following **depression** identification questions as part of a general discussion about a woman's mental health and wellbeing:

- During the past month, have you often been bothered by feeling down, depressed or hopeless?
- During the past month, have you often been bothered by having little interest or pleasure in doing things?

Also consider asking about **anxiety** using the 2-item Generalized Anxiety Disorder scale (GAD-2):

- Over the last 2 weeks, how often have you been bothered by feeling nervous, anxious or on edge?
- Over the last 2 weeks, how often have you been bothered by not being able to stop or control worrying?

NICE antenatal and postnatal mental health CG 192. 2014

Figure 13.2 NICE guidance for assessing mental health.

Managing Common Maternal Morbidities after Birth

After Pains

After pains are common and caused by involutionary uterine contractions. They last for two to three days after birth and are worse in those who are multiparous. Breastfeeding stimulates the uterus to contract and increases the severity of the pains. Non-steroidal anti-inflammatory drugs are better than placebo at relieving pain, but paracetamol is no better than placebo.

Perineal Pain

Perineal pain may be caused by trauma, stitches, infection, constipation, haemorrhoids or an anal fissure.

Perineal lacerations occur in around 90% of vaginal deliveries [26]. Obstetric anal sphincter injury causes more perineal pain than other perineal trauma. Although perineal pain affects most mothers, it usually resolves within two months of birth, but a significant minority still report perineal pain and dyspareunia at six months.

Prevention may be possible; antenatal digital perineal massage reduces the likelihood of perineal trauma (mainly episiotomies) and ongoing perineal pain and is generally well accepted [27]. The impact is more obvious for women having their first birth.

Constipation

Postnatal constipation is estimated to affect 24% of women at three months postnatal [28]. Haemorrhoids, episiotomy pain, damage to the anal sphincter or pelvic floor muscles during childbirth and iron supplementation all increase the risk. A high-fibre diet and increased fluid intake can prevent constipation, but there is a lack of good evidence about treating women; a bulk-forming laxative would be the first choice if diet and fluids are ineffective.

Haemorrhoids and fissures should be treated as in the general population.

Back Pain

Backache is reported by about 40% of women during pregnancy [29]. Factors correlated with persistent postnatal back pain may include pain before or during pregnancy, physical work and multiple pregnancy. Postnatal back pain is managed in the same way as back pain at any other time, with the appropriate care taken when prescribing analgesia for a breastfeeding woman.

Incontinence

Many women experience issues with urinary and bowel function during pregnancy and immediately after birth; for some, this will have improved by the time of the six- to eight-week check; 33% of women experience urinary incontinence after pregnancy and 20% experience faecal incontinence at some point in the first five years after a vaginal delivery. In the longer term, 33% of women have urinary incontinence and 10% experience ongoing faecal incontinence [9]. Many women with incontinence after birth do not seek any advice or treatment but GPs can be proactive in asking directly about symptoms such as urinary or faecal incontinence and incomplete bladder emptying, to identify pelvic floor dysfunction. Women with these issues in the first year postnatally should be referred to a perinatal pelvic floor service [9].

Pelvic floor muscle training (PFMT) is an effective treatment for women with persistent postnatal urinary incontinence and can also help women with faecal incontinence. Antenatal PFMT may help higher-risk women, such as women in their first pregnancy and women with a large baby. The more intensive the programme, the greater the treatment effect.

Divarication of the Recti Abdominal Muscles

Divarication of the recti abdominal muscles (DRAM) is common – it results from stretching of the linea alba during pregnancy. It usually corrects itself by eight weeks but may persist. Although most women are asymptomatic, except cosmetically, it can lead to back pain and occasionally hernias. A systematic review of various exercise regimes was inconclusive about the benefit [30], but for most women, referral to a physiotherapist for Pilates or other core-strengthening exercises is recommended. Surgery is a last-ditch cosmetic treatment which is generally not available on the NHS.

Breastfeeding Problems

In general, this is the field of expertise of midwives, health visitors and breastfeeding counsellors. However, you should know how to access the breastfeeding resources available in your locality.

Painful Nipples

Painful nipples are common and there is no evidence that specific treatments are better than applying expressed breast milk, or nothing. For most women, nipple pain reduces by 7–10 days after birth; if this does not happen, then review of the latch might be useful [31].

Mastitis

Up to 30% of lactating women get mastitis; breast abscesses are less common [32]. The usual organism is *Staphyloccocus aureus*.

Infection tends to localise to a segment (blocked milk duct) but it can spread to an entire breast quadrant. Women complain of pain, difficulty breastfeeding, engorgement, redness and cracked nipples; they may also present with fever, fatigue or rigors (sepsis), without breast localisation.

Management [32]

- Assess for red flags for sepsis and refer immediately if they are present or the woman is haemodynamically unstable (see Table 13.2).
- Continue breastfeeding, as milk stasis causes mastitis. If feeding is too painful, a woman should hand express or use a breast pump to encourage milk flow from the engorged segment.
- Treat with flucloxacillin 500 mg four times a day for 10–14 days.
- If the woman is allergic to penicillin, prescribe either erythromycin 250–500 mg four times a day or clarithromycin 500 mg twice a day for 10–14 days.

Table 13.2 Indications for hospital referral in a woman with infection [33]

Red flags or features in patients with suspected sepsis that indicate high risk of sepsis (recommend immediate management either with initiation of a sepsis bundle for inpatients or referral by blue light transfer from the community)	
Objective evidence of altered mental state	GCS < 15 or 'not alert' in Alert, Verbal, Pain, Unresponsive (AVPU) classification
Respiratory rate	≥25 breaths/min
Oxygen saturation	<94% on room air*
Heart rate	>130 bpm
Blood pressure	Systolic < 90 mmHg
Urine output	Not passed urine in >12 hours or if catheterised <0.5 mL/kg urine per hour

- Analgesia (paracetamol) and ice packs or a warm compress, bath or shower may help.
- Refer to a breastfeeding expert to check attachment and feeding technique.
- Review if symptoms are not settling after 48 hours of antibiotics or if an abscess forms.

Tiredness

Every mother is tired after birth, but most do not consult with it. Possible causes include anaemia, depression or hypothyroidism.

Anaemia

Postnatal anaemia is defined as Hb < 10 g/dL and results from postpartum haemorrhage or a low haemoglobin during pregnancy. Women should be offered iron for at least three months before having a repeat FBC and ferritin to ensure that haemoglobin and iron stores are replete. There is no indication to do a routine Hb unless there are symptoms or risk factors.

Thyroid Problems

Postnatal thyroiditis, an auto-immune disease, affects about 5% of women [34] and is the commonest cause of postnatal thyroid dysfunction. It presents with painless swelling of the thyroid gland. One-third of patients will only have a thyrotoxic phase, one-third only a hypothyroid phase and one-third will have both phases. Clinical symptoms can mimic typical fatigue following birth, as well as postnatal depression and Graves' disease. It is associated with abnormalities of thyroid hormones and positive autoantibodies. Differentiation of the hyperthyroid phase of postnatal thyroiditis from Graves' disease is important because Graves' disease requires antithyroid therapy (which does not work in postnatal thyroiditis). A low uptake on a radioisotope uptake scan confirms the diagnosis.

Mild cases need no treatment. If the hyperthyroid symptoms are troublesome, a peripherally acting beta blocker drug is indicated. Symptomatic postnatal hypothyroidism should be treated with levothyroxine. By 12–18 months most women recover, but 20% need long-term thyroid hormone replacement.

Significant Postnatal Physical Illnesses

Secondary Postpartum Haemorrhage and Genital Tract Infection

Secondary postpartum haemorrhage (PPH) is defined as abnormal or excessive bleeding between 24 hours and 12 weeks postnatally [35]. It affects 1–3% of women and is usually caused by endometritis, with or without retained products of conception. Risk factors include complicated deliveries, including caesarean section and anaemia. Most cases are caused by Group A streptococcus.

Genital tract infection is a major cause of maternal death [33,36] and should be treated aggressively with admission and intravenous antibiotics such as clindamycin and gentamicin. Surgical treatment is needed if there is excessive or continuing bleeding, irrespective of ultrasound findings.

Epilepsy

The immediate postpartum period is high risk for increased seizure frequency or for the first onset of seizures due to increased stress and anxiety, sleep deprivation, missed medication and changes in the bioavailability of medication. Women are also at risk of sudden unexpected death in epilepsy (SUDEP). They need advice about medication and breastfeeding and about reducing risk from seizures by not bathing or sleeping alone. An epilepsy specialist nurse or midwife is a useful member of the team for these patients, who should have had their pregnancy managed in a joint obstetrician/neurologist consultant-led clinic [36].

Venous Thromboembolism

Thromboembolism was the commonest cause of maternal death in 2020–2022, followed by Covid-19, cardiac disease and mental health conditions [36]. A systematic review of risk of postnatal venous thromboembolism (VTE) found that the risk varied from 21- to 84-fold compared to the non-pregnant state [37]. The absolute risk peaks in the first three weeks postnatal (421 per 100,000 person-years). A pulmonary embolism (PE) is still possible, even when a patient has had adequate thromboprophylaxis. Brief faintness and shortness of breath are common premonitory signs and buttock pain can suggest a pelvis vein thrombosis. Routine observations including temperature, pulse, blood pressure, respiratory rate and oxygen saturation are important, as well as a chest examination. Tachycardia and reduced oxygen saturation are suggestive of the diagnosis, even if the woman appears well. D-dimer and Wells scores are not validated for use in pregnant and postnatal women, so urgent diagnostic imaging is needed to exclude a PE [38].

Bereavement

One in 200 births ends in stillbirth and one in three stillbirths occurs at term. About 1 in 450 pregnancies lead to neonatal death (death in the first four weeks after pregnancy). An independent study giving a national picture of NHS care for parents of babies who died before or during birth or as newborns was published in 2014 [39]. There are several important messages for GP. Firstly, there is a high rate of anxiety and depression in both mothers and fathers. Secondly, both mothers and fathers attach value to support from GPs around 10% of parents were visited at home after the bereavement and this was especially appreciated. Thirdly, only just over half of women who had a bereavement had a six- to eight-week postnatal check; most of the rest were not invited. The GP six- to eight-week check for the woman is essential for all mothers who have given birth even if their pregnancy ended in a stillbirth, or if the infant was taken into social services care. This is an important time to check for mental health problems, to offer support, to signpost to other resources and to discuss future plans for contraception and pregnancy.

Significant Psychiatric Illness

Severe PMI, caused by severe depressive disorder or postnatal psychosis, is the leading cause of maternal death throughout the first postnatal year [36]. Nearly half of all women who die by suicide have a previous history of severe mental illness [36]. Information about past psychiatric history must be passed to the midwifery/obstetric team by the GP, even if self-booking is the norm. These women should have been referred to a perinatal psychiatrist after booking so that a care plan is in place before delivery for prevention, early detection and treatment [15].

The acute onset of postnatal psychosis (PP), one of the most severe forms of illness seen in psychiatry, is rare and a GP is likely to see a case only about once every 10 years; 50% of women who develop PP have a strong risk factor, such as previous psychosis or pre-existing bipolar disorder [40].

Most PP starts within two weeks of birth, with more than 50% starting on days 1–3; 50% of women with PP will have no significant psychiatric history and therefore have no plan in place. Sudden onset and rapid deterioration are typical; the clinical picture often changes rapidly, with wide fluctuations in the intensity of symptoms and severe mood swings. They can have mania and depression at the same time, resulting in agitation, trouble sleeping and significant change in appetite, with psychosis and suicidal thoughts.

Red Flag

Postpartum psychosis is a psychiatric emergency and requires specialist assessment and treatment within four hours [41].

Prescribing in Breastfeeding Women

Prescribing in breastfeeding needs careful consideration of risks and benefits. The British National Formulary (BNF) identifies drugs under their specific headings:

- use with caution or contraindicated in breastfeeding, such as lithium
- can be given to the breastfeeding mother because present in milk in amounts unharmful to the infant
- might be present in milk in significant amount but not harmful.

More detailed advice can be obtained from the Specialist Pharmacy Service, from the leaflets on the Best Use of Medicines in Pregnancy (BUMPS) website, or from a US site, LactMed [42,43,44].

References

[1] NICE, 'NG194. Postnatal care'. Apr. 2021. Accessed: 13 May 2024. [Online]. Available: www.nice.org.uk/guidance/ng194.

[2] NHS, 'Symptoms – postnatal depression'. Aug. 2022. Accessed: 13 May 2024. [Online]. Available: www.nhs.uk/mental-health/conditions/post-natal-depression/overview.

[3] G. Chauhan and P. Tadi, 'Physiology, postpartum changes'. StatPearls Publishing, 2024.

[4] CoSRH, 'Contraception after pregnancy'. Oct. 2020. Accessed: 13 May 2024. [Online]. Available: https://www.cosrh.org/Common/Uploaded%20files/documents/contraception-after-pregnancy-guideline-oct2020.pdf.

[5] NICE CKS, 'Contraception – assessment'. Jan. 2024. Accessed: 13 May 2024. [Online]. Available: https://cks.nice.org.uk/topics/contraception-assessment.

[6] NICE, 'QA37. Postnatal care'. Sept. 2022. Accessed: 13 May 2024. [Online]. Available: www.nice.org.uk/guidance/qs37.

[7] Healthwatch, 'Six-week postnatal checks are failing many new mothers'. Mar. 2023. Accessed: 13 May 2024. [Online]. Available: www.healthwatch.co.uk/news/2023-03-14/six-week-postnatal-checks-are-failing-many-new-mothers.

[8] National Childbirth Trust, 'NCT & Netmums research finds the six week postnatal check-up unsatisfactory'. Oct. 2014. Accessed: 13 May 2024. [Online]. Available: https://www.nct.org.uk/about-us/media/news/nct-and-netmums-less-three-minutes-for-new-mums-mental-health.

[9] NHS England, 'GP six to eight week maternal postnatal consultation – what good looks like guidance'. Dec. 2023. Accessed: 13 May 2024. [Online]. Available: www.england.nhs.uk/publication/gp-6-to-8-week-maternal-postnatal-consultation-what-good-looks-like-guidance.

[10] CoSRH, 'UK medical eligibility criteria'. Sept. 2019. Accessed: 13 May 2024. [Online]. Available: https://www.cosrh.org/Public/Public/Standards-and-Guidance/uk-medical-eligibility-criteria-for-contraceptive-use-ukmec.aspx.

[11] NICE, 'NG3. Diabetes in pregnancy: Management from preconception to the postnatal period'. Dec. 2020. Accessed: 13 May 2024. [Online]. Available: www.nice.org.uk/guidance/ng3.

[12] NICE, 'PH38. Type 2 diabetes: Prevention in people at high risk'. Sept. 2017. Accessed: 13 May 2024. [Online]. Available: www.nice.org.uk/guidance/ph38.

[13] NICE, 'NG133. Hypertension in pregnancy: Diagnosis and management'. Apr. 2023. Accessed: 13 May 2024. [Online]. Available: www.nice.org.uk/guidance/ng133.

[14] ClinRisk, 'Qrisk3'. Accessed: 13 May 2024. [Online]. Available: www.qrisk.org.

[15] NICE, 'CG192. Antenatal and postnatal mental health: Clinical management and service guidance'. Feb. 2020. Accessed: 13 May 2024. [Online]. Available: www.nice.org.uk/guidance/cg192.

[16] SIGN, '169. Perinatal mental health conditions'. Dec. 2023. Accessed: 13 May 2024. [Online]. Available: www.sign.ac.uk/media/2172/sign-169-perinatal.pdf.

[17] RCGP, 'Antenatal and postnatal mental health NICE guideline CG192: Practical implications for GPs'. Feb. 2015. Accessed: 13 May 2024. [Online]. Available: https://elearning.rcgp.org.uk/pluginfile.php/175878/mod_book/chapter/606/Perinatalmentalhealth2023.pdf.

[18] A. Bauer, M. Parsonage, M. Knapp, V. Iemmi and A. Bayo, *The Costs of Perinatal Mental Health Problems*. Centre for Mental Health and London School of Economics, 2014.

[19] RCPsych, 'Perinatal mental health services: Recommendations for the provision of services for childbearing women'. Sept. 2021. Accessed: 13 May 2024. [Online]. Available: www.rcpsych.ac.uk/docs/default-source/improving-care/better-mh-policy/college-reports/college-report-cr232–perinatal-mental-heath-services.pdf?Status=Master&sfvrsn=82b10d7e_4.

[20] A. Stein, R. M. Pearson, S. H Goodman et al., 'Effects of perinatal mental disorders on the fetus and child', *Lancet*, vol. **384**, no. 9956, pp. 1800–1891, 2014.

[21] A. L. Rodrigues, J. Ericksen, B. Watson et al., 'Interventions for perinatal depression and anxiety in fathers: A mini-review', *Front Psychol*, vol. **12**, 744921, 2022.

[22] J. F. Paulson and S. D. Bazemore, 'Prenatal and postpartum depression in fathers and its association with maternal depression: A meta-analysis', *JAMA*, vol. **303**, no. 19, pp. 1961–1969, 2010.

[23] K. P. Hirst and C. Y. Moutier, 'Postpartum major depression', *Am Fam Physician*, vol. **82**, no. 8, pp. 926–933, 2010.

[24] S. Mughal, Y. Azhar and W. Siddiqui, 'Postpartum depression'. StatPearls Publishing, 2024.

[25] L. Khan, 'Falling through the gaps: Perinatal mental health and general practice'. Centre for Mental Health, 2015. Accessed: 13 May 2024. [Online]. Available: https://www.centreformentalhealth.org.uk/wp-content/uploads/2018/09/falling.pdf.

[26] N. A. Okeahialam, A. H. Sultan and R. Thakar, 'The prevention of perineal trauma during vaginal birth', *Am J Obstet Gynecol*, vol. **230**, no. 3S, pp. S991–S1004, 2024.

[27] A. M. Abdelhakim, E. Eldesouky, I. A. Elmagd et al., 'Antenatal perineal massage benefits in reducing perineal trauma and postpartum morbidities: A systematic review and meta-analysis of randomized controlled trials', *Int Urogynecol J*, vol. **31**, no. 9, pp. 1735–1745, 2020.

[28] E. B. Turawa, A. Musekiwa and A. C. Rohwer, 'Interventions for preventing postpartum constipation', *Cochrane Database of Systematic Reviews*, vol. **8**, CD011625, 2020.

[29] N. Salari, A. Mohammadi, M. Hemmati et al., 'The global prevalence of low back pain in pregnancy: A comprehensive systematic review and meta-analysis', *BMC Pregnancy Childbirth*, vol. **23**, no. 1, 830, 2023.

[30] D. R. Benjamin, A. T. van de Water and C. L. Peiris, 'Effects of exercise on diastasis of the rectus abdominis muscle in the antenatal and postnatal periods: A systematic review', *Physiotherapy*, vol. **100**, no. 1, pp. 1–8, 2014.

[31] L. Laageide, S. Radke, D. Santillan et al., 'Postpartum nipple symptoms: Risk factors and dermatologic characterization', *Breastfeed Med*, vol. **16**, no. 3, pp. 215–221, 2021.

[32] NICE CKS, 'Mastitis and breast abscess'. Dec. 2023. Accessed: 13 May 2024. [Online]. Available: https://cks.nice.org.uk/topics/mastitis-breast-abscess.

[33] D. Lissauer, M. Morgan, A. Banerjee, F. Plaat, D. Pasupathy and the Royal College of Obstetrics and Gynaecology, 'Identification and management of maternal sepsis during and following pregnancy', *BJOG*, vol. **132**, pp. e61–e85, 2025, https://doi.org/10.1111/1471-0528.18009.

[34] S. Naji Rad and L. Deluxe, 'Postpartum thyroiditis'. StatPearls Publishing, 2024.

[35] RCOG, 'Heavy bleeding after birth (postpartum haemorrhage)'. Dec. 2016. Accessed: 13 May 2024. [Online]. Available: www.rcog.org.uk/for-the-public/browse-our-patient-information/heavy-bleeding-after-birth-postpartum-haemorrhage.

[36] MBRRACE-UKK, 'Improving mothers' care: Lessons learned to inform maternity care from the UK and Ireland Confidential Enquiries into Maternal Deaths and Morbidity 2020–22'. Oct. 2024. Accessed: 14 May 2024. [Online]. Available: www.npeu.ox.ac.uk/assets/downloads/mbrrace-uk/reports/maternal-report-2024/MBRRACE-UK%20Maternal%20MAIN%20Report%202024%20V2.0%20ONLINE.pdf.

[37] RCOG, 'Green-Top Guideline 37a. Reducing the risk of thrombosis and embolism during pregnancy and the puerperium'. Apr. 2015. Accessed: 14 May 2024. [Online]. Available: www.rcog.org.uk/guidance/browse-all-guidance/green-top-guidelines/reducing-the-risk-of-thrombosis-and-embolism-during-pregnancy-and-the-puerperium-green-top-guideline-no-37a.

[38] RCOG, 'Green-Top Guideline 37b. Thrombosis and embolism during pregnancy and the puerperium: Acute management'. Apr. 2015. Accessed: 14 May 2024. [Online]. Available: www.rcog.org.uk/guidance/browse-all-guidance/green-top-guidelines/thrombosis-and-embolism-during-pregnancy-and-the-puerperium-acute-management-green-top-guideline-no-37b.

[39] University of Oxford, National Perinatal Epidemiology Unit, 'Listening to parents after stillbirth or the death of their baby after birth'. 2014. Accessed: 14 May 2024. [Online]. Available: https://www.npeu.ox.ac.uk/listeningtoparents/report/Listening%20to%20Parents%20Report%20-%20March%202014%20-%20FINAL%20-%20PROTECTED.pdf.

[40] K. Nguyen, L. T. Mukona, L. Nalbandyan et al., 'Peripartum complications as risk factors for postpartum psychosis: A systemic review', *Cureus*, vol. **14**, no. 9, e29224, 2022.

[41] RCPsych, 'Postpartum psychosis'. Nov. 2018. Accessed: 14 May 2024. [Online]. Available: www.rcpsych.ac.uk/mental-health/mental-illnesses-and-mental-health-problems/postpartum-psychosis.

[42] Specialist Pharmacy Service, 'Safety in breastfeeding'. Accessed: 14 May 2024. [Online]. Available: www.sps.nhs.uk/home/guidance/safety-in-breastfeeding.

[43] BUMPS. Accessed: 14 May 2024. [Online]. Available: www.medicinesinpregnancy.org.

[44] National Library of Medicine, 'Drugs and Lactation Database (Lactmed)'. Accessed: 14 May 2024. [Online]. Available: www.ncbi.nlm.nih.gov/books/NBK501922.

Chapter 14

Polycystic Ovary Syndrome

Management of a Long-Term Condition in Primary Care

Anne Connolly

Key Points

- Polycystic ovary syndrome (PCOS) is a common endocrine disorder with short- and long-term health consequences; it can usually be managed in primary care.
- The condition can be diagnosed from history and examination using the updated Rotterdam criteria [1].
- Symptoms of hyperandrogenism are a common presenting feature and can usually be improved by simple treatments and weight reduction.
- Infertility is a frequent concern as anovulation is caused by the hormonal imbalance of PCOS. In most women this can be improved by weight reduction.
- Chronic anovulation is a risk factor for endometrial hyperplasia and cancer, and requires management with cyclical or continuous progestogen therapy.
- All women with PCOS require a psychological assessment and support as appropriate.
- PCOS is a long-term condition requiring regular screening to prevent the consequences of insulin resistance; that is, cardiovascular disease and diabetes.
- The diagnosis should not be confirmed within eight years of menarche [2] because of the risk of overdiagnosis. PCOS symptoms are common in adolescent women and the diagnostic findings on scan and blood tests are less sensitive and specific at this age.

Case Scenario 14.1: Shazia

Shazia, a 27-year-old classroom assistant, attends clinic, concerned about her inability to conceive over the previous 18 months. She has one child, Asha, aged three, from her first and only pregnancy. Her husband, Asif, a bus driver, is the father of her daughter.

On further questioning, Shazia reports distress about a change to her periods, which have become less frequent. The gap between her periods is now two to six months. She does frequent home pregnancy tests in the hope that the delayed period is caused by pregnancy.

Introduction

One of the commonest endocrine disorders affecting women of reproductive age [2], PCOS is a complex, long-term condition with metabolic, reproductive and psychological sequelae. Presentation is variable and includes hyperandrogenism, ovulatory dysfunction and polycystic ovarian morphology. Estimates of prevalence vary widely, from 1–2% to up to 26% [2,3], and it is likely that many women with PCOS are undiagnosed.

PCOS (initially known as Stein–Leventhal syndrome) was first described by Stein and Leventhal in 1935 [4] when they published a case series of seven patients with amenorrhoea, hirsutism and bilateral polycystic ovaries.

After years of debate to establish diagnostic criteria, a consensus workshop was held in Rotterdam in 2004, supported by the European Society of Human Reproduction and Embryology (ESHRE) and the American Society of Reproductive Medicine (ASRM). It led to the Rotterdam criteria for diagnosis of PCOS, most recently updated in 2023 [5]. The consensus criteria require two of the three key features: oligo- or anovulation, clinical and/or biochemical hyperandrogenism and polycystic ovaries on ultrasound (Table 14.1) [5]. The recent update includes the choice of using anti-Müllerian hormone (AMH) or ultrasonography to diagnose polycystic ovaries [5].

Table 14.1 Diagnosing polycystic ovary syndrome [5]

The diagnosis of PCOS can be made on the basis of two out of three of the following, assuming exclusion of other causes (e.g. congenital adrenal hyperplasia, androgen-secreting tumours or Cushing's syndrome).

- Clinical and/or biochemical signs of hyperandrogenism (acne, hirsutism or elevated testosterone).
- Ovulatory dysfunction (oligo- or anovulation).
- Polycystic ovaries on ultrasound scan or an elevated serum AMH. Polycystic ovaries are diagnosed using the following threshold:
    - ovarian volume ≥ 10 mL or
    - follicle number per section (FNPS) ≥ 10 (≥20 if older scanning technology is used).

Women with PCOS have traditionally been referred to gynaecology clinics because the underlying cause was believed to be the abnormal ovarian function, but the pathophysiology is now understood to be due to an endocrine abnormality resulting from insulin resistance [5,6,7,8]. Insulin resistance is exacerbated by weight gain, which in turn exacerbates the clinical, reproductive and metabolic features of PCOS. Most care for this long-term condition should be provided in primary care, with specialist referral for specific indications as required.

The clinical features of PCOS include [5]:

- endocrine (hyperandrogenism; acne, hirsutism, male pattern balding)
- reproductive (anovulatory infertility, irregular menstrual cycles)
- metabolic (insulin resistance, impaired glucose tolerance, adverse cardiovascular risk profile)
- psychological (increased anxiety, depression and reduced quality of life).

This condition requires a holistic life-course approach, with hyperandrogenic symptoms and infertility being more problematic in younger women and the metabolic features becoming more significant in older age groups, although this will vary for each individual woman (Figure 14.1).

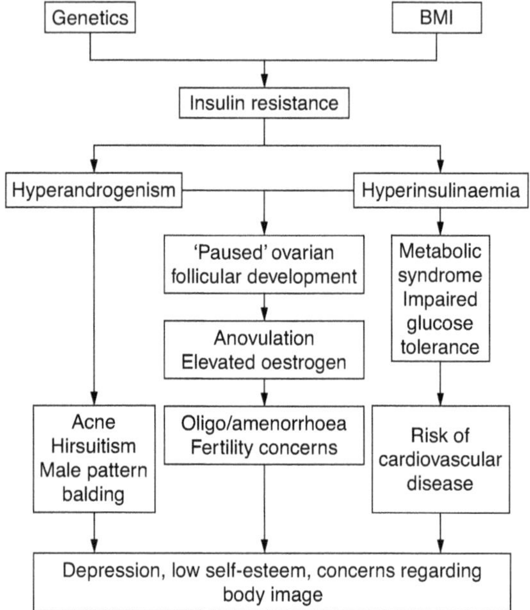

Figure 14.1 Causes and consequences of PCOS.

Pathophysiology of PCOS [9]

The current understanding of the physiology of PCOS is summarised below.

- Insulin resistance caused by genetic factors and obesity results in hyperinsulinaemia.
- Hyperinsulinaemia causes overproduction of the gonadotrophin luteinising hormone (LH), preventing the mid-cycle LH surge needed for ovulation.
- Persistently high levels of LH antagonise the action of follicle-stimulating hormone (FSH), preventing the increase in FSH necessary for normal cyclical ovarian follicular development. The numerous small antral follicles produced are 'paused follicles', which have reduced cell growth and reduced cell death. These follicles typically arrest growth at 7 mm, which is an insufficient size for ovulation (Table 14.2 and Figure 14.2).
- For normal development, the inner granulosa cells require FSH to synthesise and secrete oestradiol, whereas the thecal cells depend on LH to stimulate secretion of androgens, which are converted into oestrogen in the granulosa cells.
- The ovary requires insulin as a co-factor to augment the LH-induced thecal cell androgen secretion. Women with insulin resistance produce excessive amounts of insulin in an attempt to promote glucose uptake in muscle

Table 14.2 Consequences of PCOS

- Multiple peripheral ovarian cysts
- Menstrual irregularity
- Sub-fertility
- Mood disturbance
- Hyperandrogenism
- Obesity
- Sleep apnoea
- Acne
- Hirsutism
- Insulin resistance
- Diabetes mellitus
- Hyperlipidaemia
- Non-alcoholic steatohepatitis
- Adverse risk profile for cardiovascular disease
- Depression
- Eating disorders and impact on body image
- Endometrial hyperplasia and malignancy

and fat tissues. The ovary remains sensitive to insulin growth factor effects; resultant hyperinsulinaemia causes more androgens to be produced.

- Anovulatory cycles lack the development of the corpus luteum, which produces progesterone necessary to induce secretory endometrial changes and subsequent endometrial shedding.
- Sex hormone-binding globulin (SHBG) is the circulating protein which binds to and inhibits the effects of oestrogen and testosterone. In healthy women, 80% of circulating testosterone is bound to SHBG, 19% is bound to albumin and 1% circulates freely. It is the unbound (free) testosterone which is metabolically active.
- SHBG is inversely related to weight, so individuals with obesity or overweight produce less SHBG and have more circulating free androgens and oestrogen. As weight decreases, this effect reduces.
- Insulin is an anabolic hormone, with a role in energy storage. High insulin levels usually mean easier weight gain, which aggravates the symptoms and consequences of PCOS.
- Increased ovarian androgen production is caused by any, or a combination, of increased LH, hyperinsulinaemia and obesity. In women with obesity, insulin resistance drives the hyperandrogenism, whereas in women without obesity, elevated LH is the main cause. There is significant overlap between these distinct types of PCOS, such that 10% of women without obesity with LH-driven PCOS will have impaired glucose tolerance.

Case Scenario 14.2

As the consultation with Shazia unfolds, she becomes tearful. She knows she is putting on weight and has started shaving her upper lip and chin to try and hide the excessive hair growth which bothers her.

Symptoms of PCOS

Most women come to see their GP with concerns about the hyperandrogenism caused by PCOS.

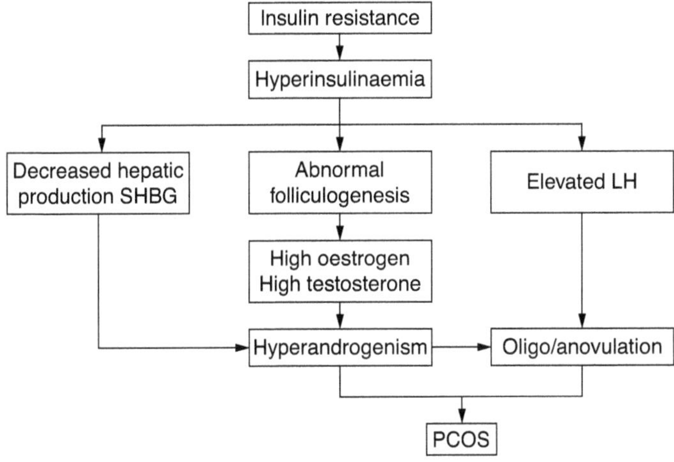

Figure 14.2 Hormonal influences on the development of PCOS.

Hirsutism is present in 65–75% of women with PCOS [10]. It may be difficult to differentiate from idiopathic hirsutism, but the hirsutism secondary to excessive androgen production is found in a male pattern hair distribution. The Ferriman and Gallwey score [11] is the most commonly used objective grading, scoring 11 different body areas (upper lip, chest, chin, lower back, upper back, lower abdomen, upper abdomen, forearm, arm, thigh and lower leg). Each area is scored 0–4 with a total score of 8 or more defining hirsutism.

Androgenic alopecia (male pattern hair loss) may also be seen in PCOS, although it is less common than hirsutism [12]; it can be very distressing.

Acne is a less specific marker of hyperandrogenism as it is common in teenagers and young women, but new-onset acne in adults is highly predictive of PCOS [13].

Signs of overt virilisation, including voice deepening, increased muscle bulk and clitoral hypertrophy, should prompt investigations including serum testosterone levels and an adrenal and ovarian ultrasound scan, to exclude an androgen-secreting tumour or late-onset congenital adrenal hyperplasia [2].

Acanthosis nigricans is also commonly found with PCOS and is dependent on the presence of insulin resistance. This skin condition is characterised by darkened velvety plaques most commonly occurring in the nape of the neck, skin folds of the axilla and groin and on pressure-bearing surfaces such as the elbows [2].

Women with PCOS also notice menstrual dysfunction. The commonest complaint is of oligo- or amenorrhoea secondary to oligo- or anovulation. Oligomenorrhoea is defined as 4–9 cycles per year with a cycle length of greater than 35 days [14,15].

Depression and anxiety are higher in women with PCOS than in the general population. Concerns about body image and appearance due to symptoms of hyperandrogenism can lead to eating disorders, and psychosexual and relationship problems, which can all be aggravated by the stress of sub-fertility [5,16].

Case Scenario 14.3

Shazia is noted to have acne and hirsutism, but no other obvious signs of virilisation. She has a Ferriman and Gallwey score of 10. She has dark pigmentation in the nape of her neck and the skin folds of her axilla. Her body mass index (BMI) is 37 kg/m^2.

The diagnosis of PCOS can be made from her history and clinical examination as she has two of the three findings to fulfil the requirements of the Rotterdam criteria; clinical signs of hyperandrogenism and oligomenorrhoea.

Shazia is informed of her diagnosis and provided with a patient information leaflet. She is also advised to consult the Verity website at www.verity-pcos.org.uk. This UK charity is for women whose lives are affected by PCOS and is a useful resource for Shazia to understand the lifestyle changes she should make [17].

Examination of a Woman with Suspected PCOS

Examination is guided by the symptoms, but should also include assessment of mood, blood pressure monitoring, BMI and ideally a waist measurement (a waist to height ratio of 0.4 - 0.49 is considered to be healthy). [29, 5]. It is important to remember that many women with PCOS find examination, and particularly waist measurement, embarrassing.

Investigations in Suspected PCOS [5]

The diagnosis of PCOS is usually made from history and clinical examination; however, it is important to exclude other conditions such as hypothyroidism, hyperprolactinaemia and premature menopause – tests would usually be guided by the clinical picture.

Blood Tests

Thyroid, Prolactin, FSH, LH

Investigations could include serology for thyroid function, prolactin, FSH and LH levels. If FSH is checked, ideally this should be done during days 2–5 of the menstrual cycle. If this is not possible because of long or absent menstrual cycles, a random sample repeated in six weeks is often the best possible option. The LH:FSH ratio is usually greater than 2:1 in PCOS.

Testosterone

Testosterone testing is complex as total testosterone levels do not demonstrate much variation due to the low circulating testosterone usually found in women. However, serum total testosterone can be useful to exclude an androgen-secreting tumour, as a level of <5.0 nmol/L is usually consistent with mild hyperandrogenism and hence PCOS, whereas a level of >5.0 nmol/L is more likely to be due to an adrenal or ovarian tumour, congenital adrenal hyperplasia or Cushing's syndrome, and requires further investigations.

Testing SHBG allows measurement of the free androgen index (FAI), if this is needed.

$$\text{FAI} = \text{total testosterone}/\text{SHBG} \times 100.$$

Anti-Müllerian Hormone (AMH)

Serum AMH is part of the latest Rotterdam criteria [5] and can be used instead of an ultrasound (both are not needed), though it is not always available in NHS primary care. It is not recommended in adolescents due to low specificity. It is essential that this result is reported using an appropriate diagnostic algorithm and not used in addition to ultrasound scanning.

AMH results are influenced by the following [19,20,21].

- Age – AMH levels usually peak between age 20 and 25.
- BMI – AMH may be reduced with higher BMI, particularly in Caucasian women.
- Hormonal contraception – AMH may be reduced in current and recent uses of combined hormonal contraception.
- Menstrual cycle – AMH levels vary across the menstrual cycle.

Blood Tests for Cardiovascular Risk

Other investigations such as HbA1c and lipids are indicated to complete a cardiovascular risk assessment – further tests such as renal or liver function may be needed if there is a diagnosis of diabetes, or concern about metabolic dysfunction-associated steatotic liver disease.

Ultrasound

Other investigations include a pelvic and transvaginal ultrasound scan (TVUS). The TVUS allows more detailed examination of ovarian pathology, particularly in women with obesity, but may not be acceptable to all women, especially those who have never been sexually active. A scan may not be necessary if the woman already meets the diagnostic criteria of PCOS without one, as demonstrated by Shazia's case study.

If a scan is done, PCOS is confirmed if there are ≥10 follicles in each ovary, measuring 2–9 mm in diameter and/or increased ovarian volume (>10 mL). The follicles tend to be peripherally sited and provide a characteristic 'string of pearls' effect. The prevalence of endometrial hyperplasia and cancer is increased in women with obesity and with oligo/anovulation caused by their elevated and unopposed circulating oestrogen levels [18]. TVUS findings of a thickened or cystic endometrium indicate the need for hysteroscopy and endometrial sampling.

Making the Diagnosis in Adolescents

The updated international evidence-based guideline for the assessment and management of PCOS [5] acknowledges the challenges of making a diagnosis of PCOS in adolescents because of the evolving diagnostic features. The recommendations include the following, which are also contained in the National Institute for Health and Care Excellence (NICE) chapter knowledge summaries (CKS) page on PCOS [6].

- Ultrasound and AMH levels are not recommended in diagnosis within eight years of menarche.
- Young women 'at risk' can be identified with follow-up assessment to reduce the risk of overdiagnosis.

Case Scenario 14.4

Shazia's main concern on this occasion is her inability to conceive. As she also has concerns about her appearance, these problems should be addressed during the management discussions.

Management

The management of PCOS is aimed at:

- helping to manage the short-term problems of hyperandrogenism, mood disturbance and fertility
- helping to reduce the long-term consequences of insulin resistance and endometrial hyperplasia.

The most important aspect of management is weight reduction by a combination of good nutrition and exercise. GLP-1 agonists may also be useful, but at the time of publication PCOS is not an indication for their provision on the NHS.

Weight loss will reduce insulin resistance, androgen levels and the systemic effects of ovarian dysfunction, resulting in improved symptoms and fertility and reduction of long-term consequences.

Other treatments should be individualised to provide appropriate symptom control. The symptoms of hyperandrogenism can be improved by any treatment to reduce circulating free androgens. Weight reduction will achieve this by increasing levels of SHBG and so will treatment with ethinyl-oestradiol, by use of any combined hormonal contraceptive, after a risk assessment.

Any combined hormonal contraceptive, used at the lowest possible dose, may help with hyperandrogenism and menstrual irregularity where use of these treatments has been balanced against the risk of potential complications, particularly thromboembolic events in women with a BMI greater than 35 kg/m^2. Oral anti-androgen therapies such as cyproterone acetate, either alone or in combination with 35 mcg ethinyl-oestradiol or alternatively a combination of ethinyl-oestradiol and the anti-androgen drosperinone, may be helpful in the treatment of those who do not respond to first-line treatment. Patients must be encouraged to continue with their medication because it may take up to nine months before they see significant improvement.

In those who have contraindications for the use of combined hormonal contraception, such as a high BMI, focal migraine or a combination of other thrombotic or cardiovascular risks (as assessed using the UK medical eligibility criteria for contraceptive use) [22], the usual treatments for acne, such as long-term oral or topical antibiotics, may be used. Oral retionid treatment, under specialist supervision, is also an option.

Once recruited, hair follicles remain active and long-term treatment for hirsutism may be required. Weight reduction and the use of anti-androgenic oral contraceptives will provide some improvement, but other women require additional symptomatic management or physical hair removal treatments such as shaving, waxing, electrolysis and laser treatments.

It is important for patients with PCOS to reduce weight to a BMI less than 30 kg/m^2 prior to conception because of the complications of pregnancy and poorer foetal outcomes which are associated with maternal obesity. Gestational diabetes mellitus (GDM) is the most frequently occurring problem, but others include pregnancy-related hypertension, preeclampsia, placental abruption and thromboembolic events [23,24]. Reliable contraception should be provided for women who do not wish to conceive, or who wish to delay conception until their BMI has reduced.

When couples present with fertility concerns, it is essential to consider other possible causes for their problem in addition to the PCOS and investigate following standard practice. Weight reduction may be sufficient to increase the chance of conception, but other investigations, including a semen analysis, should be performed, according to NICE and local guidelines [25] (Table 14.3).

The role of metformin has been controversial and generally restricted to use once diabetes has been established. The updated guideline has recommended increased use of metformin recognising the treatment benefit of improving metabolic outcomes, including insulin resistance, glucose and lipid profiles. Metformin continues to be recommended once diabetes is confirmed but the 2023 European guideline says that it can also be considered for those with a BMI over 25 kg/m^2, including adolescents, using the principles of shared decision-making and balancing the benefits against risks of adverse effects including gastro-intestinal side effects and B12 deficiency. The NICE CKS page agrees that it should be considered in women with a BMI of over 25 kg/m^2 and reminds us that metformin for this indication is off-licence, suggesting that GPs consider seeking specialist advice before initiating it in women without diabetes [6]. It is also recommended by NICE in those at risk of diabetes, if their blood sugar has deteriorated despite intensive lifestyle change, or if they are unable to participate in intensive lifestyle change, particularly if the BMI is greater than 35 kg/m^3.

Management in Pregnancy

Women with PCOS have higher-risk pregnancies and require careful monitoring throughout [27,28].

Risks include:

- higher gestational weight gain
- miscarriage
- gestational diabetes
- hypertension and pre-eclampsia
- intrauterine growth retardation
- preterm delivery.

Table 14.3 Management of women with PCOS

Problem	Management options
Obesity	Weight reduction, by diet, exercise and/or medical treatments such as GLP-1 agonists or bariatric surgery.
Hirsutism	Physical therapies – shaving, waxing, electrolysis, laser treatments. Combined hormonal contraception including ethinyl-oestradiol and cyproterone acetate or drosperinone. Other anti-androgenic treatments – spironolactone and cyproterone acetate.
Acne	Combined hormonal contraception. Topical or systemic antibiotics. Topical or systemic retinoids.
Oligo or amenorrhoea	52mg levonorgestrel intrauterine device. Combined hormonal contraception. Cyclical or continuous progestogens including desogestrel or medroxyprogesterone acetate.
Infertility	Baseline investigations, including semen analysis. Specialist management in line with local guidelines.
Insulin resistance, metabolic syndrome and cardiovascular disease	Optimise cardiovascular risk factors including: • smoking cessation • managing abnormal factors: · blood pressure · HbA1C · lipid profile.
Depression and psychosexual problems	Improve emotional wellbeing: • support • anti-depressants • counselling, including relationship counselling.

Specialist Fertility Treatments

Initial fertility advice and management is standard practice for all couples referred to specialist services and should follows NICE recommendations and local pathways [25].

This includes lifestyle advice for both partners including:

- weight optimisation
- smoking cessation
- reduction/cessation of alcohol and non-prescribed medication
- regular unprotected penetrative sexual intercourse
- stress management.

Further intervention is usually not indicated until the woman achieves her recommended BMI of <30 kg/m^2 to minimise risks to the pregnancy that are well recognised with obesity. Semen analysis and tubal patency tests are required, but, once other causes of infertility are excluded, ovulation induction treatment should be considered.

The updated international guideline [5] has amended the recommendations for ovulation induction for infertility. Letrozole (unlicensed for this indication) is recommended as the first-line pharmacological infertility treatment with higher ovulation, clinical pregnancy and live birth rates compared with clomifene alone or in combination with metformin.

Gonadotrophins alone or in conjunction with clomifene are recommended as second-line pharmacological options.

Laparoscopic ovarian drilling is a further second-line treatment option but has higher costs and risks compared with pharmacological management.

Case Scenario 14.5

The next time Shazia attends clinic, she seems low and anxious. She discloses that her husband has commented on her weight and facial hair. She has continued to gain weight and now has a BMI of 39 kg/m^2. She is reluctant to socialise normally with family and friends and has started spending time and money on make-up and hair removal treatments.

The psychological features of PCOS are often overlooked, but the impact of sub-fertility and low self-esteem with negative body image often cause depression, anxiety and relationship problems, including sexual dysfunction.

Supporting women with psychological and psychosexual concerns is an important aspect of the holistic care required. Screening should be performed at an early stage so that support can be offered. Other managements, including anti-depressants and counselling, as well as relationship counselling, should be provided as usual for any patient seen in the primary care setting.

The lifestyle changes that are essential to reduce obesity are difficult to sustain for individuals who lack self-confidence and motivation. Addressing the psychological issues can empower women to comply with the weight reduction required to reverse the metabolic and endocrine problems.

Long-Term Monitoring and Management

Women with PCOS are at increased risk of cardiovascular disease because of obesity, hyperandrogenism, hyperlipidaemia and hyperinsulinaemia [5]. Risk factors should be screened for and managed appropriately.

Women with PCOS who have oligo- or amenorrhoea are predisposed to developing endometrial hyperplasia and endometrial carcinoma due to the prolonged exposure to unopposed oestrogen. Endometrial protection can be provided by a 52mg levonorgestrel intrauterine device, combined or progestogen-only contraception (including the combined pill, patch or ring and the progestogen-only pill, implant or injection). For women who do not want to use contraception, they can have an induced withdrawal bleed, once pregnancy has been excluded, using intermittent progestogen therapy, usually medroxyprogesterone acetate 10 mg daily for 14 days or twice daily for 7–10 days every 3 months [6].

Summary

PCOS is a complex, life-long endocrine condition caused by insulin resistance. There are short- and long-term problems associated with this condition that require appropriate understanding, management and monitoring.

Patient education, psychological support and weight reduction are important elements of management that should be done in primary care.

References

[1] H. J. Teede, C. T. Tay, J. J. E. Laven et al., 'Recommendations from the 2023 international evidence-based guideline for the assessment and management of polycystic ovary syndrome', *J Clin Endocrinol Metab*, vol. **108**, no. 10, pp. 2447–2469, 2023.

[2] NICE CKS, 'Polycystic ovary syndrome'. Jan. 2024. Accessed: 19 Feb. 2024. [Online]. Available: https://cks.nice.org.uk/topics/polycystic-ovary-syndrome.

[3] S. C. Hillman and J. Dale, 'Polycystic ovarian syndrome: An under-recognised problem?', *Br J Gen Pract*, vol. **68**, no. 670, p. 244, 2018.

[4] I. Stein and M. Leventhal, 'Amenorrhoea associated with bilateral polycystic ovaries', *Am J Obstet Gynecol*, vol. **29**, pp. 181–189, 1935.

[5] Monash University, Crewhirl, CREPCOS, asrm, Endocrine Society, European Society of Human Reproduction and Embryology, European Society of Endocrinology, 'International evidence-based guideline for the assessment and management of polycystic ovary syndrome 2023 – Summary'. Accessed: 19 Feb. 2024. [Online]. Available: https://www.monash.edu/__data/assets/pdf_file/0003/3379521/Evidence-Based-Guidelines-2023.pdf.

[6] NHS, 'Polycystic ovary syndrome: Causes'. Oct. 2022. Accessed: 19 Feb. 2024. [Online]. Available: www.nhs.uk/conditions/polycystic-ovary-syndrome-pcos/causes.

[7] A. Purwar and S. Nagpure, 'Insulin resistance in polycystic ovarian syndrome', *Cureus*, vol. **14**, no. 10, e30351, 2022.

[8] C. A. Amisi, 'Markers of insulin resistance in Polycystic ovary syndrome women: An update', *World J Diabetes*, vol. **13**, no. 3, pp. 129–149, 2022.

[9] W. C. Duncan, 'A guide to understanding polycystic ovary syndrome (PCOS)', *J Plann Reprod Health Care*, vol. **40**, pp. 217–225, 2014.

[10] P. M. Spritzer, L. B. Marchesan, B. R. Santos et al., 'Hirsutism, normal androgens and diagnosis of PCOS', *Diagnostics (Basel)*, vol. **12**, no. 8, p. 1922, 2022.

[11] D. M. Ferriman and J. D. Gallwey, 'Clinical assessment of body hair growth in women', *J Clin Endocrinol*, vol. **21**, pp. 1440–1447, 1961.

[12] M. Quinn, K. Shinkai, L. Pasch et al., 'Prevalence of androgenic alopecia in patients with polycystic ovary syndrome and characterization of associated clinical and biochemical features', *Fertil Steril*, vol. **101**, no. 4, pp. 1129–1134, 2014.

[13] E. Carmina, B. Dreno, W. A. Lucky et al., 'Female adult acne and androgen excess: A report from the Multidisciplinary Androgen Excess and PCOS Committee', *J Endocr Soc*, vol. **6**, no. 3, bvac003, 2022.

[14] Y. Riaz and U. Parekh, 'Oligomenorrhea'. StatPearls Publishing, 2024.

[15] NICE CKS, 'Amenorrhoea'. Feb. 2022. Accessed: 19 Feb. 2024. [Online]. Available: https://cks.nice.org.uk/topics/amenorrhoea.

[16] A. Gnawali, V. Patel, A. Cuello-Ramírez et al., 'Why are women with polycystic ovary syndrome at increased risk of depression? Exploring the etiological maze', *Cureus*, vol. **13**, no. 2, e13489, 2021.

[17] Verity, 'Sharing the truth about PCOS'. Accessed: 19 Feb. 2024. [Online]. Available: www.verity-pcos.org.uk.

[18] Z. Haoula, M. Salman and W. Atiomo, 'Evaluating the association between endometrial cancer and polycystic ovary syndrome', *Hum Reprod*, vol. **27**, no. 5, pp. 1327–1331, 2012.

[19] V. Moy, S. Jindal, H. Lieman et al., 'Obesity adversely affects serum anti-Müllerian hormone (AMH) levels in Caucasian women', *J Assist Reprod Genet*, vol. **32**, no. 9, pp. 1305–1311, 2015.

[20] S. M. Nelson, B. J. Ewing, P. S. Gromski et al., 'Contraceptive-specific antimüllerian hormone values in reproductive-age women: A population study of 42,684 women', *Fertil Steril*, vol. **119**, no. 6, pp. 1069–1077, 2023.

[21] R. Khodavirdilou, M. Pournaghi, Y. Rastgar Rezaei et al., 'Does anti-Müllerian hormone vary during a menstrual cycle? A systematic review and meta-analysis', *J Ovarian Res*, vol. **15**, p. 78, 2022.

[22] CoSRH, 'UK medical eligibility criteria for contraceptive use'. Sept. 2019. Accessed: 5 Dec. 2025. [Online]. Available: https://www.cosrh.org/Public/Public/Standards-and-Guidance/uk-medical-eligibility-criteria-for-contraceptive-use-ukmec.aspx.

[23] J. Z. Qin, L. H. Pang, M. J. Li et al., 'Obstetric complications in women with polycystic ovary syndrome: A systematic review and meta-analysis', *Reprod Biol Endocrinol*, vol. **11**, p. 56, 2013.

[24] RCOG Green-Top Guideline 72, 'Care of women with obesity in pregnancy'. Nov. 2018. Accessed: 19 Feb. 2024. [Online]. Available: www.rcog.org.uk/guidance/browse-all-guidance/green-top-guidelines/care-of-women-with-obesity-in-pregnancy-green-top-guideline-no-72.

[25] NICE CKS, 'Infertility'. Jul. 2023. Accessed: 19 Feb. 2024. [Online]. Available: https://cks.nice.org.uk/topics/infertility.

[26] NICE, 'Type 2 diabetes: Prevention in people at high risk'. Sept. 2017. Accessed: 19 Feb. 2024. [Online]. Available: www.nice.org.uk/guidance/PH38.

[27] S. Kamalanathan, J. P. Sahoo and T. Sathyapalan, 'Pregnancy in polycystic ovary syndrome', *Indian J Endocrinol Metab*, vol. **17**, no. 1, pp. 37–43, 2013.

[28] National Institute of Child Health and Human Development, 'Does PCOS affect pregnancy?' Jan. 2017. Accessed: 19 Feb. 2024. [Online]. Available: www.nichd.nih.gov/health/topics/pcos/more_information/FAQs/pregnancy.

[29] NICE guidance on obesity Available: https://www.nice.org.uk/guidance/ng246/.

Chapter 15

Management of Premature Ovarian Insufficiency (POI) in Primary Care

Timothy Hillard, Amanda Hillard and Abbie Laing

Key Points

- Consider premature ovarian insufficiency (POI) in women under 40 presenting with more than three months of oligo or amenorrhoea.
- Elicit family history of early menopause, autoimmune conditions, genetic conditions such as fragile X syndrome and a personal history of potential iatrogenic causes, such as chemo or radiotherapy.
- Untreated POI increases the lifetime risk of osteoporosis, cardiovascular disease, dementia, cognitive decline and parkinsonism.
- Treatment should be with hormone replacement therapy (HRT) or combined oral contraceptive pill (COCP) until at least the average age of menopause at 51.
- Emphasise the importance of hormone replacement at least up until the age of natural menopause: for most women the benefits of treatment far outweigh any risks.
- Patient preference for method of administration must be considered when prescribing, as should their contraceptive needs.
- Women with POI represent a different cohort to women who have menopause at the average age so the risks of cancer and stroke routinely quoted for HRT do not apply to these younger women.
- Spontaneous POI is associated with 5–10% pregnancy rate so the potential need for ongoing contraception should be discussed.
- Lifestyle modification including regular weight-bearing exercise, limiting caffeine and alcohol intake, smoking cessation, maintaining healthy body weight, and a healthy diet containing adequate calcium and vitamin D.
- Be aware of the psychosocial and psychosexual impact of the diagnosis of POI and provide appropriate support.
- Consider referring people with POI to healthcare professionals with the relevant experience to help them manage all aspects of physical and psychosocial health related to their condition.

Introduction

Premature ovarian insufficiency (POI) is a potentially life-changing condition which is often under-recognized and incompletely managed. It describes the loss of ovarian function in women younger than 40 years which causes amenorrhoea and sex steroid deficiency, with sustained elevation of gonadotropins (luteinising hormone (LH) and follicle-stimulating hormone (FSH)). Without appropriate treatment it can have significant long-term health consequences. It is not a homogeneous condition; for some there is a genetic or congenital cause, while it may be iatrogenic or secondary to other conditions (Table 15.1). No cause is found in 75–90%.

The management of this group of women can be complex and made difficult by the paucity of research studies in this area. The study of this condition is complicated by its low incidence and lack of agreed nomenclature and diagnostic criteria. This chapter is based on up-to-date (2024) internationally agreed recommendations.

Definition and Nomenclature

The nomenclature in this area can be confusing and the terms and definitions have been applied inconsistently. In the past, numerous terms have been used to describe the condition including premature ovarian failure, premature menopause and premature ovarian senescence; however, POI is now the preferred and accepted term.

The median age of menopause in the Western world is 51 but may be lower in some countries. Approximately 5% of women will undergo menopause between the ages of 40 and 45 which is referred to as ‘early menopause’. Premature menopause, now called POI, is reserved for women who undergo menopause before the age of 40. The age of 40 years is used as the cut-off as this represents two standard deviations below the mean age of natural menopause.

This condition affects about 1 in 100 women under 40, 1 in 1,000 women under the age of 30 and 1 in 10,000 women under the age of 20. It accounts for 10–28% of women with primary amenorrhoea and 4–18% of those with secondary amenorrhoea. However, with the number of survivors from childhood cancers increasing, these traditional figures may be an underestimate.

The term 'menopause' denotes an irreversible condition. However, in women with spontaneous onset of POI, it is possible that there may be some return of ovarian function and even fertility restored so the term premature ovarian insufficiency is preferred.

Causes and Risk Factors

POI is either iatrogenic or spontaneous. Iatrogenic POI occurs in around 11% of cases and may be due to surgery, chemotherapy or radiotherapy (Table 15.1). In many cases the cause of POI remains elusive, despite the numerous conditions that are associated with it (Table 15.1). Spontaneous POI occurs in around 85–90% of cases. Chromosomal abnormalities can be identified as the cause of POI in approximately 10–13% of cases and autoimmune ovarian damage in up to 10% of cases. With improvement in cancer therapy, there is an increasing number of young female cancer survivors with iatrogenic POI. Management of POI in this group of patients is an important cancer survivorship issue that is often overlooked. In women presenting with spontaneous POI, no cause is usually found in 70–90% of cases. However, the discovery of novel candidate genes through mapping of the genomic landscape of POI is revealing that many of these cases may be genetic in origin.

Table 15.1 Known causes and risk factors for POI

Primary	Examples
Congenital	Absent/infantile ovaries
Chromosome abnormalities	Turner syndrome, fragile X, other x linked mutations, Downs syndrome
Other genetic cause	FSH receptor gene mutations BRCA1
Enzyme deficiency	Galactosaemia
Autoimmune diseases	Addison's disease, Hashimoto's thyroiditis, type 1 diabetes, adrenal insufficiency, Sjogren's syndrome, rheumatoid arthritis, inflammatory bowel disease, multiple sclerosis, coeliac disease, myasthenia gravis,
Family history of early menopause	Inheritable genetic causes; an increasing number of candidate genes are being identified
Secondary	
Chemotherapy and radiotherapy	-
Surgical removal of ovaries	-
Previous hysterectomy or other procedures where ovarian blood supply may be compromised	
Uterine artery embolisation	-
Severe endometriosis	-
Infections	Mumps, tuberculosis, HIV

Presentation

Spontaneous POI commonly presents with menstrual disturbances such as amenorrhoea and oligomenorrhoea together with symptoms of oestrogen deficiency, such as hot flushes and night sweats, vaginal dryness, low libido, low energy levels, sleep disturbance, lack of concentration, stiffness, skin/hair changes and mood swings. However, these symptoms may be atypical and presenting in a younger woman may not automatically be considered to be menopausal. The presence and severity of menopausal symptoms vary immensely, with 12–14% of women with POI not experiencing any symptoms. Others may have fluctuation of their symptoms due to the intermittent production of ovarian hormones. Conversely, women with iatrogenic POI often have more severe symptoms. Other more subtle presentations which may be missed include pubertal delay, oligomenorrhoea, menstrual dysfunction and infertility.

Diagnosis

A comprehensive gynaecological and obstetrics history should be taken, including a detailed menstrual history. While the type and severity of menopausal symptoms may vary, menstrual disturbances such as amenorrhea or oligomenorrhea are a consistent feature. While vigilance for a possible diagnosis is important, it is also important that POI is not overdiagnosed in those with no history of relevant menstrual disturbance.A full family history is important as between 4% and 31% of cases of spontaneous POI appear to be inherited. An autoimmune aetiology may be suspected from a family history of autoimmune diseases (Table 15.1). A detailed contraceptive history should be taken, as combined pill use, for example usually produces a regular cycle and could mask evidence of POI that may have occurred some years earlier. In young women and adolescents, consider a physical examination to confirm normal secondary sexual characteristics and breast development.

Updated international guidelines (ESHRE 2024) have agreed that the diagnosis of POI should be based on irregular menstrual cycles and elevated FSH levels (>25 IU/L), measured twice four to six weeks apart. The diagnosis of POI is frequently delayed as it often presents a fluctuating clinical picture with ovarian dysfunction preceding failure. If there is still some menstruation, FSH tests should be performed on days 2–3 of the cycle. Women should not be informed they have POI based on the results of one test due to the fluctuation in FSH levels. Taking hormone treatments with high-dose progestogens or oestradiol can lead to suppression of FSH levels. Other initial investigations should include measurement of serum oestradiol, prolactin, androgens and thyroid function tests.

Further Investigations

Once POI is suspected, further tests should be considered particularly in the younger patient. These should include karyotyping, genetic studies, autoimmune antibodies, pelvic ultrasound and a DEXA scan for bone mineral density (BMD). The extent to which POI is investigated will depend on a number of factors including the age of the patient, family history and the potential desire for future fertility.

The most clinically significant autoimmune association of POI is with adrenal insufficiency. Testing for adrenal cortex or 21-hydroxylase antibodies is the most sensitive test. Thyroid peroxidase autoantibodies and thyroid function should also be tested for due to the frequent co-existence of autoimmune thyroid disorders. Ovarian antibody testing is not recommended.

Autosomal genetic testing is not at present indicated in women with POI, unless there is evidence suggesting a specific mutation. Ideally all women with spontaneous POI where the cause is unknown should be offered referral for genetic tests; however, where resources are limited, women with early POI <30 years, those with learning difficulties and those with a family history of POI should be prioritised. Currently, the only genetic tests routinely performed in non-syndromic POI are FMR1 premutation and cytogenetics, the latter specifically for X-chromosome abnormalities.

There is no role for tests of ovarian reserve such as anti-Müllerian hormone (AMH) in primary care. These tests are expensive, unreliable and need cautious interpretation.

Measurement of BMD around the time of the initial diagnosis of POI should be considered for all women, but especially when there are additional risk factors for osteoporosis. A transvaginal ultrasound scan might be helpful if there is a suspicion of any urogenital tract anatomical abnormalities.

Consequences

POI and early menopause, whether spontaneous or induced, are associated with significant long-term health risks, mainly associated with oestrogen deficiency. Oestrogen replacement mitigates some, but not all, of these consequences. Untreated POI is associated with a 50% higher mortality than woman who undergo menopause at the average age. There are also significantly increased risks of cardiovascular disease (80%), dementia, cognitive decline and parkinsonism.

Menopausal symptoms can have a profound effect on a woman's quality of life and self-esteem at any age, but this may be particularly pronounced in the younger age group. These women may also suffer significant psychosexual dysfunction and mood disorders. Sexual dysfunction, fertility concerns and psychological problems are the issues that disturb women the most.

In some with autoimmune-associated POI, thyroid and rarely adrenal dysfunction can develop. POI is also associated with a reduction in the risk of breast cancer. Published evidence in this area is mainly derived from cohort studies of women with surgical menopause. There is much less data on the long-term outcome of spontaneous POI or the effect of hormone replacement in this group of women.

Bone

Prolonged premature oestrogen deficiency has a potentially devastating effect on bone, with a reduction in BMD starting at an early age leading to osteoporosis and an increased risk of fracture.

Individual long-term strategies for the monitoring and prevention of osteoporosis should be established with the patient.

Measurement of BMD at initial diagnosis of POI with DEXA should be considered for all women, but especially when there are additional risk factors. If the BMD is normal and adequate systemic oestrogen replacement is commenced, the value of repeated DEXA scan is low. If a diagnosis of low bone density or osteoporosis is made and oestrogen replacement or other therapy initiated, then BMD measurement should be repeated within five years. A decrease in BMD should prompt review of oestrogen replacement therapy and of other potential factors. The assessment of bone health in young women with POI can been problematic because maximal bone density is not achieved until the mid- to late 20s. Specialist input is recommended if there is any doubt. The importance of other factors such as regular weight-bearing exercise and an adequate calcium and vitamin D intake should be emphasized.

Cardiovascular Disease

Given the cardiometabolic consequences associated with POI, annual assessment of cardiovascular risk markers is recommended. This might include blood pressure, BMI, HbA1c and lipid profiles and a review of smoking status.

Fertility

For many women, the loss of fertility that comes with a diagnosis of POI can be devastating. However, unless they have had a bilateral oophorectomy, women with POI should not automatically be considered infertile. In 50% of women with spontaneous POI there is some background ovarian activity with a spontaneous pregnancy rate of 5–10%. Unfortunately it is not possible to predict the likelihood of a pregnancy in individuals; therefore if pregnancy is not desired, contraceptive use is essential. The use of the COCP as replacement treatment is potentially useful in this situation as HRT is not a contraceptive. Alternatively, the 52 mg LNG-IUD can be used alongside a separate oestrogen. Conversely, for those who do wish for a pregnancy, referral to fertility services is recommended. The use of assisted reproductive techniques does not improve the conception rate in this group of women, thus the only realistic treatment option is in vitro fertilisation with donor oocytes and her partner's sperm. There are many psychological and ethical implications involved, and appropriate counselling before embarking on such treatment is mandatory. The availability and costs of such treatment vary widely, although it is becoming more widely used in some European countries. Prior cryopreservation of oocytes is an option if a woman is about to lose her ovaries through surgery or radiotherapy and such discussions should be had proactively. For women with POI as a result of cancer treatment, pregnancy may carry increased risk of preterm deliveries, intrauterine growth retardation and miscarriages. Other options such as adoption and surrogacy should also be discussed.

Counselling/Emotional Support

POI can be a very difficult diagnosis for a woman to accept. The impact of such a diagnosis on a young woman's view of her sexuality, femininity and self-image can be devastating. The resulting infertility can be the hardest aspect to come to terms with, and this doesn't necessarily depend on whether or not she already has children.

Women with POI have an increased incidence of sexual dysfunction, depression and a sense of isolation. The younger the woman, the more likely she is to have psychosexual problems. These women need holistic care and specialised support, ideally from a multidisciplinary team, which includes counselling and support from professionals with experience in POI. They need adequate information given in a sensitive way and should be encouraged to seek additional support through national support groups such as the Daisy Network (www.daisynetwork.org.uk). Specific genetic counselling may also be needed, depending on the aetiology of the POI.

Hormone Replacement

POI is an endocrine condition of oestrogen deficiency and the appropriate treatment is replacement of the missing hormones. Thus oestrogen or HRT is recommended to treat the symptoms of POI and prevent the long-term adverse effects of oestrogen deficiency. This is the recommendation from all national and international menopause societies and the National Institute for Health and Care Excellence (NICE) guidance. HRT should be continued at least until the natural age of menopause, at around 51. Other treatments such as SSRIs have much poorer efficacy, offer no long-term protections for cardiovascular and bone health and are not recommended unless there is evidence of clinical depression. Long-term use of bisphosphonates in young women for prevention of bone loss has not been well studied, may be harmful and is not recommended. Bisphosphonates can remain incorporated in bone matrix for a long period of time. In addition, a theoretical concern exists over possible over-suppression of bone turnover with long-term bisphosphonate treatment, resulting in brittle skeleton and atypical fractures. Caution is also applicable to other bone-sparing agents in younger women such as denosumab and selective oestrogen receptor modulators. These too have a lack of data for efficacy and long-term safety in young women.

There is relatively little research done on the optimal treatment regimen for POI. Currently most clinics use oestradiol-based HRT (with a progestogen if the uterus is present) or the COCP as replacement therapy. There is emerging evidence that oestradiol-based HRT may give superior long-term benefits when compared to synthetic-oestrogen-containing COCP. HRT may be more beneficial in improving bone health and cardiovascular markers compared to the COCP. However, in this group of women, where long-term replacement is necessary, compliance is important and the COCP may be a better choice. It is very popular among younger patients as it is a medication that they and their peers are familiar with, provides contraception and does not carry the negative connotations that may be associated with HRT. If the COCP is given in a conventional 21/7 or 24/4 regimen, symptoms can recur during the hormone-free interval and valuable treatment time for primary prevention is lost. The pill-free week amounts to three months of oestrogen deficiency per year so if prescribed, it should be taken continuously. Newer COCP formulations with oestradiol maybe an alternative option. There is a large randomised trial (POISE) underway assessing the merits of different treatments.

Management of young women presenting with primary amenorrhea requires close collaboration with paediatric endocrinologists. In such cases, proper induction of puberty with optimal breast and uterine development is very important. Puberty should be induced or progressed with 17-b oestradiol, starting with a low dose at the age of 12 years with a gradual increase over 2–3 years. The oral contraceptive pill is contraindicated for puberty induction.

Specific Considerations

Women with POI who take HRT often need a higher dose of oestrogen to control their symptoms compared to women in their 50s; 100 mcg transdermal oestradiol or 3–4 mg oral oestradiol or even higher doses may be necessary. Oral oestradiol (2–4 mg day) can be safely used in non-obese women thought not to be at increased risk of thrombosis. Ethinyl oestradiol (10 mcg) is likely to offer an equivalent dose of oestrogen replacement to 1–2 mg of oestradiol. Modern COCP regimens that deliver 17b-estradiol rather than ethinylestradiol can also be used, although experience is limited.

Specialist help should be sought if symptoms prove hard to control. Although these doses may seem high, it should be remembered that with fully functioning ovaries the circulating oestradiol levels would be much higher through the cycle. Vaginal oestrogens may be needed in addition to systemic HRT to control symptoms of urogenital atrophy. Symptoms related to urogenital atrophy have been reported in 40–50% of women with POI.

Women with POI may report reduced libido or sexual function, despite apparently adequate doses of oestrogen replacement. This is more common in oophorectomised women. The use of additional testosterone should be considered in such cases.

There are very few absolute contraindications to HRT in young women with POI. For the vast majority, the benefits of oestrogen replacement will outweigh any risks. Although the data is limited, the use of HRT does not increase the risk of breast cancer when compared to normally menstruating women. The joint position statement from the British Menopause Society (BMS), the Royal College of Obstetricians and Gynaecologists (RCOG) and the Society of Endocrinology indicates: 'women with POI and early menopause (40–45 years old) should be advised that HRT is unlikely to increase risk of breast cancer in younger menopausal women under the age of 50'. Women with the BRCA gene mutations undergoing prophylactic bilateral salpingo-oophorectomy (BSO) can still be candidates for hormone replacement as this does not appear to attenuate the benefits of surgery.

Some of the negative publicity around HRT in recent years has resulted in some women being worried or anxious about taking HRT. They should be specifically reassured that any such concerns do not usually apply to women with POI and, up until the age of 51, HRT is simply replacing the hormones they would have produced if their ovaries had still been functioning.

Women with POI should be reviewed annually and advised to lead a healthy lifestyle to improve cardiovascular and bone health. These include weight-bearing exercise, limiting caffeine and alcohol intake, smoking cessation and maintaining healthy body weight. Referral to a specialist menopause service should be considered especially in younger women, those with other risk factors and those in whom there is difficulty controlling symptoms.

Conclusion

POI can be a devastating diagnosis for a young woman. It potentially has wide-ranging implications for her quality of life and long-term physical and mental health. Its treatment and management are long term. HRT or the COCP are the mainstays of treatment up until the age of natural menopause, but the risks and sequelae of POI may be life-long. Although some aspects of the care will require specialist medical, diagnostic and counselling input, the role of the GP is central to the overall management of such a long-term condition. The GP is ideally placed to provide ongoing support for the woman and her family, and monitoring for associated morbidity such as subsequent development of osteoporosis and autoimmune diseases.

References

[1] NICE Guideline NG23, 'Menopause: Diagnosis and management'. 2015. Accessed 12 Nov. 2025. [Online]. Available: www.nice.org.uk/guidance/ng23.

[2] T. Hillard, K. Abernethy, H. Hamoda et al., *Management of the Menopause*. 6th ed. British Menopause Society, 2017.

[3] N. Panay and A. J. Vincent, 'Updated premature ovarian insufficiency guideline', *Climacteric*, vol. 27, no. 6, 509, 2024, https://doi.org/10.1080/13697137.2024.2408922.

[4] N. Panay, R. A. Anderson, R. Nappi et al., 'Premature ovarian insufficiency: An International Menopause Society white paper', *Climacteric*, vol. **23**, no. 5, pp. 426–446, 2020.

[5] L. Lambrinoudaki, S. A. Paschou, M. A. Lumsden et al., 'Premature ovarian insufficiency: A toolkit for the primary care physician', *Climacteric*, vol. **24**, no. 5, pp. 425–437, 2021.

[6] R. J. Baber, N. Panay, A. Fenton et al., 'IMS recommendations on women's midlife health and menopausal hormone therapy', *Climacteric*, vol. **19**, no. 2, pp. 109–150, 2016.

[7] W. A. Rocca, M. M. Mielke, L. Gazzuola Rocca and E. A. Stewart, 'Premature or early or bilateral oophorectomy', *Climacteric*, vol. **24**, no. 5, pp. 466–473, 2021.

[8] N. Panay, 'Progress in understanding and management of premature ovarian insufficiency', *Climacteric*, vol. **24**, no. 5, pp. 423–424, 2021.

[9] H. Hamoda, N. Panay, H. Pedder, R. Arya and M. Savvas, 'The British Menopause Society and Women's Health Concern 2020 recommendations on hormone replacement therapy in menopausal women', *Post Reproductive Health*, vol. **26**, no. 4, pp. 181–209, 2020.

Chapter 16

Premenstrual Disorders (PMD)

A Practical Approach in Primary Care

Angela Wright

Key Points

- The diagnosis should be made by analysing the patient's daily recordings of the frequency and severity of symptoms over two cycles.
- A woman may be suffering from core premenstrual disorder (PMD) or one of its variants.
- All women should be advised of general lifestyle changes that could improve symptoms.
- Cognitive behavioural therapy has been shown to be effective in the treatment of PMD.
- Agnus castus is a recommended treatment. Other complementary therapies for which there is some evidence of effectiveness include magnesium, calcium and vitamin D, isoflavones, and St John's Wort.
- Evidence-based therapies focus on ovarian suppression and include combined drosperinone-containing pills, transdermal oestradiol, SSRIs and GnRH analogues.
- Progestogens and progesterone can induce symptoms in sensitive women.
- Any specific treatment may take up to three months to be effective. If a woman's symptoms are severe, the more aggressive treatment options should be started earlier rather than later.
- Hysterectomy and bilateral oophorectomy can be offered in severely resistant cases.
- The National Association for Premenstrual Syndrome provides support for sufferers, their loved ones and the health professionals who care for them. The International Association for Premenstrual Disorders (IAMPD) offers useful resources on their website, www.IAMPD.org, including webinars and other educational content for members.

It's like somebody else has taken over my body, mind and soul. There is a demon spirit inside me, telling me to do inappropriate things, prompting me to say hurtful, offensive words, urging me to be the meanest bitch that ever walked the earth.

Quote from The Twenty-Eighth Day *by Catherine Barry, an Irish poet and novelist, portraying the experience of a PMD sufferer. Published by the National Association for Premenstrual Syndrome.*

Introduction

Most women are aware of physical and/or psychological changes during their menstrual cycle. For a significant number, these symptoms are troublesome and impact their daily activities. A recent meta-analysis [1] suggested that premenstrual syndrome affects approximately half of women of reproductive age worldwide. It is estimated that 5–8% of women have severe symptoms, and that this group may fulfil the American Psychiatric Association criteria for premenstrual dysphoric disorder, as detailed in the *Diagnostic and Statistical Manual* (DSM), Version IV [2].

There have been many different definitions and terms used to describe this cyclical menstrual disorder, namely premenstrual syndrome, premenstrual tension and premenstrual dysphoric disorder. During 2008, a group of international experts (the International Society for Premenstrual Disorders or ISPMD) met in Montreal, Canada [3]. Their aim was to reach a consensus on the definition and diagnostic criteria of premenstrual disorders.

This consensus was in part responsible for premenstrual dysphoric disorder (PMDD) being added to the fifth edition of the DSM in 2013 as a mood disorder [4]. In 2019 PMDD was also included in the World Health Organization's International Classification of Diseases (11th ed.; ICD-11) [5], shown as both a genitourinary and depressive disorder. These diagnostic classifications allowed more patients to access an accurate diagnosis and treatment. They also formed the backbone for more research into the condition.

The ISPMD also developed clinical standards for managing PMDD [6], which underpin the guidelines by the Royal College of Obstetrics and Gynaecology released in 2013 [7] (Figure 16.1).

Making the Diagnosis

The key to effective management of PMDD and other premenstrual disorders is to achieve a precise diagnosis. The symptoms should be present over at least two consecutive cycles, to confirm:

- cyclicity with respect to the luteal phase
- relief of symptoms after onset or menses, with a symptom-free period
- impact on daily functioning.

Distinguishing PMDD from premenstrual exacerbation of an existing mood disorder is often challenging. Many primary mood and anxiety disorders overlap with PMDD, as can emotionally unstable personality disorder and trauma-related disorders. The late luteal phase is a vulnerable time in many mental disorders and symptoms which are manageable at other times in the month may become unstable. A symptom-free period after menstruation is the key to a diagnosis of PMS or PMDD.

All PMD diagnoses require symptoms to be severe enough to affect daily functioning or interfere with work, school performance or interpersonal relationships. A 2022 survey showed that 34% of PMDD sufferers will attempt suicide at least once [8]. This confirms the findings of a 2020 systematic review and meta-analysis [9] which suggested that PMDD is a strong risk factor for suicide attempt and ideation, increasing the likelihood by seven- and four-fold, respectively. Women with PMDD should be considered to be at high risk for suicidality. Loss of impulse control and impaired interpersonal functioning are likely to contribute to the vulnerability to suicide of women with PMDD.

Core and Variant PMD

The ISPMD classification divides premenstrual disorders into core PMD associated with ovulatory cycles and variant PMDs.

Core Premenstrual Disorder (Premenstrual Syndrome or Premenstrual Dysphoric Disorder)

Symptoms occur regularly in ovulating women during the luteal phase of the cycle, resolve by the end of menstruation and are followed by a symptom-free interval.

About 200 possible physical and psychological symptoms have been described, but the diagnostic criteria do not require specific symptoms to be present. The most frequently encountered physical symptoms are breast tenderness, bloating and headaches. Anxiety, depression and mood swings are the commonest psychological symptoms.

Variant Premenstrual Disorder

The variant PMDs do not meet the criteria for core PMDs. There are four subtypes, as follows.

Premenstrual Exacerbation of an Underlying Physiological or Medical Condition

Physical conditions, such as asthma and epilepsy, and psychological conditions, such as depression, anxiety, eating disorders or obsessive-compulsive disorder (OCD), can all worsen premenstrually.

Premenstrual Symptoms in the Absence of Menstruation

This may happen when amenorrhoea has been induced by insertion of a progestogen-releasing intrauterine device, following an endometrial ablation or hysterectomy with conservation of the ovaries.

Progestogen-Induced Premenstrual Syndrome

In susceptible women, giving cyclical progestogen in the form of sequential hormone replacement therapy (HRT) or combined hormonal contraceptives can induce symptoms.

Non-ovulatory Premenstrual Disorders

This disorder is poorly understood but it is thought that, in some women, follicular activity can precipitate symptoms even if ovulation does not occur.

Aetiology

There are four main areas of research with regard to the aetiology of the premenstrual disorders.

The influence of luteal phase hormonal fluctuations is not in doubt – these conditions do not occur before menarche, during pregnancy or after menopause. Women with PMDD cannot be distinguished from asymptomatic women in terms of peripheral ovarian hormone levels [10] so it is not hormonal fluctuations per se that are responsible

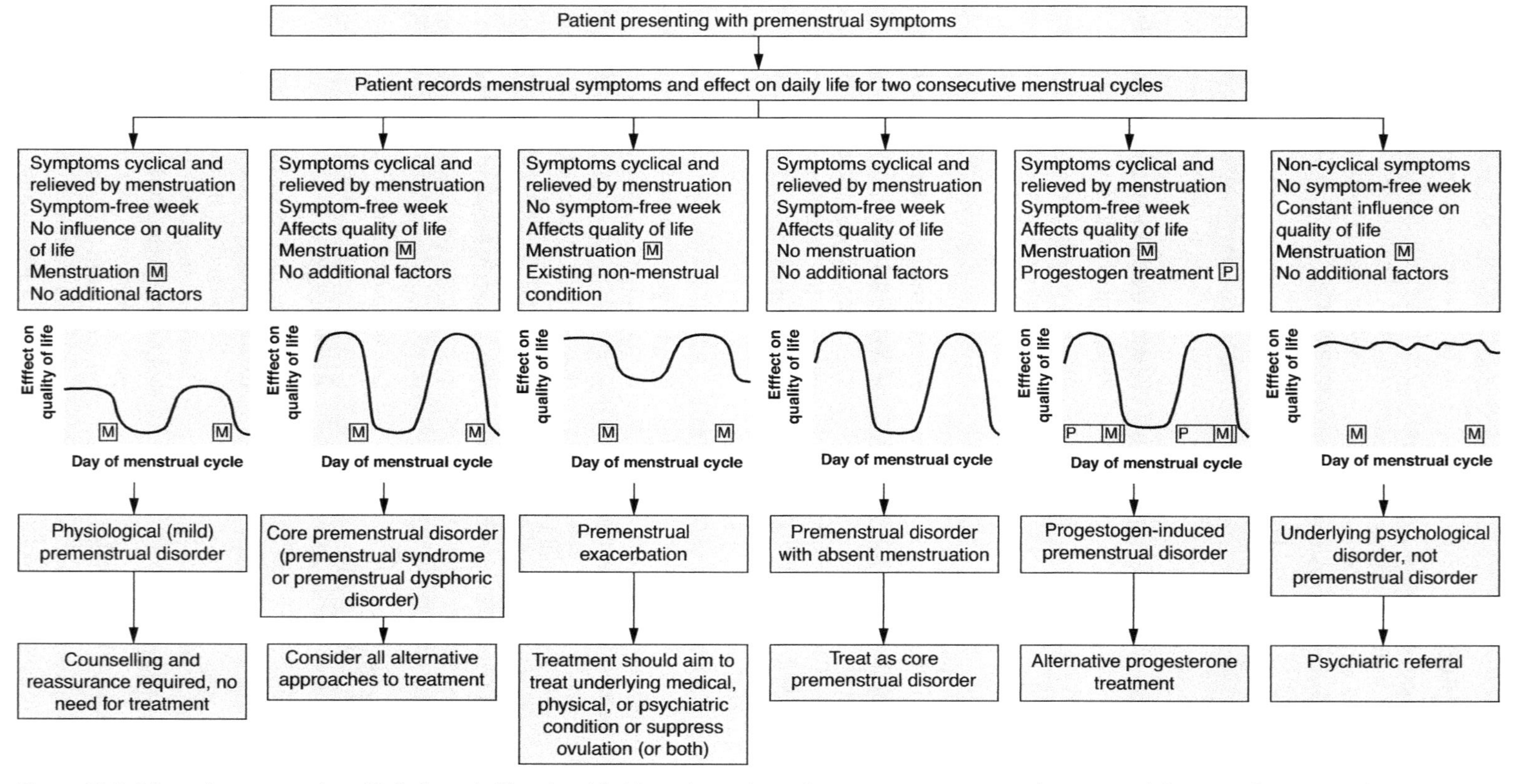

Figure 16.1 Schematic representation of Daily Record of Severity of Problems charts obtained on patients presenting with a presumed diagnosis of premenstrual disorder [7].

for PMDD symptoms but rather women's response to them.

PMDD is therefore an abnormal brain response to normal menstrual hormonal fluctuations. Overlapping genetic and environmental factors seem to feed into a state of neurobiological vulnerability. It can be very validating for women to understand the biological nature of their problem – particularly because our society still perpetuates negative tropes about women being 'hormonal'.

Genetics

PMDD appears to have heritability between 30% and 80% [4]. Research has suggested that polymorphism in the oestrogen receptor alpha (ESR1 gene) may confer different sensitivity to hormones in women with PMDD. Studies are also being carried out on serotonin gene polymorphism and serotonin transporter genotype.

Dysregulation in the Serotonergic System

A study using positron emission tomography (PET) scans found that serotonin 1 A receptor (5-HT_{1A}) availability in the brainstem is higher in the late luteal phase in controls but not individuals with PMDD [11]. This may explain why SSRIs are helpful in managing PMDD.

Allopregnanolone

There has been intense interest in recent years in the role of the main neuroactive metabolite of progestogen, allopregnanolone (ALLO), in the aetiology of PMDD. Progesterone is converted to ALLO via 3-and-5 alpha-reductase enzymes. ALLO acts as a neuromodulator at GABA-$_A$ receptors which are mainly found in the amygdala where they help regulate emotional responses. ALLO modulation of GABA-$_A$ receptors usually has an anxiolytic, mood-enhancing effect. In PMDD, ALLO appears to have a paradoxical effect on GABA-$_A$ receptors producing negative rather than positive mood symptoms at endogenous luteal phase levels. This is felt to be due to plasticity of the GABA-$_A$ receptors [12].

Stress and Inflammation

A history of stress and trauma exposure has also been implicated in the aetiology of PMDD. A study of almost 4,000 women found that trauma and PTSD were independently associated with PMDD [13]. Another study of approximately 3,000 women found a strong correlation between physical and emotional abuse and moderate to severe PMS/PMDD [13]. The mechanism linking stress and PMDD remains unclear but may involve allopregnanolone [15]. As well as stress, inflammation is thought to be another predisposing factor to PMDD. The luteal phase has been shown to be a pro-inflammatory state, and one study has shown a relative increase in inflammatory markers in women with PMDD vs controls [16].

Women who suffer with a premenstrual disorder also have a higher prevalence of postnatal depression and low mood during their menopause transition. They may also experience negative mood impact when using prescribed hormones as contraception or HRT.

Guidelines reviewing the diagnosis and management of premenstrual disorders are available from the Royal College of Obstetrics and Gynaecology (RCOG) [7]. The National Association for Premenstrual Syndrome (NAPS) guidelines are also available to download from its website [17].

Diagnosis of Premenstrual Disorders

Case History 16.1

Rachel is 34 years old. She is married to Tom and has two children: Bethany, aged six, and Charlie, aged four. She works part-time selling greetings cards. Her work involves regular visits to local retailers to present the company's products and secure business deals. Tom is a self-employed joiner.

At the start of the consultation, she bursts into tears, saying that she cannot cope. On questioning, she explains that she has had symptoms of anxiety, low mood and emotional lability and has been having difficulty concentrating. These symptoms start about a week before her period is due and she usually feels better one to two days after her bleeding starts.

During this time her symptoms are so severe that she occasionally has to cancel some of her appointments at work. She has a good relationship with her husband, but when she has symptoms, she finds fault, and arguments follow.

The Initial Consultation

I would ask Rachel about the nature and severity of her symptoms and the degree to which they impact her relationships at work and at home. I would assess her physical health, significant past medical history and current regular medication, including contraceptive use. Many women will report certain contraceptives that had a negative impact on mood. I would also ask about lifestyle factors, including diet, exercise, alcohol intake, smoking status and stress levels.

On questioning, Rachel describes moderately severe anxiety for about 10 days leading up to her period and for the first 2 or 3 days of bleeding. She has no features of an endogenous depression or suicidal intent. She eats a healthy, balanced diet, but for a few days before her period, she craves chocolate. She drinks about 20 units of alcohol a week and does find that she uses alcohol as a way of 'unwinding' after the children have gone to bed. She enjoys exercise and tries to go to the gym about three times a week, but sometimes this is not possible due to work and family commitments. Her body mass index (BMI) is 29. She has no significant past medical history, has never smoked and uses condoms for contraception.

Making the Diagnosis

It is important to try and secure the diagnosis at an early stage, before specific treatments are initiated. The best way to do this is by asking the patient to prospectively record the frequency and severity of the symptoms on a daily basis over two cycles, using either the Daily Record of Severity of Problems [18,19] or the menstrual chart, available to download on the NAPS website [20]. Retrospective recording is unreliable.

I would therefore tell Rachel that I think she has PMD, and I would suggest a prospective symptom diary over two cycles.

I would discuss the benefits of a healthy lifestyle (level 2 evidence) including good nutrition, regular exercise, avoiding sleep deprivation, moderating her alcohol intake and minimising stress where possible. With respect to diet, I would advise regular meals and snacks with a low glycaemic index to avoid the effects of low blood sugar. The diet should be low in fat and refined carbohydrates, and high in fruit and fibre.

I would direct her to the NAPS or IAMPD websites where she could find details of the various treatment options available, their guidelines and a free menstrual diary to download (Figure 16.2).

Case History 16.2

Rachel returns two months later. She has completed a menstrual chart, which shows a pattern typical of core premenstrual disorder. She has made some lifestyle modifications and has noticed a slight improvement in her symptoms but is still not coping with work and family commitments. She has read the NAPS guidelines and wants to know which complementary therapies I would recommend. She is not keen on taking anti-depressants or hormone treatment.

Treatment of Premenstrual Disorders

Cognitive Behavioural Therapy

Cognitive behavioural therapy, including relaxation, stress management and assertiveness training, has been shown in multiple studies to be effective. In one head-to-head trial, it was found to be as effective as fluoxetine [21].

The availability of psychological services varies from area to area, but women could also be directed to internet-based resources and reading material.

Complementary Therapies

It is difficult to assess the true value of the following interventions. They are freely available with little regulation. Research studies are limited, and side effects and interactions may be underestimated.

Reflexology and Acupuncture

Some studies have shown benefit from these interventions, but further research is needed [22].

Calcium and Vitamin D

Some evidence suggests that they are useful in menstrual migraine and PMDs [23].

Agnus Castus (Evidence Level 1 [24])

A systematic review has supported the use of Vitex agnus castus [24]. It comes from the fruit of the chaste tree and contains a mixture of iridoids and flavonoids. Adverse effects are uncommon, but it should not be used with SSRIs.

Magnesium

There is evidence for the use of magnesium in PMS [25].

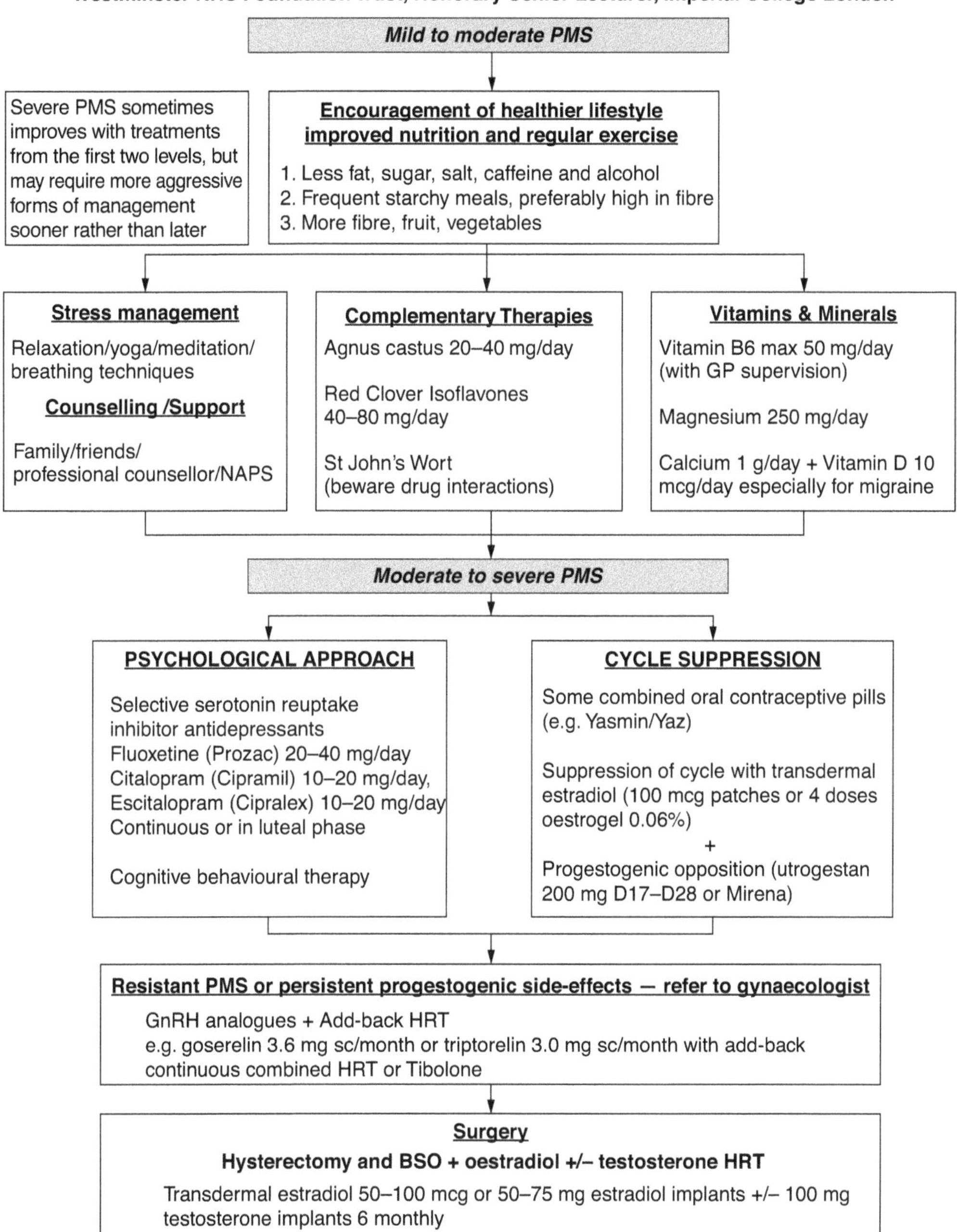

Figure 16.2 Treatment guidelines for PMS.

Isoflavones

There is some evidence for the benefits of isoflavones, but further studies are needed [26].

Vitamin B6

It is often used to treat PMD, but with little evidence for its effectiveness and mixed results from studies. There is a risk of peripheral neuropathy with higher doses [27,28].

Evening Primrose Oil

Some studies have shown that it may alleviate symptoms of breast tenderness, but that it is not helpful for other premenstrual symptoms [29].

Others

Research has also been carried out on St John's Wort [30,31] (caution is needed because of interactions with conventional medicines), but further work needs to be undertaken before recommendations can be made.

Case History 16.3

You explain to Rachel some of the options and where evidence is lacking. You also tell her that the Medicines and Healthcare Products Regulatory Agency (MHRA) has a quality mark for complementary medicine, the Traditional Herbal Registration (THR); if she is going to go down this route, she might want to look for a product with a THR mark [32,33]. Rachel decides to take agnus castus. She comes back three months later. Again, she has noticed some improvement in her symptoms and reports that she is much calmer and less confrontational with her husband. However, she is still having problems with anxiety. Having read about the different treatment options, she would like to try an SSRI. She expresses two concerns about starting an SSRI. Firstly, she is not keen to take it all the time when she is only symptomatic for part of the month. Secondly, she and her husband are considering having another baby and she asks whether taking an SSRI has been shown to be harmful in early pregnancy.

Selective Serotonin Reuptake Inhibitors

There is a good body of evidence for the use of SSRIs in the treatment of PMD; studies have also suggested some benefit with serotonin and noradrenaline reuptake inhibitors (SNRIs) [34].

SSRIs may work differently in women with PMDD than in women with depression, having a very rapid onset of action. This may be because they target 5-HT receptors and interaction with allopregnanolone levels in the brain, thus indirectly modulating the function of GABA-a receptors. Symptoms may improve within 48 hours of starting treatment. They can therefore be taken only when a woman is symptomatic; that is, during the luteal phase of the cycle. All the SSRIs appear to be equally effective, but adverse effects are relatively frequent and only 50% of patients using SSRIs for PMDD persist for over six months [35]. They may also have sexual side effects such as reduced libido and delayed or absent climax [36].

Perinatal SSRI exposure does not increase the risk of major malformations or gestational diabetes, after accounting for confounders due to the underlying maternal illness [37]. No SSRIs are safer than any others, but perinatal psychiatrists may favour sertraline because of its low secretion into the breast milk and fluoxetine because of the amount of data available about its use. Patients who wish to know more could be signposted to the Best Use of Medicines in Pregnancy (BUMPS) website [19].

Conclusion

Rachel could be advised to start the SSRI at symptom onset, or 24–48 hours before symptoms usually start, through to day 3 of her next cycle, when her symptoms would usually resolve. Gradual withdrawal is unnecessary if treatment is with low-dose luteal phase and side effects are less common.

Case History 16.4

Karen is 42 years old. She attends the surgery for advice about contraception; she is divorced, and her ex-husband had a vasectomy so she hasn't needed contraception for some years. She has just started a new relationship. On questioning, she explains that her cycle has become more irregular recently and her periods heavier. For years she has noticed that she is more emotionally labile a few days before her period, but she has never sought help for this. In recent months this has worsened, and she is having difficulty coping with daily activities in the days leading up to her period. She has also noticed occasional hot flushes and night sweats. She has no significant past medical history and has never smoked. She has a BMI of 22. Her mother went through the menopause at the age of 40, but she has no other family history of note.

The Initial Consultation and Diagnosis

It is likely that Karen is starting to go through the perimenopause, a time during which premenstrual symptoms can worsen. Even though Karen's fertility will be declining, she still requires contraception until two years after her last natural period. After a full history, it would be appropriate to counsel about dietary and lifestyle changes and discuss options for contraception and HRT, focusing on regimes that may also alleviate her premenstrual and menopausal symptoms.

Combined Hormonal Contraceptives

Early studies showed mixed results with respect to the effect of the combined pill on PMD. Combined hormonal methods do suppress ovulation, but symptoms can be induced by exogenous hormones (such as the second-generation progestogens norethisterone and levonorgestrel) and can be precipitated by fluctuations in hormone levels around the time of the hormone-free interval.

Further research has focused on some of the newer combined pills, in particular those pills containing the progestogen drospirenone, which has anti-mineralocorticoid and anti-androgenic properties [39]. Pills containing 20 and 30 mcg ethinylestradiol are available, some of which are licensed for menstrual symptoms.

There is evidence to support the use of extended regimes, reducing the pill-free interval. In one study the participants took an ethinylestradiol/drospirenone pill on a 168-day regime. There was a significant reduction in premenstrual symptoms compared with the standard 21/7 regime.

A combined pill in an extended regime would be an option for Karen, as she has no contraindications to its use. In addition, treating her with oestrogen may also help her mild menopausal symptoms.

Progestogens and Natural Progesterones

There is insufficient data to recommend the routine use of progestogens or natural progesterone in the treatment of PMD [41,42]. Indeed, in sensitive women, progestogens may precipitate and worsen symptoms [43].

However, some studies [44,45] have shown a lower prevalence of premenstrual symptoms in women using injectable progestogens.

Natural progesterone may have anxiolytic and mild diuretic effects. Cyclogest (a progesterone pessary) is the only product licensed for treatment of PMD in the UK.

Non-oral Oestradiol with Progestogenic Opposition

There is some evidence for this option [46]; the progestogen includes the LNG-IUD or a newer form of 4 mg drosperinone-only pill (Slynd). It is also possible to use micronised progesterone in a sequential or continuous regimen.

Both the LNG-IUD and Slynd also provide contraception and may provide options where the combined oral contraceptive pill (COCP) is contraindicated (e.g. with elevated BMI, in smokers and migraineurs).

There is no data on the safety of these regimes with respect to the long-term effects on breasts and endometrium. However, it is reassuring that when the cycle is adequately suppressed, oestradiol levels should be no higher overall than the expected levels during a woman's natural menstrual cycle.

- Evidence-based regimes:
  - Oestradiol patches: 75–100 mcg patch, twice weekly.
  - Progestogens and natural progesterones that provide endometrial protection and minimise side effects given for a minimum of 12 days per 28-day cycle:
    - the progestogen-releasing intrauterine device (LNG-IUD)
    - the 4 mg drosperinone pill (discarding the four sugar pills in each pack)
    - natural micronised progesterone: 200 mg a day either orally or per vagina
    - vaginal progesterone gel, crinone 8%: one applicator/alternate days for 12 days/28 day cycle; that is, six applications
    - cyclogest pessaries 400 mg a day: one/day for 12 days/28 day cycle. Usually used vaginally but use rectally if vaginal infection, postpartum or using barrier contraception.

Danazol

Studies have shown the benefit of danazol for breast tenderness [47]. However, its use is restricted because of potential irreversible virilising effects and teratogenicity. For these reasons it should only be used under the supervision of a specialist. It is not a contraceptive.

GnRH Analogues and Hysterectomy and Bilateral Oophorectomy

In the most resistant and severe cases of PMD, referral to a specialist is indicated and consideration can be given for treatment with GnRH analogues. GnRH analogues cause profound cycle suppression and elimination of premenstrual symptoms [48,49]. A lack of effectiveness when using this treatment would challenge the accuracy of the diagnosis rather than the efficacy of the medical treatment [48,49].

To reduce the loss of bone mineral density, treatment should be combined with HRT (continuous combined therapy or tibolone in preference to a cyclical progestogen therapy, to minimise progestogen intolerance). Women on long-term treatment should have bone densitometry on an annual basis.

Hysterectomy and removal of the ovaries is occasionally performed, but only after very detailed counselling [50]. It should always be preceded by a course of GnRH analogues to confirm the diagnosis. HRT, including consideration of testosterone therapy, is needed after the operation, as premenstrual symptoms are often replaced with menopausal symptoms.

Adverse effects include the risks of surgery, and the fact that this induces a hypo-oestrogenic state, which can cause hot flushes, night sweats and an increased risk of osteoporosis.

Transdermal oestradiol and an LNG-IUD would be a good treatment option for Karen.

Conclusion

The two case histories illustrate features of core premenstrual disorder. The same treatment options can be applied to any of the variant premenstrual disorders. When severe psychopathology is suspected, it is important to consider incorporating the support of local psychiatric services.

It is appropriate for most women to be managed in a primary care setting, but women at the severe end of the spectrum should be preferentially referred into specialist hospital services with a multidisciplinary team. This team should include a psychologist, dietitians and a gynaecologist with expertise in the management of this common and at times challenging medical condition.

References

[1] A. Direkvand-Moghadam, K. Sayehmiri, A. Delpisheh et al., 'Epidemiology of premenstrual syndrome (PMS): A systematic review and meta-analysis study', *J Clin Diagn Res*, vol. **8**, no. 2, pp. 106–109, 2014.

[2] American Psychiatric Association, 'Premenstrual dysphoric disorder'. In *Diagnostic and Statistical Manual of Mental Disorders*, 4th ed., American Psychiatric Press, 2000, pp. 771–774.

[3] P. M. S. O'Brien, T. Backstorm, C. Brown et al., 'Towards a consensus on diagnostic criteria, measurement and trial design of the premenstrual disorders: The ISPMD Montreal consensus', *Arch Womens Ment Health*, vol. **14**, pp. 13–21, 2011.

[4] American Psychiatric Association, *Diagnostic and Statistical Manual of Mental Disorders*, 5th ed. American Psychiatric Press, 2013.

[5] ICD-11, 'Premenstrual dysphoric disorder'. 2024. Accessed: 3 Feb. 2025. [Online]. Available: https://icd.who.int/browse/2024-01/mms/en#1526774088.

[6] E. Ismaili, S. Walsh, P. M. S. O'Brien et al. (Consensus Group of the International Society for Premenstrual Disorders), 'Fourth consensus of the International Society for Premenstrual Disorders (ISPMD): Auditable standards for diagnosis and management of premenstrual disorder', *Arch Womens Ment Health*, vol. **19**, no. 6, pp. 953–958, 2016.

[7] RCOG, 'Premenstrual syndrome, management (Green-Top Guideline No. 48)'. 2016. Accessed: 3 Feb. 2025. [Online]. Available: www.rcog.org.uk/guidance/browse-all-guidance/green-top-guidelines/premenstrual-syndrome-management-green-top-guideline-no-48.

[8] T. Eisenlohr-Moul, M. Divine, K. Schmalenberger et al., 'Prevalence of lifetime self-injurious thoughts and behaviors in a global sample of 599 patients reporting prospectively confirmed diagnosis with premenstrual dysphoric disorder', *BMC Psychiatry*, vol. **19**, no. 22(1), 199, 2022.

[9] E. Osborn, J. Brooks, P. M. S. O'Brien et al., 'Suicidality in women with premenstrual dysphoric disorder: A systematic literature review', *Arch Womens Ment Health*, vol. **24**, no. 2, pp. 173–184, 2021.

[10] T. Bäckström, D. Sanders, R. Leask et al., 'Mood, sexuality, hormones, and the menstrual cycle. II. Hormone levels and their relationship to the premenstrual syndrome', *Psychosom Med*, vol. **45**, no. 6, pp. 503–507, 1983.

[11] H. Jovanovic, A. Cerin, P. Karlsson et al., 'A PET study of 5-HT1A receptors at different phases of

the menstrual cycle in women with premenstrual dysphoria', *Psychiatry Res*, vol. **148**, nos. 2–3, pp. 185–193, 2006.

[12] L. Andréen, S. Nyberg, S. Turkmen et al., 'Sex steroid induced negative mood may be explained by the paradoxical effect mediated by GABAA modulators', *Psychoneuroendocrinology*, vol. **34**, pp. 1121–1132, 2009.

[13] C. E. Pilver, B. R. Levy, D. J. Libby et al., 'Posttraumatic stress disorder and trauma characteristics are correlates of premenstrual dysphoric disorder', *Arch Womens Ment Health*, vol. **14**, pp. 383–393, 2011.

[14] E. R. Bertone-Johnson, B. W. Whitcomb, S. A. Missmer et al., 'Early life emotional, physical, and sexual abuse and the development of premenstrual syndrome: A longitudinal study', *J Womens Health (Larchmt)*, vol. **23**, pp. 729–739, 2014.

[15] L. Hantsoo and C. Neill Epperson, 'Allopregnanolone in premenstrual dysphoric disorder (PMDD): Evidence for dysregulated sensitivity to GABA-A receptor modulating neuroactive steroids across the menstrual cycle', *Neurobiol Stress*, vol. **12**, 100213, 2020.

[16] L Hantsoo and C. Neill Epperson, 'Premenstrual dysphoric disorder: Epidemiology and treatment', *Curr Psychiatry Rep*, vol. **17**, no. 11, 87, 2015.

[17] National Association for Premenstrual Syndrome, 'Treatment guidelines for premenstrual syndrome'. Accessed: 3 Feb. 2025. [Online]. Available: www.pms.org.uk/support.

[18] IAPMD, 'Provider resources for PMDD and PME'. Accessed: 3 Feb. 2025. [Online]. Available: https://iapmd.org/provider-resources.

[19] J. Endicott, J. Nee and W. Harrison, 'Daily record of severity of problems: Reliability and validity', *Arch Womens Ment*, vol. **9**, no. 1, 43, 2006.

[20] National Association for Premenstrual Syndrome, 'Support/menstrual diary'. Accessed: 3 Feb. 2025. [Online]. Available: https://www.pms.org.uk/support/menstrual-diary/.

[21] M. Hunter, J. Ussher, M. Cariss et al., 'Medical (fluoxetine) and psychological (cognitive behavioural therapy) treatment for premenstrual dysphoric disorder: A study of treatment processes'. *J Psychosom Res*, vol. **53**, pp. 811–817, 2002.

[22] M. Armour, C. C. Ee, J. Hao et al., 'Acupuncture and acupressure for premenstrual syndrome', *Cochrane Database Syst Rev*, vol. **14**, no. 8, CD005290, 2018.

[23] A. Arab, N. Rafie, G. Askari et al., 'Beneficial role of calcium in premenstrual syndrome: A systematic review of current literature', *Int J Prev Med*, vol. **11**, 156, 2020.

[24] M. Rafieian-Kopaei and M. Movahedi, 'Systematic review of premenstrual, postmenstrual and infertility disorders of vitex agnus castus', *Electron Physician*, vol. **9**, no. 1, pp. 3685–3689, 2017.

[25] F. Parazzini, M. Di Martino and P. Pellegrino, 'Magnesium in the gynecological practice: A literature review', *Magnes Res*, vol. **30**, no. 1, pp. 1–7, 2017.

[26] I. Kang, C. H. Rim, H. S. Yang et al., 'Effect of isoflavone supplementation on menopausal symptoms: A systematic review and meta-analysis of randomized controlled trials', *Nutr Res Pract*, **16** (Suppl. 1), pp. S147–S159, 2022.

[27] K. Wyatt, P. Dimmock, P. Jones et al., 'Efficacy of vitamin B6 in the treatment of premenstrual syndrome: Systematic review', *BMJ*, vol. **318**, pp. 1375–1381, 1999.

[28] P. O. Chocano-Bedoya, J. E. Manson, S. E. Hankinson et al., 'Dietary B vitamin intake and incident premenstrual syndrome', *Am J Clin Nutr*, vol. **93**, no. 5, pp. 1080–1086, 2011.

[29] M. Mahboubi, 'Evening primrose (*Oenothera biennis*) oil in management of female ailments', *J Menopausal Med*, vol. **25**, no. 2, pp. 74–82, 2019.

[30] S. H. Jang, D. I Kim and M. S. Choi, 'Effects and treatment methods of acupuncture and herbal medicine for premenstrual syndrome/premenstrual dysphoric disorder: Systematic review', *BMC Complement Altern Med*, vol. **14**, 11, 2014.

[31] B. Peterson and H. Nguyen, 'St. John's Wort'. StatPearls Publishing, 2025.

[32] MHRA, 'The Traditional Herbal Registration (THR) Certification Mark: Guidance for business'. Accessed: 3 Feb. 2025. [Online]. Available: https://assets.publishing.service.gov.uk/media/5fef1924e90e0776aa141302/The_Traditional_Herbal_Registration__THR__Certification_Mark_Guidance_for_Business.pdf.

[33] MHRA, 'Herbal medicines granted a traditional herbal registration (THR)'. Aug. 2024. Accessed: 3 Feb. 2025. [Online]. Available: www.gov.uk/government/publications/herbal-medicines-granted-a-traditional-herbal-registration-thr.

[34] C. Jespersen, M. P. Lauritsen, V. G. Frokjaer et al., 'Selective serotonin reuptake inhibitors for premenstrual syndrome and premenstrual dysphoric', *Cochrane Database Syst Rev*, vol. **8**, no. 8, CD001396, 2024.

[35] E. Cary and P. Simpson, 'Premenstrual disorders and PMDD – A review', *Best Pract Res Clin Endocrinol Metab*, vol. **38**, no. 1, 101858, 2024.

[36] J. Rothmore, 'Antidepressant-induced sexual dysfunction', *Med J Aust*, vol. **212**, no. 7, pp. 329–334, 2020.

[37] UKTIS, 'Use of selective serotonin reuptake inhibitors in pregnancy'. June 2022. Accessed: 3 Feb. 2025. [Online]. Available: https://uktis.org/monographs/use-of-selective-serotonin-reuptake-inhibitors-in-pregnancy.

[38] BUMPS – Best Use of Medicines in Pregnancy. Accessed: 3 Feb. 2025. [Online]. Available: www.medicinesinpregnancy.org.

[39] S. Ma and S. J. Song, 'Oral contraceptives containing drospirenone for premenstrual syndrome', *Cochrane Database Syst Rev*, vol. **6**, no. 6, CD006586, 2023.

[40] A. L. Coffee, T. J. Kuehl, S. Willis et al., 'Oral contraceptives and premenstrual symptoms: Comparison of a 21/7 and extended regimen', *Am J Obstet Gynecol*, vol. **195**, no. 5, pp. 1311–1319, 2006.

[41] K. Wyatt, P. Dimmock, P. Jones et al., 'Efficacy of progesterone and progestogens in management of premenstrual syndrome: Systematic review', *BMJ*, vol. **323**, pp. 1–8, 2001.

[42] O. Ford, A. Lethaby, H. Roberts et al., 'Progesterone for premenstrual syndrome', *Cochrane Database of Systematic Reviews*, vol. 2012, no. 3, CD003415, 2012.

[43] S. Modzelewski, A. Oracz, S. Żukow et al., 'Premenstrual syndrome: New insights into etiology and review of treatment methods', *Front Psychiatry*, vol. **15**, 1363875, 2024.

[44] L. Hourani, H. Yuan and R. M. Bray, 'Psychosocial and lifestyle correlates of premenstrual symptoms among military women', *J Women's Health (Larchmt)*, vol. **13**, pp. 812–821, 2004.

[45] C. Sadler, H. Smith, J. Hammond et al. (Southampton Women's Survey Study Group), 'Lifestyle factors, hormonal contraception, and premenstrual symptoms: The United Kingdom Southampton Women's Survey', *J Womens Health (Larchmt)*, vol. **19**, no. 3, pp. 391–396, 2010.

[46] B. Naheed, J. H. Kuiper, O. A. Uthman et al., 'Non-contraceptive oestrogen-containing preparations for controlling symptoms of premenstrual syndrome', *Cochrane Database of Systematic Reviews*, vol. **2017**, no. 3, CD010503, 2017.

[47] P. M. O'Brien and I. Abukhalil, 'Randomized controlled trial of the management of premenstrual syndrome and premenstrual mastalgia using luteal-phase only danazol', *Am J Obstet Gynecol*, vol. **180**, pp. 18–23, 1999.

[48] K. Wyatt, P. Dimmock, K. Ismail et al., 'The effectiveness of GNRHa with and without "add back" therapy in treating premenstrual syndrome: A meta-analysis', *BJOG*, vol. **111**, pp. 585–593, 2004.

[49] M. Wagner-Schuman, A. Kania, J. C. Barone et al., 'What's stopping us? Using GnRH analogs with stable hormone addback in treatment-resistant premenstrual dysphoric disorder – Practical guidelines and risk-benefit analysis for long-term therapy', *J Clin Psychiatry*, vol. **84**, no. 4, 22r14614, 2023.

[50] W. Cronje, A. Vashisht and J. Studd, 'Hysterectomy and bilateral oopherectomy for severe premenstrual syndrome', *Hum Reprod*, vol. **19**, pp. 2152–2155, 2005.

Chapter 17

Non-menstrual Vaginal Bleeding Management in Primary Care

Carys Sonnenberg

Key Points

- Fluctuations in endogenous hormones can cause non-menstrual bleeding but pathology must be excluded by performing a speculum and pelvic examination.
- Consider hormonal contraceptives or hormone replacement therapy (HRT) as a cause of abnormal vaginal bleeding; this is common in the first three to six months of treatment, or after a change in regime, but should be investigated if persistent.
- Women aged under 25 with abnormal bleeding do not need a cervical smear test, but should always be examined and investigated.
- Women with postmenopausal bleeding usually need urgent referral to exclude malignancy, after an assessment and examination.
- A transvaginal pelvic ultrasound scan is advised if routinely referring a woman with intermenstrual bleeding.
- Cervical ectropion can cause abnormal bleeding; if persistent, the patient should be referred. An asymptomatic ectropion does not require referral.
- Always exclude sexually transmitted infections and pregnancy in women with postcoital bleeding.

Vaginal bleeding that is unrelated to menstruation is a common symptom in primary care. The causes vary with age, although overlap occurs between age groups. In young women (<35), malignancy is uncommon, and bleeding may be more likely related to contraceptive use, particularly progestogen-only contraception. The likelihood of gynaecological cancer increases with age, as do other diseases such as uterine fibroids and polyps. Abnormal bleeding can cause anxiety and should be approached sensitively.

Pathophysiology of Uterine Bleeding

The uterine and ovarian arteries become the arcuate arteries, which send radial branches that supply the two layers of the endometrium, the stratum functionalis and stratum basalis. Progesterone levels fall at the end of the menstrual cycle, causing enzymatic breakdown of the functionalis layer, leading to blood loss and sloughing during menstruation. Functioning platelets, thrombin and vasoconstriction of the arteries to the endometrium control blood loss. Altered uterine structure (such as fibroids, polyps, adenomyosis, malignancy or hyperplasia), derangements to clotting pathways or disruption of the hypothalamic-pituitary-ovarian axis can affect menstruation and lead to abnormal uterine bleeding [1].

The causes of non-menstrual vaginal bleeding are listed in Box 17.1.

Box 17.1 Causes of Non-menstrual Vaginal Bleeding [2]

- Physiological; spotting can occur around ovulation or during perimenopause.
- Exogenous hormones (contraception or HRT).
- Endometriosis or adenomyosis.
- Endometrium – endometritis, endometrial polyps, endometrial hyperplasia, endometrial cancer.
- Benign or malignant lesions of the vagina or vulva.
- Genitourinary syndrome of menopause (GSM).
- Trauma from piercings or female genital mutilation (FGM).
- Foreign body (e.g. retained tampon).
- Intrauterine devices – copper (Cu-IUD) and levonorgestrel (LNG-IUD).
- Bleeding disorders.
- Pregnancy.
- Sexually transmitted infection (STIs).
- Cervical causes (cervical ectropion, polyp, cervical intraepithelial neoplasia (CIN) or cancer).
- Ovarian causes (e.g. ovarian cancer).

Case Scenario 17.1

Anna is a 22-year-old student. She is worried as she has started bleeding after sex – this has happened twice and does not happen every time that she has sex. She has a new partner, stopped taking the combined pill six months ago and is currently using condoms for contraception. She is otherwise well.

History and Examination

Postcoital bleeding (PCB – non-menstrual bleeding that occurs immediately after sexual intercourse) has a prevalence of 0.7–9% of menstruating women [3]. It can be a symptom of a gynaecological malignancy (e.g. cervical cancer), but commonly is caused by cervical ectropion or cervical polyps. Other causes include cervicitis, endometrial polyps, vaginal cancer, trauma, sexual abuse or atrophic change. No cause is found in 50% of women [4]. Box 17.2 outlines the important points to consider in the history. As Anna is young, it is important to check her history of human papilloma virus (HPV) vaccination. See Box 17.3 for more information on HPV vaccination and Box 17.4 for points on the examination.

Box 17.2 Non-menstrual Vaginal Bleeding: History Points

- Menstrual history:
  - duration, frequency and severity of abnormal bleeding, to include PCB and intermenstrual bleeding (IMB)
  - last menstrual period date, regularity and heaviness of periods.
- Pregnancy risk.
- Exogenous hormone therapy (contraception or HRT and adherence to this).
- Infection risk – sexual history, past STIs or recent screening of patient and partner.
- Abnormal vaginal discharge.
- Cervical smear history, colposcopy and past treatment.
- Relevant past medical/surgical history (including diabetes and coagulation disorders).
- Past gynaecological and obstetric history including polycystic ovarian syndrome (PCOS), obesity, GSM and treatment of any premalignant or malignant lesions.
- Other symptoms including dyspareunia, pain and symptoms of the gastrointestinal or urinary tract.
- History of sexual abuse, FGM, foreign body, trauma or piercings.
- Family history including of cancers and Lynch or Cowden syndrome.
- Current and past medication history including over-the-counter medication and supplements which might interact with contraception, such as enzyme inducing medication, St John's Wort, tamoxifen or unopposed oestrogen HRT.
- Smoking history.

Box 17.3 Notes on HPV Vaccination [5,6,7]

- It has been found that 99.7% of cervical cancer is caused by HPV infection, with HPV subtypes 16 and 18 accounting for around 70% of all invasive cervical cancers.
- HPV is a double-stranded DNA virus which infects the basal cells of the squamous epithelia.
- Girls aged 12–14 have been vaccinated in the UK since 2008, with boys being added to the programme in 2019; since 2022 the Gardasil 9® vaccine has been used, giving protection against nine subtypes (6, 11, 16, 18, 31, 33, 45, 52, 58).
- From September 2023, the vaccine programme changed from two doses to one.

Investigation

Investigations during examination should include a pregnancy test in women of reproductive age and swabs for STIs.

The following pathologies are found in women with PCB – cervical polyps (5–13%), cervical ectropion (34%), cervicitis due to an STI (2%), cervical intraepithelial neoplasia (7–17%) and invasive cervical cancer (0.6–4%) [2]. Cervical, vaginal or endometrial cancer is the cause in less than 1% of women [8]. Cervical ectropion is related to the hormone oestrogen, and is therefore common in young women,. pregnant women and those using combined hormonal contraception [9].

Management

Management of postcoital bleeding depends on the cause. It is always important to rule out red flags, such as a suspicious-looking cervical, vulval or vaginal lesion which requires an urgent referral on the suspected cancer pathway.

In Anna's age group, checking for STIs and excluding pregnancy and cervical pathology are likely to be the main priorities. Local pathways and the availability of ultrasound and procedures such as polyp removal in primary care may guide referral decisions. Any infection found should be treated, and the patient must be informed to come back if the bleeding doesn't stop after treatment.

Benign Pathology

Cervical ectropion is a common cause of postcoital bleeding. The cervix has two types of cells; squamous epithelium, covering the outer part of the cervix, and dark-red vascular columnar/glandular epithelium, lining the inside of the cervix. These cells meet at the squamocolumnar junction (SCJ). At birth, the SCJ is positioned at or within the cervical opening. After puberty, increased oestrogen causes the rim of the cervix to roll outwards and more vascular red columnar cells are visible on the cervix, forming an ectropion. Cervical ectropion can also be caused by hormonal changes (including contraception) and pregnancy. It is not linked to cervical cancer or any other malignancy and it usually resolves without treatment. It can, however, cause a discharge, pain or bleeding during or after sex, or pain during a cervical smear. If the ectropion is symptomatic, symmetrical and even, a routine referral to gynaecology can be made for it to be treated with outpatient cryotherapy or electrocautery. A smear should be taken prior to referral, if due, and infection should be excluded. If there is any doubt about its benign nature, a suspected cancer referral should be made – it is not always easy to visually distinguish between ectropion and malignancy.

A cervical polyp may also cause postcoital bleeding. These may be removed in primary care and sent for histology or, more commonly, referred for removal in an outpatient setting. The vast majority of cervical polyps are benign – malignancy is rare.

Occasionally, a chronic yeast infection or eczema-like dermatosis can cause fissures and inflammation that can bleed during or after sex because of friction. Treatment with soap substitutes and anti-fungals can help with chronic yeast infections. Eczema and dermatitis are treated with emollients and topical steroids.

Anna is at risk of an STI because of a recent change in partner. STIs can cause bleeding from cervicitis and/or endometritis. Epithelial damage, usually caused by *Neisseria gonorrhoeae* and *Chlamydia trachomatis*, may allow opportunistic entry of other micro-organisms, causing pelvic inflammatory disease, the clinical features of which are listed in Box 17.5. PID is diagnosed clinically; treatment should not be deferred to

Box 17.4 Examination

- General inspection:
  - body mass index (BMI), pallor, blood pressure and pulse if concerned about haemodynamic stability
  - if relevant from the history, examine for signs of systemic disease such as diabetes, thyroid dysfunction, hyperprolactinaemia, hyperandrogenism or coagulopathy
  - abdominal palpation – iliac fossae tenderness, pelvic masses, abdominal distension.
- Pelvis:
  - inspect the vulva, looking for suspicious lesions and signs of trauma, skin changes, inflammation, scarring, ulceration or fissuring. Consider whether the woman has GSM
  - speculum examination, noting suspicious cervical lesions, ectropion or contact bleeding. Take a cervical smear test if it is due and the woman is not currently bleeding
  - assess any discharge and take appropriate swabs
  - look for blood and a site of origin.
- Bimanual examination:
  - palpate the cervix and assess uterine size and adnexal regions for tenderness or masses
  - check for cervical excitation by gently moving the cervix.

Box 17.5 Symptoms and Signs of Pelvic Inflammatory Disease (PID) [11]

- Symptoms:
  - lower abdominal pain – usually bilateral
  - abnormal vaginal bleeding – intermenstrual, postcoital or menorrhagia
  - abnormal vaginal discharge – can be purulent
  - deep dyspareunia.
- Signs:
  - fever
  - lower abdominal tenderness
  - cervix motion tenderness (cervical excitation)
  - adnexal tenderness on bimanual pelvic examination.

wait for swab results [10]. Delay in treatment can increase the risk of tubal damage and subsequent ectopic pregnancy, infertility and chronic pelvic pain. Antibiotic regimes should be according to local or national guidelines [10,11]. Partner screening is required.

Case Scenario 17.1 – Feedback

Anna's examination demonstrated a normal cervix, with a small central ectropion. Her pregnancy test and swabs were negative. While waiting for the swab results she had no further bleeding. She was reassured that there are no signs of pathology and advised to return if she has any further postcoital bleeding as this would require a referral to gynaecology clinic for colposcopy.

Case Scenario 17.2

Hana is a 44-year-old-healthcare assistant. She has noticed bleeding in between her periods for the last four months. It is light and she finds it more of a nuisance than anything else. She has two children, and her family is complete.

History

A thorough history of her bleeding problem is important – refer to Box 17.1.

As Hana is of reproductive age, it is important to ask about use of contraception, pregnancy risk and change in sexual partner, as well as assessing her risk of cervical or endometrial malignancy. Does she have red flags in her history (see Box 17.6)? Red flags should prompt consideration of malignancy – every year in the UK there are over 250 cases of vaginal cancer, 1,000 cases of vulval cancer, 3,000 cases of cervical cancer, 7,000 cases of ovarian cancer and 8,000 cases of endometrial cancer [12]. Some red flags should lead directly to a suspected cancer referral, while for others, initial investigation in primary care is appropriate.

Causes of intermenstrual bleeding include can be summarised using the abbreviation PALM-COEIN, used by the International Federation of Obstetrics and Gynaecology (FIGO) [13].

- Polyp
- Adenomyosis
- Leiomyoma
- Malignancy and hyperplasia
- Coagulopathy
- Ovulatory dysfunction
- Endometrial
- Iatrogenic
- Not otherwise classified

Box 17.6 'Red Flags' and Gynaecological Malignancy Details to Consider Alongside Clinical Judgement and Examination Findings [14]

Ovary:

- Ascites and/or a pelvic/abdominal mass which is not obviously fibroids.
- The following symptoms occurring more than 12 times/month:
  - persistent abdominal distension/bloating
  - early satiety or loss of appetite
  - pelvic or abdominal pain
  - increased urinary urgency or frequency.
- Unexplained weight loss, fatigue or changes in bowel habit.
- Serum CA125 result 35 IU/mL or higher.

Endometrium:

- Unexplained vaginal discharge in a woman aged 55 or over which is either new or is associated with thrombocytosis or haematuria.
- Visible haematuria with anaemia, thrombocytosis or raised blood sugar.
- Postmenopausal bleeding (more than 12 months after menstruation has stopped).

Cervix:

- Appearance of the cervix consistent with cancer.

Vulva:

- Unexplained vulval lump, ulceration or bleeding.

Vagina:

- Unexplained palpable mass in or at the entrance to the vagina.

Examination

Pelvic and speculum examinations are required, with screening for STIs.

The Relevance of BMI

The incidence of endometrial cancer is increasing, mainly due to increasing obesity rates and an ageing population. It is the commonest gynaecological cancer and the fourth commonest cancer in women [15]. Other risk factors include diabetes, PCOS with fewer than four periods per year and the use of tamoxifen, or unopposed oestrogen HRT.

Women with obesity have an increased risk of developing endometrial hyperplasia and malignancy because of increased exposure to oestrogen. Adipose tissue is the major site of conversion of androstenedione to oestrone, and plasma levels of sex hormone-binding globulin (SHBG), which binds oestradiol (E2), are lower in women with obesity, so higher levels of serum oestradiol and oestrone are available to target-sensitive tissues such as the endometrium.

Investigations

Given Hana's age, and the history of new bleeding, it is important to exclude malignancy. If there are any red flags then appropriate investigations should be done, or a direct referral made – depending on local pathways, it may be appropriate for the GP to arrange an ultrasound before/at the same time as the referral, or not at all if the receiving clinic has a 'one stop shop' approach which includes a scan.

Blood Tests

Bleeding disorders may be related to platelet number (e.g., idiopathic thrombocytopenic purpura) or function (e.g., Von Willebrand disease). They usually present with menorrhagia rather than intermenstrual bleeding, but if there is any suggestion of this aetiology, then a full blood count and coagulation screen are recommended, with referral to haematology if required. In the context of heavy menstrual bleeding, the National Institute for Health and Care Excellence (NICE) advise testing for coagulation disorders if a woman has had heavy bleeding since the menarche and has a personal or family history suggesting a coagulation disorder [16].

Pregnancy Test

Hana is still fertile; pregnancy-related bleeding must be excluded. Early pregnancy bleeding is very common and if the pregnancy test is positive, she needs a referral to an early pregnancy assessment unit. If she has had recent unprotected sex, a pregnancy test may be falsely negative and she should be advised to repeat it at least three weeks after the last episode of unprotected sex.

Transvaginal Ultrasound

Transvaginal ultrasound (TVUS) is the first-line imaging modality, with indications varying between guidelines. Abnormal or inconclusive physical examination is considered an indication in the NICE guidelines [16]. TVUS is reliable in identifying structural abnormalities of the uterine corpus but may be less reliable in the detection of intracavitary lesions such as polyps and sub-mucous fibroids. If intracavitary lesions are suspected, hysteroscopy is the preferred investigation. The endometrial thickness measurement which would raise concern for pathology in a pre-menopausal woman is not clear, as endometrial thickness varies throughout the cycle [17].

If the ultrasound shows benign pathology, a routine referral for hysteroscopic examination would usually be appropriate. This referral is also necessary with a normal ultrasound if she continues to experience intermenstrual bleeding, but any new red flags might prompt a suspected cancer referral. Hysteroscopy is the gold-standard investigation, allowing direct visualisation of the endometrium, including any endometrial or endocervical polyps not seen on ultrasound; suspicious-looking lesions can be biopsied. Small polyps may also be removed in the outpatient hysteroscopy clinic, with larger lesions requiring removal under general anaesthesia.

The ultrasound may indicate endometrial thickening or abnormal cystic appearances suggestive of endometrial hyperplasia. This is caused by greater than normal proliferation during the menstrual cycle. It is confirmed by an endometrial biopsy sample; histology may be benign proliferative, secretory or atrophic. There may also be hyperplasia with or without atypia, or endometrial adenocarcinoma.

Hyperplasia is classified according to the presence of atypia on histopathology. For simple hyperplasia without atypia, the risk of progression to carcinoma is 1%; these patients can be managed medically with high-dose oral or intrauterine progestogens to maintain a thin endometrium. Where there is complex hyperplasia or atypia, the risk is increased up to around 29% for complex hyperplasia with atypia – this is often managed surgically [18].

Differential Diagnoses

Bleeding on Hormonal Contraception

Hana might be using hormonal contraception, as she is of reproductive age and has completed her family. Exogenous hormones influence endometrial pathology – the mechanism is not fully understood, but there may be changes in blood vessel fragility and other factors that influence bleeding [19]. Frequent and irregular bleeding are common in the first three months after starting any hormonal method of contraception.

Irregular bleeding is more likely if pills are not taken consistently. Bleeding with the combined contraceptive pill may result because of insufficient sex steroid concentrations to maintain the endometrium – this may require dose adjustment if continuing after the initial three months. Bleeding with the progestogen-only pill or implant may result from partial suppression of ovulation. It is unpredictable and often difficult to improve.

If a woman has previously experienced a regular bleeding pattern (or amenorrhoea) while using a form of contraception and is taking it regularly, any change in bleeding pattern should be investigated.

Hormonal contraception reduces but does not abolish the risk of endometrial cancer. An endometrial biopsy should always be performed in women over the age of 45 with persistent intermenstrual bleeding using hormonal contraception and in women under the age of 45 with severe or persistent symptoms and/or risk factors for endometrial cancer. If in doubt, College of Sexual and Reproductive Healthcare (CoSRH) guidance on problematic bleeding with hormonal contraception should be followed [19].

Physiological Causes

If all investigations are normal, there may be a physiological explanation for intermenstrual bleeding. During the menstrual cycle, oestradiol levels increase in the follicular phase, resulting in endometrial proliferation. Progesterone secretion in the luteal phase is anti-oestrogenic, inhibiting endometrial growth and glandular differentiation. Withdrawal of both hormones results in menstruation. If there is an excessive fall in oestrogen after the follicular phase peak, there is premature shedding of the endometrium, causing intermenstrual bleeding. As the corpus luteum forms, oestrogen and progesterone levels rise again and so bleeding stops. This is most common in younger women. In this situation, cyclical progesterones or the combined oral contraceptive may be considered if management is required.

Case Scenario 17.2 – Feedback

Hana has a BMI of 34 kg/m^2, she is up to date with her cervical screening and infection was excluded. She has not been using any contraception as her partner had a vasectomy five years previously. There were no abnormal findings on speculum or pelvic examination, so a TVUS was organised. This reported an area of thickened endometrium at the fundus, suggestive of an endometrial polyp, and she was referred to the local gynaecology department for hysteroscopy.

Case Scenario 17.3

Mai is a 65-year-old woman who attended for her annual diabetes review appointment with the nurse and mentioned that she had experienced some vaginal bleeding. She is now very anxious as she has waited in surgery to be seen in an extra urgent appointment.

History

As previously, the history is important to determine what exactly she means by 'bleeding'. In postmenopausal women, malignancy should be at the forefront of the differential diagnosis; risk factors for gynaecological malignancy, in addition to her age, should be considered.

As of early 2026, cervical screening is performed at regular intervals (3–5 years depending on country of the UK) and stops at 65 (unless a woman has a recent abnormal result or has not been screened since the age of 50).

Risk factors for endometrial cancer include obesity, diabetes mellitus, PCOS, taking unopposed oestrogen, use of tamoxifen, previous atypical endometrial hyperplasia, Lynch syndrome and Cowden syndrome [16].

Other possible causes of postmenopausal bleeding include the use of HRT – previous and current HRT, recent dose changes or poor adherence should be explored. Bleeding irregularity can be normal following change to the dose or formulation. Additionally, the use of sequential combined HRT for more than five years is associated with a small increase in risk of endometrial cancer, whereas continuous combined HRT is associated with a neutral risk when compared to placebo [20].

Tamoxifen has anti-oestrogenic effects on breast tissue but oestrogenic effects on the endometrium, causing an increase in risk of endometrial cancer.

A postmenopausal woman is also at risk of ovarian cancer – the history must include family history of ovarian cancer, early satiety, loss of appetite, abdominal or pelvic pain, weight loss, feeling bloated, changes in bowel habit or new urinary frequency [14].

Examination

A pelvic examination is essential, where it can be tolerated – speculum and bimanual pelvic examination can help to stratify the likelihood of malignancy and the urgency of any referral. Vulval examination includes looking for ulcers and skin changes. Atrophic labia are thin and may be pale or inflamed in patches. Lichen sclerosis can cause pale white scarring and labial fusion. Vulval intraepithelial neoplasia (VIN) may result in lesions that are white, red, grey or raised.

A speculum examination should be performed if tolerated. Atrophic vaginal skin can look thin and dry, with tiny clusters of blood vessels resulting in patchy redness. Stretching of tight skin can cause fissures that can bleed during examination. Vaginal cancer is rare, but lesions are most commonly found in the posterior wall of the upper third of the vagina.

Management

The frequency of spontaneous postmenopausal bleeding is widely accepted to be around 10%, more common in the first year after menopause [21]. Postmenopausal bleeding is defined as bleeding after 12 consecutive months of amenorrhoea for which there is no other physiological or pathological cause and in the absence of intervention.

In postmenopausal women, exclusion of cancer is the primary objective, so investigations and referral must be made as per local guidelines and NICE recommendations [14]. In women presenting with postmenopausal bleeding, the most common findings in one study were endometrial polyps (38%), atrophic tissue (31%) and malignancy or atypical hyperplasia (6.8%) [22]; another meta-analysis put the risk of endometrial malignancy at 9% [23].

Atrophic endometrial changes are a common cause of postmenopausal bleeding, but cannot be confirmed as the sole cause of the bleeding until other more serious causes are excluded.

TVUS is the investigation of choice; a uniform, thin, distinct endometrial echo will accurately identify the 40% of women in whom atrophy is the cause of the bleeding. If the echo is clearly and succinctly visualised in its entirety and is 4 mm or less, no further investigations are necessary in the average-risk woman [22]. A thickened endometrium is an indication for further investigations. Endometrial cancer incidence increases with age to a peak at 75–79 years, after which the incidence declines [15].

A general rule is that the thicker the endometrium of a postmenopausal woman on ultrasound, the higher the likelihood of endometrial cancer being present. The endometrial thickness at which a biopsy is done varies, dependent on local criteria in the UK, ranging from 3 to 5 mm; a thickness of 4 mm or less has a negative predictive value for endometrial cancer of greater than 99% [24].

The pelvic ultrasound scan will also examine the ovaries. Ovarian volume is reduced in the menopause. If there are any concerns about the ovarian appearance on ultrasound, such as the appearance of a cyst, or if there are symptoms and signs suggestive of ovarian cancer, then CA125 should be requested [14,25]. Ovarian malignancies that secrete oestrogen, such as granulosa cell tumours, can result in vaginal bleeding.

If examination raises suspicion of another gynaecological cancer, such as of the vagina or vulva, the woman should be referred on the local suspected cancer pathway [14].

GSM is due to lack of oestrogen post-menopause and can be managed in primary care. It can also be iatrogenic, for example due to the injectable progestogen-only contraceptive, GnRH analogues or post-oophorectomy. A lack of oestrogen causes thinning of the vaginal epithelium and can lead to an overgrowth of Gram-negative bacteria, such as *Escherichia coli*, which can cause urinary tract infections. Atrophic vaginitis can be treated with topical oestrogens (pessaries, rings or cream) or with systemic HRT, or a combination of both if required. Long-term data shows that there are no adverse effects on the endometrium from topical oestrogens [20] as systemic absorption is very low. Plasma oestrogen levels rise initially, before settling – they never exceed normal postmenopausal levels, so no endometrial protection is required, even with long-term use. In women who have had oestrogen-dependent malignancies and other contraindications to oestrogen therapy, refer to the British Gynaecological Cancer Society and British Menopause Society guidelines 'Management of menopausal symptoms following treatment of gynaecological cancer' and the British Society of Sexual Medicine 'Position Statement for Management of Genitourinary Syndrome of the Menopause (GSM)' [26,27]. Non-hormonal vaginal moisturisers and lubricants can also be used, either with or instead of hormonal treatment.

Case Scenario 17.3 – Feedback

Mai presented with a history of vaginal bleeding which had lasted for three days and required her to use a sanitary towel. She had also noticed a similar episode two weeks previously, but this settled after 24 hours so she had not thought it important.

Examination revealed a dry atrophic vagina with a normal postmenopausal cervix. Bimanual examination was normal. Mai was referred to the gynaecology department using the fast-track form. She was seen in the one-stop hysteroscopy service within 10 days and had a reassuringly normal TVUS, with a thin endometrium of 3 mm. She was reassured and returned to the clinic a few days later, where she was prescribed a course of topical oestrogen to use long term.

Conclusion

Non-menstrual bleeding is a common presentation in primary care. A logical and individualised approach to history-taking, examination, investigations and management should be taken.

References

[1] E. Davis and P. B. Sparzak, 'Abnormal uterine bleeding'. StatPearls Publishing, 2023. Accessed 13 Nov. 2025. [Online]. Available: www.ncbi.nlm.nih.gov/books/NBK532913.

[2] A. M. Lumsden, A. Gebbie and C. Holland, 'Managing unscheduled bleeding in non-pregnant premenopausal women', *BMJ*, vol. **346**, f3251, 2013.

[3] C. M. Tarney and J. Han, 'Postcoital bleeding: A review on etiology, diagnosis, and management', *Obstet Gynecol Int*, vol. **2014**, 192087, 2014.

[4] B. Sahu, R. Latheef and S. Aboel Magd, 'Prevalence of pathology in women attending colposcopy for postcoital bleeding with negative cytology', *Arch Gynecol Obstet*, vol. **276**, no. 5, pp. 471–473, 2007.

[5] UK Health Security Agency, 'HPV vaccination guidance for healthcare practitioners'. Jun. 2023. Accessed 24 Jan. 2024. [Online]. Available: www.gov.uk/government/publications/hpv-universal-vaccination-guidance-for-health-professionals/hpv-vaccination-guidance-for-healthcare-practitioners.

[6] K. S. Okunade, 'Human papillomavirus and cervical cancer', *J Obstet Gynaecol*, vol. **40**, no. 5, pp. 602–608, 2020.

[7] C. K. Chan, G. Aimagambetova, T. Ukybassova et al., 'Human papillomavirus infection and cervical cancer: Epidemiology, screening, and vaccination – Review of current perspectives', *J Oncol*, vol. **2019**, 3257939, 2019.

[8] P. M. Casey, M. E. Long and M. L. Marnach, 'Abnormal cervical appearance: What to do, when to worry?', *Mayo Clin Proc*, vol. **86**, no. 2, pp. 147–150, 2011.

[9] P. Aggarwal and A. Ben Amor, 'Cervical ectropion'. StatPearls Publishing, 2024.

[10] NICE CKS, 'Pelvic inflammatory disease'. Oct. 2023. Accessed 24 Jan. 2024. [Online]. Available: https://cks.nice.org.uk/topics/pelvic-inflammatory-disease.

[11] BASHH, 'United Kingdom national guideline for the management of pelvic inflammatory disease'. 2019. Accessed 24 Jan. 2024. [Online]. Available: https://www.bashh.org/resources/6/pid_2019/.

[12] NICE CKS, 'Gynaecological cancers – recognition and referral'. Accessed 24 Jan. 2024. [Online]. Available: https://cks.nice.org.uk/topics/gynaecological-cancers-recognition-referral.

[13] M. G. Munro, H. O. Critchley, M. S. Broder et al. (FIGO Working Group on Menstrual Disorders), 'FIGO classification system (PALM-COEIN) for causes of abnormal uterine bleeding in nongravid women of reproductive age', *Int J Gynaecol Obstet*, vol. **113**, no. 1, pp. 3–13, 2011.

[14] NICE NG12, 'Suspected cancer: Recognition and referral'. Oct. 2023. Accessed 24 Jan. 2024. [Online]. Available: www.nice.org.uk/guidance/ng12.

[15] Cancer Research UK, 'Uterine cancer statistics'. Accessed 24 Jan. 2024. [Online]. Available: www.cancerresearchuk.org/health-professional/cancer-statistics/statistics-by-cancer-type/uterine-cancer.

[16] NICE, 'NG88: Heavy menstrual bleeding: Assessment and management'. Accessed 24 Jan. 2024. [Online]. Available: www.nice.org.uk/guidance/ng88.

[17] C. Saccardi, G. Spagnol, G. Bonaldo et al., 'New light on endometrial thickness as a risk factor of

cancer: What do clinicians need to know?', *Cancer Manag Res*, vol. **14**, pp. 1331–1340, 2022.

[18] G. Singh and Y. Puckett, 'Endometrial hyperplasia'. StatPearls Publishing, 2024.

[19] CoSRH, 'Clinical guideline: Problematic bleeding with hormonal contraception'. 2015. Accessed 24 Jan. 2024. [Online]. Available: https://www.cosrh.org/Public/Public/Standards-and-Guidance/Problematic-Bleeding.aspx.

[20] British Menopause Society, 'BMS & WHC's 2020 recommendations on hormone replacement therapy in menopausal women'. 2021. Accessed 24 Jan. 2024. [Online]. Available: https://thebms.org.uk/wp-content/uploads/2025/09/02-BMS-ConsensusStatement-BMS-WHC-2020-Recommendations-on-HRT-in-menopausal-women-SEPT2025-A.pdf.

[21] S. Sung, K. Carlson and A. Abramovitz, 'Postmenopausal bleeding'. StatPearls Publishing, 2024.

[22] D. Black, 'Diagnosis and medical management of abnormal premenopausal and postmenopausal bleeding', *Climacteric*, vol. **26**, no. 3, 22, 2023.

[23] M. A. Clarke, B. J. Long, A. Del Mar Morillo et al., 'Association of endometrial cancer risk with postmenopausal bleeding in women: A systematic review and meta-analysis', *JAMA Intern Med*, vol. **178**, no. 9, pp. 1210–1222, 2018.

[24] E. Dreisler, 'Postmenopausal bleeding: Which endometrial thickness is safe in menopausal hormone therapy users?' *Case Rep Womens Health*, vol. **35**, e00431, 2022.

[25] RCOG, 'Ovarian cysts in postmenopausal women' (Green-Top Guideline No. 34). 2016. Accessed 2 Jan. 2024. [Online]. Available: www.rcog.org.uk/guidance/browse-all-guidance/green-top-guidelines/ovarian-cysts-in-postmenopausal-women-green-top-guideline-no-34.

[26] https://thebms.org.uk/publications/bms-guidelines/management-of-menopausal-symptoms-following-treatment-of-gynaecological-cancer/.

[27] https://bssm.org.uk/wp-content/uploads/2024/03/BSSM-Position-statement-for-management-of-genitourinary-syndrome-of-the-menopause-GSM.pdf.

Chapter 18

Management of the Patient with Suspected Endometriosis in Primary Care

Keith A. Louden and Alice E. J. Stickland

Key Points

- Endometriosis is a benign condition affecting women in their reproductive years and is defined by the presence of endometrial glands and stroma outside the uterus.
- Endometriosis is common, and may have a major impact on a woman's quality of life.
- Endometriosis is often diagnosed late, sometimes more than a decade after the onset of symptoms, by which time significant pelvic organ damage may have occurred.
- Chronic inflammatory changes in the pelvis lead to severe pain and infertility.
- An awareness of the symptoms and signs of endometriosis will help timely referral and improved outcomes.

Case Scenario 18.1

Mia is 31 years old and presents to her GP with a longstanding history of heavy and painful periods. She is in a relationship and wants to have children. She takes paracetamol and ibuprofen but often needs to take time off work due to the pain. She finds intercourse very painful and reports her symptoms are having a negative impact on her quality of life.

Introduction

Endometriosis is a common benign condition affecting women in their reproductive years, and is defined by the presence of endometrial glands and stroma outside the uterus.

It affects 10–15% of women of reproductive age and 35–50% of women with chronic pain and infertility, peaking between 25 and 35 years of age [1,2].

Endometriosis is more commonly seen in patients with a positive family history involving a first-degree relative, as well as in those with early menarche, late menopause, delayed first pregnancy and rarely congenital abnormalities which prevent menstrual outflow. Half of the variation in endometriosis risk is inherited [3].

Symptoms include dysmenorrhoea, dyspareunia, dyschezia (rectal pain) and infertility, leading to adverse effects on personal relationships, quality of life and work productivity [4].

There are three recognised morphological lesions: superficial peritoneal implants, ovarian endometriomas ('chocolate cysts') and deep infiltrating lesions (DIE) affecting the rectum, bladder and uterosacral ligaments. Pathogenesis remains unclear, with competing theories including retrograde menstruation, impairment of the immune system, enhanced angiogenesis and metaplasia of normal tissues.

The major challenge in general practice is the timing of the referral decision. There is international evidence of unacceptable diagnostic delay of 8–12 years (especially in teenagers) from the onset of symptoms to the diagnosis of endometriosis. However, the prevalence of simple dysmenorrhoea amongst healthy young women is high, and there is considerable symptomatic overlap between endometriosis and other causes of pelvic pain, such as irritable bowel syndrome (IBS) [5]. A UK study of primary care found that women with endometriosis were 3.5 times more likely to have had an initial diagnosis of IBS and 6.4 times more likely to have had a diagnosis of pelvic inflammatory disease compared with controls [6]. One-third of patients consulted their GP six times or more before referral to secondary care. Earlier diagnosis and treatment are likely to be the best way to prevent severe and debilitating disease and to protect fertility. To avoid this diagnostic delay, consideration should be given to referral criteria for suspected endometriosis that encompasses symptoms, physical signs and imaging findings.

Case Scenario 18.2

Mia's history reveals a pattern of painful periods dating back to menarche with maximal pain mid-cycle. She has tried taking the combined oral contraceptive pill (COCP) with a monthly withdrawal bleed but this did not improve her symptoms. She takes paracetamol, ibuprofen and codeine for the pain.

History

Pain is the most likely presenting symptom of endometriosis, and a detailed pain history is particularly important. The index of suspicion of underlying endometriosis is raised when simple treatment strategies such as using the COCP and non-steroidal anti-inflammatory drugs (NSAIDs) such as mefenamic acid have been unsuccessful. There is little advantage to be gained by swapping one COCP or NSAID for another unless there is a problem with tolerability. These treatment strategies would be expected to be effective in the majority of women with dysmenorrhoea, so a failure of conservative treatment should lead to active consideration of endometriosis as the underlying diagnosis.

The patient's description of pain, as well as timing, may also offer important clues. While patients with simple dysmenorrhoea describe pain with the onset of menstrual flow, patients with endometriosis often describe premenstrual pain for days or even a week or more before menstruation. Mid-cycle pain is also common with endometriosis. The timing of the pain may reflect the underlying anatomical pathology. For example, if an ovary is adherent to the lateral pelvic sidewall (secondary to the inflammatory nature of endometriosis, with its propensity for scarring and adhesions), then the description of mid-cycle pain around the time of ovulation can be understood. Peritoneal lesions in the pouch of Douglas become more florid during the luteal phase, as both the normal endometrium and the endometriotic deposits undergo cyclical proliferation, and this is consistent with the description of premenstrual pain symptoms. Over years, symptoms may change from cyclical to a more chronic or indeed acyclical pattern. This may reflect the chronic inflammatory changes in the pelvis, with the development of adhesions, scarring and deep nodular disease, which can ultimately result in a 'frozen pelvis'. In a situation with a fixed retroverted uterus, bilateral endometriotic cysts kissing in the midline and obliteration of the pouch of Douglas, pain will likely be constant.

Endometriosis may be found in the rectovaginal septum, infiltrating the wall of the rectum or sigmoid colon, or invading the bladder. These more severe forms of endometriosis may present with specific and anatomically understandable symptoms. The most important of these is cyclical dyschezia: the description of rectal pain during defecation at the time of menstruation. This pain is often described as knife-like, and can be very severe. It may, however, be a symptom which the patient does not disclose unless directly questioned. A rectal nodule which extends through into the mucosa of the bowel has the potential for cyclical rectal bleeding, but this bleeding pattern is more commonly observed with simple internal haemorrhoids. Similarly, endometriotic lesions within the bladder wall may cause cyclical dysuria, and sometimes cyclical haematuria if the nodule is full thickness and reaches the bladder mucosa.

Patients with rarer extra-pelvic endometriosis may present with cyclical pain in the region of hernial orifices or the tip of the shoulder, reflecting endometriosis within a small hernial sac, or on the peritoneum overlying the diaphragm, respectively. A painful, cyclical blue-black swelling or bleeding from the umbilicus, pfannenstiel or episiotomy scar may be caused by endometriosis. Even recurrent respiratory symptoms, such as pneumothorax or haemoptysis may be attributed to endometriosis; the crucial aspect of diagnosis is the recognition that the symptoms are cyclical.

Endometriotic lesions are most commonly found in the pouch of Douglas, affecting the peritoneal surfaces, the uterosacral ligaments and the ovaries. As a result, deep dyspareunia may occur because of the intimate anatomical relationship between the posterior fornix of the vagina and the peritoneum of the pouch of Douglas. This also explains why some women will describe deep dyspareunia, which may be relieved by changing position.

If the patient presents with heavy and painful periods, and the uterus is enlarged and tender on examination, then there may be underlying adenomyosis, with presence of endometrial glands and stroma within the myometrium. This condition is often difficult to diagnose as ultrasound findings may be subtle: there may be evidence of small myometrial areas of cystic change, and the myometrium may be described as inhomogenous.

Box 18.1 Symptoms Associated with Endometriosis

- Dysmenorrhoea.
- Deep dyspareunia.
- Cyclical/mid-cycle/premenstrual pain.
- Cyclical bowel and bladder symptoms of pain or bleeding.
- Infertility.

MRI is now being increasingly used for diagnosis of adenomyosis. The condition, which may occur alongside endometriosis, has been shown to be effectively managed with the levonorgestrel-releasing intrauterine device (IUD) (Box 18.1).

Case Scenario 18.3

The notes show that Mia has never had a vaginal examination. She is very reluctant to be examined and explains that she finds intercourse very painful. She has stopped taking the COCP because she wants to start a family, but she is distressed that she is unable to tolerate intercourse. There are no other psychological or relationship concerns.

Classification

Perhaps surprisingly, there is not always a correlation between the severity of pain symptoms and the reported stage of endometriosis. Several different classification systems have been developed to describe disease severity. These include the Revised American Society of Reproductive Medicine (rASRM) which grades endometriosis as severity I–IV and is straightforward to use [7]. However, its predictive value regarding fertility outcome and clinical presentation is limited, and it does not take into account deep infiltrating endometriosis involving retroperitoneal structures. The Endometriosis Fertility Index (EFI) was developed to better evaluate fertility. This combines the rASRM score with fertility history and macroscopic assessment of fallopian tubes and ovaries in terms of function.

The #Enzian classification, created through a consensus process in 2021, is a comprehensive system for complete mapping of endometriosis, including anatomical location, size of the lesions, adhesions and degree of involvement of the adjacent organs, and can be used with both diagnostic and surgical methods [8].

Endometriosis and associated chronic pain can adversely affect quality of life. The impact of endometriosis may be reflected by time off school or work, with reduced exercise and social activity. The condition may be challenging both to work performance and personal relationships. These factors are of major importance to patients, often over and above specific pain and fertility issues, and are not necessarily reflected in the classification of disease.

Examination

The limitations of pelvic examination in terms of diagnosis for ovarian cysts, for example are well known. However, in the context of a patient in whom endometriosis is suspected, important diagnostic information may be revealed. Pelvic tenderness is most likely demonstrated, but the location of endometriotic deposits and the consequent chronic inflammatory changes with scarring and nodule formation may be detected on bimanual examination. The uterus may be in a fixed, retroverted position, with reduced mobility, secondary to scarring. There may be palpable tender nodularity of the uterosacral ligaments. Occasionally, a deep deposit of rectovaginal endometriosis may be palpable in the posterior fornix of the vagina, and may even be visible on speculum as a blue-black lesion penetrating the vaginal mucosa. An adnexal mass may be palpated if there is an endometrioma present. Abnormal pelvic examination findings should lead to further investigation with transvaginal ultrasound, and prompt referral to secondary care.

Case Scenario 18.4

An attempt at pelvic examination fails because of pain and apparent vaginismus. A scan is requested. This has to be transabdominal as Mia is unable to consent to the preferred transvaginal route. The result is normal, with no abnormality demonstrated.

Adolescent Presentations

Adolescents presenting with possible endometriosis can be challenging. There is often a reluctance to refer teenagers when endometriosis is suspected because the incidence of primary dysmenorrhoea is so high, and it might seem inappropriate to consider early laparoscopy. It should be remembered that endometriosis does affect teenagers; the long diagnostic delays which patients experience often extend back to their teenage years. Failure of conservative management, even in this younger patient population, should prompt referral. Medical therapy may be preferable in this population; however, surgery may be considered in certain cases. Earlier diagnosis and appropriate medical treatment may reduce the need for extensive surgery in later life [9].

Investigations

Transvaginal ultrasound is the imaging modality of choice for suspected endometriosis, as ovarian endometriomas have a characteristic ground glass appearance. It may be difficult to make the diagnosis between a small corpus luteum, haemorrhagic cyst and a small endometrioma, but a rescan three months later allows time for a corpus luteum cyst to resolve, while an endometrioma will remain. Aside from the finding of an endometrioma, a normal transvaginal ultrasound does not exclude the diagnosis of endometriosis, as peritoneal and uterosacral disease may escape detection. In specialist centres, there is some evidence that transvaginal ultrasound may be able to predict severe disease with rectal involvement [10]. Further imaging with MRI may be undertaken in secondary care to better map the disease before surgery.

Serum CA125 has been shown to be elevated with endometriosis, particularly with endometrioma formation, but as a potential screening tool it has been found to be of no clinical value.

In general practice, a definitive diagnosis will not always have been confirmed in the absence of positive findings on imaging or at laparoscopy. Hence, treatment efforts focus on the practical management of a patient with a set of symptoms which may reflect underlying endometriosis, but might also reflect IBS, pelvic inflammatory disease, primary dysmenorrhoea, interstitial cystitis or chronic pelvic pain.

Case Scenario 18.5

There are no symptoms suggestive of IBS, and Mia describes normal bowel and bladder function. Her pain symptoms are severe and significantly impacting her quality of life. She is referred by her GP to secondary care, for review in the pelvic pain clinic.

Medical Treatment

If symptoms are mild to moderate, and there are no signs of endometriosis to suggest nodular DIE or an endometrioma, then a three-month trial of medical treatment may be indicated when endometriosis is suspected [11]. However, some patients may wish to have a definitive diagnosis, particularly if there is associated infertility.

Choice of analgesia usually rests with paracetamol and NSAIDs. Opiates may be required, but with symptoms of this severity, referral should be considered.

Beyond analgesia, medical strategies involve hormonal suppression of ovarian activity, preventing the cyclical proliferative changes in the endometriotic implants, hence relieving symptoms. The COCP and progestogens are most commonly prescribed, with no clear superiority of one treatment over the other. A principle of treatment is that cycle suppression should aim for amenorrhoea, so the COCP should be used continuously, as long as breakthrough bleeding allows. However, this strategy may be limited by side effects including weight gain, bloating, low libido and breast tenderness, seen in 14% of women [12].

The IUD has been found to be effective in the treatment of endometriosis. It is a good choice in those presenting with dysmenorrhoea and menorrhagia, as long as contraception is acceptable for the woman. The IUD may also offer benefit in those women with underlying adenomyosis. Furthermore, the IUD will commonly be offered to patients as an adjunct to surgical treatment.

The progesterone-only pill or the subcutaneous progestogen-releasing implant may be used, although there are limited studies demonstrating effectiveness in endometriosis patients. Similarly, depo provera and oral progestogens such as medroxyprogesterone acetate have been employed. However, 100 mg of medroxyprogesterone acetate daily may be associated with side effects including acne and fluid retention.

The use of gonadotrophin-releasing hormone analogues, which are effective at suppressing ovarian activity, is limited by the side effects of vasomotor symptoms and bone demineralisation with prolonged use. The use of add-back hormone replacement therapy greatly increases tolerability and reduces the risk of bone demineralisation, but long-term studies are lacking.

Box 18.2 Indications for Referral

- Failure of conservative treatment.
- Pelvic mass.
- Endometrioma on transvaginal ultrasound.
- Physical signs of endometriosis, such as palpable nodularity in the pouch of Douglas.
- Severity of pain symptoms.

The limitations of medical therapy include the side-effect profile, the associated contraception and the duration of treatment. While medical treatment can suppress the cyclical activity of individual lesions, it is unable to resolve issues of the formation of chronic inflammatory nodules, with the associated scarring and adhesions. The practicality of maintaining cycle suppression and amenorrhoea in the long term is considerable. When hormonal therapy is discontinued, the endometrial deposits become active again, and symptoms may recur.

If symptoms are severe or medical treatment is unsuccessful or not accepted by the patient, referral to secondary care is indicated. Similarly, patients with endometriosis symptoms and fertility concerns require referral. Ideally, such a referral should be made to a local specialist endometriosis centre (Box 18.2).

Surgical Management

In secondary care, patients may be offered laparoscopy to confirm the diagnosis, assess the stage and perform excision of disease. This procedure should be undertaken by a surgical team who are able to offer a 'see and treat' approach for mild to moderate disease, following appropriate preoperative counselling. In a minority of patients there may be unexpectedly severe disease, such as a deep rectal nodule, diagnosed at initial laparoscopy, that may require repeat surgery after further counselling, multi-disciplinary team (MDT) involvement and bowel prep. The concept of the 'diagnostic laparoscopy' without the facility for treatment is no longer acceptable [13].

The British Society for Gynaecological Endoscopy (BSGE) has established a network of endometriosis centres of excellence for the surgical treatment of DIE. This ensures appropriate caseload, audit and MDTs operating for complex cases often involving the bowel and the bladder. In 2018 a landmark paper was published in *BMJ Open*. This large, multicentre prospective cohort study concluded that women who underwent laparoscopic excision of deep rectovaginal endometriosis in a BSGE Endocentre saw a significant improvement in their symptoms and quality of life, and these improvements were sustained at two years [14]. All women with rectovaginal endometriosis who are managed in BSGE Endocentres are asked to complete standardised symptom questionnaires regarding chronic pelvic pain, bladder and bowel symptoms, analgesia use and quality of life (EuroQol). These are completed prior to surgery and at 6, 12 and 24 months postoperatively. The results are entered onto the national BSGE database.

The surgical principle for the management of endometriosis-related pain is the surgical excision of all disease, almost invariably through a minimal access approach, either laparoscopically or robotically. Peritoneal and uterosacral disease is excised. Endometriomas are separated from their attachments to the lateral pelvic sidewall, opened, drained and the cyst lining carefully stripped, ablated or coagulated. Simple fenestration is insufficient because of high recurrence rates. Great care must be taken to minimise ovarian injury to preserve function; meticulous surgical technique and the avoidance of excessive diathermy are important. DIE is a common finding in association with an endometrioma, hence these patients are best managed in a specialist centre.

The most severe cases may involve surgical 'shaving' of a deep nodule off the anterior surface of the rectum, and the excision of full thickness lesions from the posterior fornix of the vagina or bladder. Disc resection of the rectum or even segmental bowel resection may be needed. Ureteric lesions may require excision and reanastamosis. Hence, there is a requirement for multidisciplinary teamworking in the BSGE centres.

Fertility and Endometriosis

Recent evidence suggests that viable intrauterine pregnancy rates were significantly increased after laparoscopic surgery for endometriosis. This was based mainly on peritoneal endometriosis. Therefore, operative laparoscopy may be offered as a treatment option for endometriosis-associated infertility. Surgical treatment of an endometrioma may also successfully treat pain symptoms as well as increasing natural pregnancy chances. There is a lack of data to conclude if surgical treatment of severe deep endometriosis improves fertility [15].

For women with subfertility, the probability of pregnancy three years following surgery for endometriosis has been shown to be 47% [16]. Specialist fertility advice and referral should be offered to patients and a multidisciplinary approach taken with regard to their care.

A difficulty may arise when a patient has a laparoscopy for suspected endometriosis and only minor disease is found. It is known that there is a poor correlation between the stage of endometriosis and the severity of pain symptoms. The excision of peritoneal disease may be very minimal, but the patient may interpret this operative finding as a revelation in a long search for an explanation for her symptoms. There may be brief symptomatic improvement as a consequence, with a placebo-type effect, followed by return of symptoms which the patient may interpret as recurrent endometriosis. It is important, therefore, to be cautious in the postoperative explanation of the surgical treatment of mild endometriosis, as sequential laparoscopic treatments for minor disease carry risks and may not improve the pain long term.

Case Scenario 18.6

In secondary care, Mia is seen in a specialist endometriosis clinic. She is counselled about treatment options including laparoscopic surgery and excision of endometriosis if found. She decides to proceed with surgery.

Awareness of Endometriosis

There has been a huge increase in the number of women and those assigned female at birth with endometriosis: it is estimated to affect 1.5 million in the UK. However, despite this, it is not well reported and research funding globally is lacking [17].

Recently, awareness of the disease has been raised through social media as well as groups including Endometriosis UK (www.endometriosis-uk.org), the Royal College of Obstetricians and Gynaecologists (www.rcog.org.uk/globalassets/documents/patients/endometriosis.pdf) and NHS Direct (www.nhs.uk/conditions/endometriosis/Pages/Introduction.aspx). In September 2020, menstrual wellbeing became part of primary and secondary school education in England. This aims to teach young people more about menstrual cycles, and how and when to seek help.

The BSGE project to create specialist centres for the surgical treatment of DIE and the publication of the *BMJ Open* paper has been an important step forward [14]. The key to improving outcomes for endometriosis patients is through earlier suspicion of the diagnosis and referral to secondary care, ideally to a BSGE endometriosis centre, where multidisciplinary discussion and operating are available.

Case Scenario 18.7

At laparoscopy, Mia has extensive endometriosis involving both uterosacral ligaments, and both ovaries are adherent to the lateral pelvic sidewalls. There is a full thickness vaginal nodule penetrating into the pouch of Douglas, and the rectum has been pulled up onto the back of the cervix. The endometriotic tissue is excised, the ovaries released and the vaginal defect sutured, leaving no visible or palpable disease. Mia describes an 80% improvement in her pain and her quality of life. In terms of fertility, she goes on to conceive two children.

References

[1] B. Smolarz, K. Szyłło and H. Romanowicz, 'Endometriosis: Epidemiology, classification, pathogenesis, treatment and genetics (review of literature)', *Int J Mol Sci*, vol. **22**, no. 19, 10554, 2021. http://doi.org/10.3390/ijms221910554. PMID: 34638893; PMCID: PMC8508982.

[2] S. Ozkan, W. Murk and A. Arici, 'Endometriosis and infertility: Epidemiology and evidence based treatments', *Ann NY Acad Sci*, vol. **1127**, pp. 92–100, 2008.

[3] S. A. Treoar, D. T. O'Connor, V. M. O'Connor and N. G. Martin, 'Genetic influences on endometriosis in an Australian twin sample', *Fertil Steril*, vol. **71**, pp. 701–710, 1999.

[4] A. A . DeGraaff, T. M. D'Hooghe, G. A. Dunselman et al., 'The significant effect of endometriosis on physical, mental and social wellbeing: Results from an international cross-sectional survey', *Hum Reprod*, vol. **28**, pp. 2677–2685, 2013.

[5] K. Ballard, K. Lowton and J. Wright, 'What's the delay? A qualitative study of women's experiences of reaching a diagnosis of endometriosis', *Fert Steril*, vol. **86**, pp. 1296–1301, 2006.

[6] Z. Pugsley and K. Ballard, 'Assessment of endometriosis in general practice: The pathway to

diagnosis', *Br J Gen Pract*, vol. **57**, no. 539, pp. 470–476, 2007.

[7] A. Fruscalzo, A. Dayer, A. P. Londero et al., 'Endometriosis and infertility: Prognostic value of #Enzian classification compared to rASRM and EFI score', *J Pers Med*, vol. **12**, no. 10, 1623, 2022.

[8] J. Keckstein, E. Saridogan, U. A. Ulrich et al., 'The #Enzian classification: A comprehensive non-invasive and surgical description system for endometriosis', *Acta Obstet Gynecol Scand*, vol. **100**, pp. 1165–1175, 2021.

[9] L. Lazzeri, K. Andersson, S. Angioni et al., 'How to manage endometriosis in adolescence', *JMIG*, vol. 30, pp. 616–626, 2023.

[10] T. K. Holland, J. Yazbek, A. Cutner et al., 'Value of transvaginal ultrasound in assessing severity of pelvic endometriosis', *Ultrasound Obstet Gynaecol*, vol. **36**, no. 2, pp. 241–248, 2010.

[11] National Institute for Health and Care Excellence (NICE), 'Endometriosis: Diagnosis and management'. NG73. 2017. Accessed: 13 Nov. 2025. [Online]. Available: www.nice.org.uk/guidance/ng73/resources/endometriosis-diagnosis-and-management-pdf-1837632548293.

[12] P. Vercellini, G. Frontino, O. De Giorgi et al., 'Continuous use of an oral contraceptive for endometriosis-associated recurrent dysmenorrhoea that does not respond to a cyclic pill regimen', *Fertil Steril*, vol. **80**, no. 3, pp. 560–563, 2003.

[13] J. M. N. Duffy, K. Arambage, F. J. S. Correa et al., *Laparoscopic Surgery for Endometriosis*. The Cochrane Library. Issue 4. John Wiley and Sons, 2014.

[14] D. Byrne, T. Curnow and P. Smith on behalf of BSGE Endometriosis Centres et al., 'Laparoscopic excision of deep rectovaginal endometriosis in BSGE endometriosis centres: a multicentre prospective cohort study', *BMJ Open*, vol. **8**, e018924, 2018.

[15] C. Becker, A. Bokor, O. Heikinheimo et al., 'ESHRE Endometriosis Guideline Group'. ESHRE Guideline: Endometriosis. *Human Reproduction Open*, vol. **2022**, no. 2, hoac009, 2022, https://doi.org/10.1093/hropen/hoac009.

[16] P. Vercellini, L. Fedele, G. Aimi et al., 'Reproductive performance, pain recurrence and disease relapse after conservative surgical treatment for endometriosis: The predictive value of the current classification system', *Hum Reprod*, vol. **21**, pp. 2679–2685, 2006.

[17] N. Hudson, 'The missed disease? Endometriosis as an example of "undone science"', *Reprod Biomed Soc Online*, vol. **14**, pp. 20–27, 2021.

Chapter 19

Management of the Patient with Heavy Menstrual Bleeding in Primary Care

Anne Connolly

Key Points

- Heavy menstrual bleeding (HMB) affects around 25% of women aged 30–50 years old and can significantly reduce quality of life.
- All women with HMB should have a full blood count.
- Consider an endometrial biopsy in women with risk factors for endometrial hyperplasia/malignancy; these include age >45 years, polycystic ovary syndrome (PCOS) and obesity.
- Women without risk factors for structural or histological abnormalities should be offered medical treatment for HMB at their initial assessment.
- The National Institute for Health and Care Excellence (NICE) recommends the 52 mg levonorgestrel-releasing intrauterine device (LNG-IUD) as first-line treatment for HMB in women without significant structural or histological pathology and in whom hormonal treatment is acceptable. For brevity, the term 'LNG-IUD' in this chapter should be assumed to refer to any brand of 52 mg device, but not the lower-dose devices.
- Endometrial ablation is less invasive and lower risk than a hysterectomy but gives fewer quality-of-life years (QALYs).
- Newer, less invasive treatment options are available for fibroids, including medical management, transcervical resection of fibroids and uterine artery embolisation for women wanting to preserve fertility.

Case Scenario 19.1

Lisa, 42, attends the surgery with worsening HMB. Lisa is a flight attendant and mother to 10-year-old Thomas and 12-year-old Emily. Her periods are regular, lasting six days, with the first four being very heavy with clots and flooding. They impact on her quality of life at home and at work.

Introduction

Heavy menstrual bleeding (HMB) is defined clinically as excessive menstrual blood loss, interfering with a woman's physical, social, emotional and/or material quality of life. It can occur alone or with other symptoms [1].

HMB affects around 25% of women aged 30–50 years old – the prevalence may be as high as 37% in adolescents [2]. It can significantly reduce quality of life, and many women will see their GP. In England and Wales, an estimated 50,000 women are referred to secondary care for HMB every year and approximately 28,000 women undergo surgical treatment [3].

The management of HMB has changed in the last few decades, with the introduction of the 52 mg LNG-IUD, hysteroscopic surgery including endometrial ablation and uterine artery embolisation. These techniques have drastically reduced the percentage of women who have a hysterectomy for HMB, down from 60% in the early 1990s [4].

Aetiology

In 2011 the International Federation of Gynaecology and Obstetrics (FIGO) published the PALM-COEIN classification system for the causes of abnormal uterine bleeding (AUB), which includes HMB [6] (Table 19.1).

Structural Causes

Around half of all women with HMB will have no structural cause. Many will have leiomyoma (fibroids), endometrial polyps or adenomyosis, but these structural pathologies may not be causing the HMB. For example, 70% of white women and more than 80% of black women have at least one fibroid by the age of 50 [7], but at least 50% of these are asymptomatic [8]. It is generally accepted that intracavity fibroids, or those which contain a submucosal

Table 19.1 Causes of heavy menstrual bleeding

Structural	Non-Structural
Polyps	**C**oagulopathy
Adenomyosis	**O**vulatory disorder
Leiomyoma	**E**ndometrial
Malignancy or hyperplasia	**I**atrogenic
–	**N**ot yet classified

component, are the most likely to contribute to heavy or abnormal bleeding [6].

Endometrial Hyperplasia and Malignancy

Endometrial hyperplasia is the proliferation of glands making them irregular in size and shape, with an increase in the gland-to-stroma ratio. Hyperplasia is classified as with or without atypia. If left untreated, hyperplasia without atypia has a 1–3% risk of progressing to malignancy, compared to 30–60% if atypia is present [9].

The incidence of endometrial hyperplasia and malignancy increases with age. It is also associated with conditions resulting in higher circulating levels of oestrogen (e.g. obesity and PCOS), which causes over-proliferation of the endometrium. Hyperplasia is not a common cause of HMB, but the consequences of a missed or delayed diagnosis could be significant, so it must be considered.

Risk factors for endometrial hyperplasia and malignancy include:

- age over 45 years
- obesity
- diabetes
- PCOS (unopposed oestrogens from anovulatory cycles)
- nulliparity
- unopposed oestrogen therapy with an intact uterus
- tamoxifen in postmenopausal women
- endogenous oestrogens, such as ovarian granulosa cell neoplasm
- family history of breast, endometrial or colonic cancer.

Non-structural Causes

- The term coagulopathy encompasses the many disorders of systemic haemostasis which may contribute to HMB.
- The endometrial category in the PALM-COEIN system refers to disorders of the mechanisms controlling local endometrial haemostasis, for example inhibited production of local vasoconstrictors or accelerated clot lysis due to excessive production of plasminogen activator.
- Iatrogenic HMB may be due to the copper-intrauterine device (Cu-IUD) or the use of anticoagulant medication.

Initial Assessment

To determine the likely cause and management of Lisa's HMB, a thorough initial assessment needs to be undertaken.

History

The history should identify symptoms suggestive of structural causes and any risk factors for malignancy; it should also determine the effect on Lisa's life.[6]

Important aspects to clarify include:

- How is HMB affecting her physically, emotionally and socially?
- Does she have intermenstrual or postcoital bleeding, dysmenorrhoea or pelvic pain?
- Does she need contraception?
- Has she completed her family?
- Is she up to date with her cervical screening?
- Does she have a history suggestive of a clotting disorder?
- Does she have any significant family history?
- Has she tried any previous treatments for HMB and did they help?

Although gynaecological malignancy is rare in premenopausal women such as Lisa, it is crucial to be aware of the possibility and to act on any red flag symptoms. Postcoital bleeding and persistent intermenstrual bleeding may warrant a referral under the suspected cancer pathway, once pregnancy and sexually transmitted infections are excluded.

Examination

Women presenting with HMB should have a body mass index recorded. Obesity is an important risk factor for endometrial hyperplasia and malignancy.

The purpose of a physical examination is to detect underlying pathology to inform management. Many women will not have a structural or histological cause for their symptoms. The NICE guideline [1] therefore advises that it is not necessary to examine if the history does not suggest a structural or histological abnormality. However, women who are not up to date with their cervical screening should have cervical screening offered and women who choose an LNG-IUD will need a physical examination at the time of fitting. Women should also have a physical examination before any referral or investigations.

Case Scenario 19.1 Feedback

As Lisa has no symptoms or risk factors to suggest a structural or histological abnormality, it would be reasonable not to examine her at the initial appointment. Should she have had a history suggestive of a structural or histological abnormality, for example intermenstrual bleeding, dysmenorrhoea or any pelvic pressure symptoms, an abdominal examination, speculum examination and bimanual examination would be an important part of the initial assessment.

Blood Tests

A full blood count is recommended in all women with HMB, because many have an insidious onset of anaemia [1]. If iron deficiency anaemia is present, treatment should be provided in parallel with investigation of the HMB.

Thyroid function testing is not recommended in the absence of other signs or symptoms of thyroid disease. Hormone testing is not indicated in women with HMB and no associated menstrual irregularity. Coagulation testing is only recommended in women with HMB since menarche, who have a personal or family history suggestive of a clotting disorder.

Further Investigations

Women who are identified from the history or examination as being at risk of structural causes or hyperplasia/malignancy should be investigated as follows. Investigations may also be needed if initial empirical medical management fails.

Investigations for Structural Pathology

An ultrasound scan is the preferred investigation where the history or examination suggests larger fibroids (e.g. pressure symptoms or a palpable uterus), or where examination is inconclusive or difficult because of obesity [1].

An ultrasound scan is also recommended in women with HMB who are suspected to have adenomyosis because of significant dysmenorrhoea, or a bulky tender uterus on examination.

Transvaginal ultrasound scanning is preferrable as it is more accurate; however, if this is not acceptable for the woman, then consider transabdominal scanning [1].

Investigations for Histological Pathology

Direct visualisation by hysteroscopy is the preferred investigation if the history suggests submucosal fibroids, endometrial polyps or other endometrial pathology (because of symptoms such as persistent intermenstrual bleeding, or risk factors for endometrial pathology) [1].

Case Scenario 19.1 Feedback

As Lisa has no risk factors for structural or histological pathology, she does not require any further investigations at this stage.

Medical Management

Women without risk factors for structural or histological abnormalities should be offered medical treatment at their initial assessment. Those who are being referred for investigations or to secondary care should be offered treatment with tranexamic acid or a non-steroidal anti-inflammatory drug (NSAID) while waiting for a definitive treatment plan.

Non-hormonal Treatment

Tranexamic Acid

Tranexamic acid is an anti-fibrinolytic drug which works by inhibiting the breakdown of fibrin in preformed clots in the spiral endometrial arterioles. It does not affect coagulation within healthy blood vessels and is not associated with any increase in arterial thrombosis. The increased risk of venous thrombosis (VTE) is small – one study showed that 78,549 women would need to be treated for five days to be associated with one extra VTE [10]. The treatment dose for HMB is 1 g three to four times daily from the onset of the heavy bleeding for a maximum of four consecutive days. Trials have shown that tranexamic acid can reduce menstrual blood loss (MBL) by up to 58% [11] and that it improves quality of life when used for HMB [12]. It has no effect on dysmenorrhoea or cycle regularity and is less cost-effective than the LNG-IUD.

Non-steroidal Anti-inflammatory Drugs (NSAIDs)

NSAIDs affect prostaglandin synthesis. Prostaglandins are involved in the local pathways affecting both uterine bleeding and uterine cramps, as well as generalized pain pathways. NSAIDs should be taken regularly from the onset of the bleeding until the bleeding has settled. NSAIDs are less effective at reducing MBL when compared with tranexamic acid (reductions of around 30%) [13] but have the advantage of also treating dysmenorrhoea.

Hormonal Treatments

Levonorgestrel Intrauterine Device (LNG-IUD)

The LNG-IUD releases levonorgestrel, which acts locally to prevent endometrial proliferation, to thicken cervical mucus and, in some women, to prevent ovulation. The licences of the different LNG-IUDs vary; however, College of Sexual and Reproductive Healthcare (CoSRH) guidance on the intrauterine device (IUD) does not distinguish between the different brands of 52 mg devices [14]. A device can be left in situ for longer than the licensed recommendation if only used for HMB and still providing benefit [15]. Training is required for insertion and removal of an IUD.

The LNG-IUD may take up to six months to reach full effect; over that time women can experience unscheduled bleeding which is usually light, but may be persistent. Systemic absorption of progesterone from the LNG-IUD is minimal, but some women experience hormonal side effects, including acne, breast tenderness, headache and mood changes; they tend to be mild and transient, decreasing with duration of use [14].

A LNG-IUD can reduce MBL by 90% [16]. It is the most cost-effective pharmaceutical treatment option and is recommended by NICE as a first-line treatment for HMB in women without significant structural or histological pathology as well as for women with fibroids less than 3 cm in diameter that are not causing distortion of the uterine cavity and for women with suspected or diagnosed adenomyosis [1].

Combined Hormonal Contraceptives (CHCs)

CHCs contain oestrogen and a progestogen and act on the hypothalamic-pituitary axis to suppress ovulation and prevent endometrial proliferation. CHCs have traditionally been taken as a 21-day treatment cycle followed by a 7-day break during which a withdrawal bleed occurs. Tailored regimes can also be used, including continuous use, shorter breaks of 4 days or tricycling regimens followed by a 4 or 7 day break. These potentially eliminate or reduce the frequency of the withdrawal bleed and any related symptoms, which may be helpful in women experiencing painful or heavy periods. However, these extended regimens are off licence and may lead to unscheduled bleeding. There is currently insufficient data to recommend one regimen over another – it is advised that all women using a CHC for contraception have both traditional and tailored regimes discussed [17]. The combined pill has been shown to give a 12–77% reduction in MBL [18].

Oral High-Dose Progestogens

Norethisterone 15 mg daily given from days 5 to 26 of the cycle has been found to reduce MBL but is often limited by tolerability [3].

At doses of 5 mg or more, norethisterone and norethisterone acetate are partly metabolised to ethinylestradiol (EE). The conversion equates to an oral dose of 4 mcg of EE per 1 mg of norethisterone, thus therapeutic doses of norethisterone (15 mg daily) should be viewed similarly to a combined oral contraceptive pill with regards to the risks of VTE [19].

Medroxyprogesterone acetate is not metabolised to EE and is therefore an alternative for HMB, with a usual dose of 10 mg once daily (cyclically as above). The dose can be increased to 20–30 mg daily if not effective. Medroxyprogesterone acetate may be as effective as norethisterone, but supporting data is not available [19].

Progesterone-Only Injectable Contraceptive

There is no evidence directly assessing the use of injected progestogens for HMB. However, the contraceptive injection, depot medroxyprogesterone acetate (DMPA), often causes amenorrhoea as a side effect and thus may be useful for HMB. Patient using DMPA may experience progestogenic side effects, including weight gain,

Table 19.2 Efficacy of pharmaceutical treatments [1]

Method	Percentage decrease in menstrual blood flow
LNG-IUD	Up to 95%
Oral progestogen high dose	Up to 80%
CHC	Up to 40%
Tranexamic acid	Up to 58%
NSAIDs	Up to 50%

breast tenderness, acne and mood changes [20] (Table 19.2).

Oral Desogestrel and the Progestogen Contraceptive Implant

Both the desogestrel progestogen-only pill and the progestogen contraceptive implant inhibit ovulation. As a result of this, a proportion of women will become amenorrhoeic. However, both can also be associated with variable unpredictable bleeding, which may be frequent or prolonged [21,22]. Neither method has any supporting evidence for use in managing HMB, or a licence for this indication, and neither method is included in the NICE guidelines [1].

Medical Management of HMB – Summary

Pharmaceutical treatment can be used in primary care in women without structural or histological abnormalities, or for women with fibroids smaller than 3 cm which are causing no distortion of the uterine cavity.

NICE recommend that an LNG-IUD is considered as first-line treatment in this group, as well as in those with structural or diagnosed adenomyosis. If this is declined, or not suitable, they advise any of the following pharmacological treatments:

- Non-Hormonal:
  - Tranexamic acid
  - NSAIDs.
- Hormonal:
  - CHC
  - Cyclical oral progestogens.

Case Scenario 19.1 Feedback

Lisa requires contraception and is interested in initially managing her HMB medically. Having outlined the treatment options, she is keen to think about it. You send her a link to the NICE-endorsed shared decision-making aid for HMB [1] and prescribe tranexamic acid in the interim.

Lisa returns, having decided that she would like an LNG-IUD. You examine her and find no abnormalities; as a qualified fitter of intrauterine devices, you counsel her fully and arrange this for her.

Surgical Management

For women who have had unsuccessful medical treatment, or who choose not to have medical management, surgical treatment may be an option. This includes endometrial ablation, hysterectomy and the surgical treatment of fibroids.

Endometrial Ablation

For women who have a normal-sized uterus, or small uterine fibroids, endometrial ablation or resection can be offered as an initial treatment option, or after failed medical management. Endometrial ablation is less invasive than a hysterectomy and associated with fewer complications; it can be performed in the out-patient setting under local anaesthetic.

The principle is to destroy or remove the endometrium, along with the superficial myometrium, resulting in the destruction of most or all of the glands from which the endometrium develops. There are several different ablation methods available.

Endometrial ablation (or resection) is not a fertility-conserving treatment, nor is it a method of contraception. Women must be advised to use adequate contraception; pregnancy following endometrial ablation or resection can be life-threatening for both fetus and mother. All women considering endometrial ablation should be counselled about their contraceptive options (which may include tubal ligation), in parallel to discussing surgical treatment for HMB.

Ninety per cent of women experience a significant reduction in blood loss after endometrial ablation and around 50% of women have no bleeding when reviewed one year after the procedure [1].

Hysterectomy

Hysterectomy is the surgical removal of the uterus. There are different methods available, including abdominal, vaginal and laparoscopic. All are considered to be major surgery and require considerable physical recuperation with at least several weeks off work [23]. NICE states that hysterectomy should not be used as a first-line treatment solely for HMB, but that referral to consider surgical options, including hysterectomy, should be considered if other treatment is unsuccessful or declined, or if symptoms are severe [1].

Women considering hysterectomy should be fully informed of the risks and complications of surgery – these include the following:

- sexual feelings
- impact on fertility
- bladder function
- need for further treatment
- treatment complications, including a risk of haemorrhage or damage to other abdominal organs
- her expectations
- alternative surgery
- psychological impact
- possible loss of ovarian function and consequences, even if ovaries are retained during hysterectomy.

The woman's expectations should be fully explored, and all other treatment options discussed. A cost-effective analysis found that although hysterectomy is more expensive than endometrial ablation, it produces more QALYs for women with HMB and is thus more cost-effective than endometrial ablation [24].

Treatment of Uterine Fibroids

For women with large fibroids (>3 cm in diameter) and HMB which is having a severe impact on quality of life, consider interventions for the treatment of fibroids. The type of treatment should consider the location and number of fibroids and whether women wish to conserve their fertility.

Medical Management Initiated in Secondary Care

Ulipristal acetate (UPA) is a selective progesterone receptor modulator which has a licence to treat moderate to severe symptoms of fibroids in women of reproductive age. This can be provided as intermittent treatment, taking 5 mg daily for three months, with repeated courses or more definitive treatment to follow [25].

UPA should only be considered if surgery or uterine artery embolisation is not suitable, has been declined or has failed [1].

Women considering use of UPA must be advised that:

- UPA can be associated with serious liver injury and the signs and the symptoms to look out for.
- They require liver function testing before starting UPA, monthly for the first two courses and once before each new treatment course.
- Any signs and symptoms of liver failure require UPA treatment to be discontinued with urgent liver function testing to be arranged.

In addition to this advice in the NICE guidance, a drug safety update advises that liver function also be tested two to four weeks after each treatment course ends and that the drug not be started in women who have liver enzymes which are more than twice the upper limit of normal [26].

A number of GnRH antagonist medications are in development; some are available for specialist initiation for treatment of fibroids. All GnRH antagonists require hormone replacement add-back therapy to prevent menopausal symptoms and complications such as osteoporosis. Some products are combination GnRH antagonist and hormone replacement, while others require the hormone replacement therapy (HRT) prescribed separately [27].

Radiological Management

Uterine artery embolisation is a radiological technique performed under local anaesthetic. It can be offered to women who wish to retain their uterus and can be effective for multiple fibroids. Particles are used to block the uterine arteries; this causes the fibroids to shrink with no known permanent effect on the rest of the uterus.

Surgical Management

Myomectomy may be offered for treatment of large focal fibroids and can be done hysteroscopically or laparoscopically, by removal or morcellation (cutting the fibroids into smaller pieces to allow for vaginal or laparoscopic removal) [28]. Laparoscopic or open myomectomy can be undertaken for women with intramural or subserosal fibroids, but this may not significantly improve HMB if the fibroids are not distorting the endometrial cavity. Although myomectomy can be considered a fertility-sparing option, it is important to note the risk of bleeding and subsequent hysterectomy as a complication. In women who wish to maintain fertility, the benefits versus risks of any surgery on the uterus need to be carefully considered and discussed.

For women who have HMB related to fibroids and have completed their family, a hysterectomy is a curative treatment option.

Case Scenario 19.1 Feedback

Unfortunately, after 12 months of use, the LNG-IUD is not successful in treating Lisa's HMB. Primary care management has failed so you arrange a referral. Lisa is keen for a definitive treatment as she has completed her family and potentially has over a decade of menstrual cycles ahead of her. Hysteroscopy confirms no cause for her HMB. Following a discussion regarding the risks and benefits of endometrial ablation versus laparoscopic hysterectomy, she elects to go ahead with endometrial ablation because of the lower risks and faster recovery time.

Conclusion

HMB is a common problem which can have a considerable effect on a woman's quality of life. A careful history of the problem and examination, where appropriate, helps determine whether further investigations are required.

The NICE guidance on HMB [1] gives GPs a logical and evidence-based pathway of care, the majority of which can be provided in a primary care setting.

References

[1] NICE, 'NG88: Heavy menstrual bleeding – assessment and management'. 2021. Accessed: 29 Jan. 2024. [Online]. Available: www.nice.org.uk/guidance/ng88.

[2] NICE CKS, 'Menorrhagia (heavy menstrual bleeding)'. Mar. 2023. Accessed: 29 Jan. 2024. [Online]. Available: https://cks.nice.org.uk/topics/menorrhagia-heavy-menstrual-bleeding.

[3] R. S. Geary, I. Gurol-Urganci, A. Kiran et al., 'Factors associated with receiving surgical treatment for menorrhagia in England and Wales: Findings from a cohort study of the National Heavy Menstrual Bleeding Audit', *BMJ Open*, vol. **9**, no. 2, e024260, 2019.

[4] S. Mayor, 'NICE says hysterectomy must be last option for heavy menstrual bleeding'. *BMJ*, vol. **334**, no. 7586, 175, 2007.

[5] NICE, 'QS47: Heavy menstrual bleeding'. 2020. Accessed: 29 Jan. 2024. [Online]. Available: www.nice.org.uk/guidance/qs47.

[6] M. Munro, H. O. Critchley, M. S. Broder et al. (FIGO Working Group on Menstrual Disorders), 'FIGO classification system (PALM-COEIN) for causes of abnormal uterine bleeding in nongravid women of reproductive age', *Int J Gynaecol Obstet*, vol. **113**, no. 1, pp. 3–13, 2011.

[7] M. A. Lumsden, I. Hamoodi, J. Gupta et al., 'Fibroids: Diagnosis and management', *BMJ*, vol. **351**, h4887, 2015.

[8] H. Divakar, 'Asymptomatic uterine fibroids', *Best Pract Res Clin Obstet Gynaecol*, vol. **22**, no. 4, pp. 643–654, 2008.

[9] R. J. Kurman, M. L. Carcangiu, C. S. Herrington et al. (eds.), *WHO Classification of Tumours of Female Reproductive Organs*, 4th ed. IARC, 2014.

[10] A. Meaidi, L. Mørch, C. Torp-Pedersen et al., 'Oral tranexamic acid and thrombosis risk in women', *EClinicalMedicine*, vol. **35**, 100882, 2021.

[11] N. C. Gleeson, F. Buggy, B. L. Sheppard et al., 'The effect of tranexamic acid on measured menstrual loss and endometrial fibrinolytic enzymes in dysfunctional uterine bleeding', *Acta Obstet Gynecol Scand*, vol. **73**, no. 3, pp. 274–277, 1994.

[12] U. H. Winkler, 'The effect of tranexamic acid on the quality of life of women with heavy menstrual bleeding', *Eur J Obstet Gynecol Reprod Biol*, vol. **99**, no. 2, pp. 238–243, 2001.

[13] J. Potter, Z. Sari and A. J. Lindblad, 'NSAIDs for heavy menstrual bleeding', *Can Fam Physician*, vol. **67**, no. 8, 598, 2021.

[14] CoSRH, 'CoSRH Clinical Guideline: Intrauterine contraception'. 2023. Accessed: 14 Nov. 2025. [Online]. Available: https://www.cosrh.org/Common/Uploaded%20files/documents/fsrh-clinical-guideline-intrauterine-contraception-mar-23-amended.pdf.

[15] PCWHS. 10 top tips for the use of intrauterine devices. https://www.pcwhs.co.uk/resources/115/10_top_tips_for_the_use_of_intrauterine_devices.

[16] M. Bofill Rodriguez, A Lethaby and V. Jordan, 'Progestogen-releasing intrauterine systems for heavy menstrual bleeding', *Cochrane Database of Systematic Reviews*, vol. **6**, CD002126, 2020.

[17] CoSRH, 'CoSRH Clinical Guideline: Combined hormonal contraception'. 2023. Accessed: 14

Nov. 2025. [Online]. Available: https://www.cosrh.org/Public/Documents/fsrh-guideline-combined-hormonal-contraception.aspx

[18] A. Lethaby, M. R. Wise, M. A. J. Weterings et al., ‘Combined hormonal contraceptives for heavy menstrual bleeding’, *Cochrane Database of Systematic Reviews*, vol. **2**, CD000154, 2019.

[19] D. Mansour, ‘Safer prescribing of therapeutic norethisterone for women at risk of venous thromboembolism’, *J Fam Plann Reprod Health Care*, vol. **38**, pp. 148–149, 2012.

[20] CoSRH, ‘CoSRH Clinical Guideline: Progestogen only injectable’. 2023. Accessed: 14 Nov. 2025. [Online]. Available: https://www.cosrh.org/Public/Documents/fsrh-ceu-guidance-progestogen-only-injectables.aspx.

[21] CoSRH, ‘CoSRH Clinical Guideline: Progestogen only implant’. 2023. Accessed: 14 Nov. 2025. [Online]. Available: www.cosrh.org/Common/Uploaded%20files/documents/fsrh-guideline-progestogen-only-implants.pdf.

[22] CoSRH, ‘CoSRH Clinical Guideline: Progestogen only pill’. 2023. Accessed: 14 Nov. 2025. [Online]. Available: www.cosrh.org/Common/Uploaded%20files/documents/fsrh-ceu-clinical-guideline-progestogen-only-pills-aug22-amended-11july-2023-.pdf.

[23] NHS, ‘Hysterectomy – recovery’. 2022. Accessed: 2 Feb. 2024. [Online]. Available: www.nhs.uk/conditions/hysterectomy/recovery.

[24] T. E. Roberts, A. Tsourapas, L. J. Middleton et al., ‘Hysterectomy, endometrial ablation, and levonorgestrel releasing intrauterine system (Mirena) for treatment of heavy menstrual bleeding: cost effectiveness analysis’, *BMJ*, vol. **342**, d2202, 2011.

[25] J. Donnez, R. Hudecek, O. Donnez et al., ‘Efficacy and safety of repeated use of ulipristal acetate in uterine fibroids’, *Fertil Steril*, vol. **103**, no. 2, pp. 519–527, 2015.

[26] MHRA, ‘Esmya (ulipristal acetate) and risk of serious liver injury: New restrictions to use and requirements for liver function monitoring before, during, and after treatment’. 2018. Accessed: 2 Feb. 2024. [Online]. Available: https://www.gov.uk/drug-safety-update/esmya-ulipristal-acetate-and-risk-of-serious-liver-injury-new-restrictions-to-use-and-requirements-for-liver-function-monitoring-before-during-and-after-treatment.

[27] A. Di Spiezio Sardo, F. Ciccarone, L. Muzii et al., ‘Use of oral GnRH antagonists combined therapy in the management of symptomatic uterine fibroids’, *Facts Views Vis Obgyn*, vol. **15**, no. 1, pp. 29–33, 2023.

[28] Royal College of Obstetricians and Gynaecologists, ‘Morcellation for myomectomy or hysterectomy’. 2019. Accessed: 2 Feb. 2024. [Online]. Available: www.rcog.org.uk/for-the-public/browse-our-patient-information/morcellation-for-myomectomy-or-hysterectomy.

Chapter 20

Management of the Patient with Continence Problems in Primary Care

Abigail Macleod-Thompson

Key Points

- Urinary incontinence is a debilitating, chronic condition of multiple aetiologies. It can affect a patient's quality of life, sexuality and relationships.
- The prevalence of urinary incontinence is increasing alongside our rising ageing population, making it essential for clinicians to understand the impact of the condition and management in both primary and secondary care settings.
- Urinary incontinence can be classified into three main types: stress, urge and mixed urinary incontinence.
- Pelvic floor muscle training, vaginal devices and surgical interventions are the mainstay treatments for stress urinary incontinence symptoms. Surgical interventions involving vaginal mesh have stopped post the high-vigilance restrictions that were put in place in July 2018 by NHS England and NHS Improvement.
- Behavioural, lifestyle and pharmacological therapies are the basis of treating urge urinary incontinence symptoms.
- Genitourinary syndrome of menopause (GSM) can be a major contributor to bladder symptoms, therefore vaginal oestrogens should be part of first-line treatment in perimenopausal and menopausal women.
- Multidisciplinary teams, including community-based continence teams, GPs, urologists and urogynaecologists, play an invaluable role in treating patients with urinary incontinence.

Case Scenario 20.1

Jane is a 52-year-old who complains that every time she coughs, laughs or does any exercise she leaks small volumes of urine. She states she has reduced her activities to reduce the amount of 'accidents' she has on a daily basis. She also complains of urinary urgency and frequency up to ten times during the day and three times at night.

Jane has had three vaginal deliveries (one forceps delivery) and no other medical problems or current medication. She has a body mass index (BMI) of 39 and smokes 10 cigarettes/day.

Introduction

Urinary incontinence (UI) is a common debilitating condition that patients are embarrassed to disclose to healthcare professionals and their families. It is difficult to ascertain the true prevalence due to patients' under-reporting their symptoms. Some research suggests that it affects around 50% of women at some point in their lives [1].

A UK-based cross-sectional postal study of 1,415 women showed the prevalence of UI was 39.9%. Stress urinary incontinence was the most common type of incontinence occurring in 24%; 7% had overactive bladder symptoms and urge incontinence and 20% had mixed urinary incontinence. It also showed that more severe incontinence affected older patients likely due to associated co-morbidities [2].

UI is defined by the International Continence Society as 'the complaint of any involuntary loss of urine' and is broadly subcategorised as:

- *Stress urinary incontinence (SUI)* – complaint of involuntary loss of urine on effort or physical exertion including sporting activities or on sneezing or coughing. It can be associated with bladder neck weakness, obesity, poor pelvic floor muscle strength or nerve damage.
- *Urgency urinary incontinence (UUI)* – complaint of involuntary loss of urine associated with urgency (a sudden compelling desire to urinate that is difficult to delay).
- *Mixed urinary incontinence (MUI)* – involuntary urine leakage associated with

urgency and physical exertion, coughing or sneezing [3].

- *Overactive bladder (OAB)* – urinary urgency, usually accompanied by increased daytime frequency and/or nocturia. It can be subclassified as 'OAB wet' and 'OAB dry', depending on whether or not the urgency is associated with incontinence. These combinations of symptoms are suggestive of the urodynamic finding of detrusor overactivity (DO) [4].
- *Functional* (unable to reach toilet in time), *overflow* (bladder outlet obstruction from uterine prolapse or previous surgery) and *extra-urethral loss incontinence* (due to fistulas) are rare types of UI which need excluding.

Social and Financial Implications of UI

The impact of UI is considerable for both the patient and the NHS as a whole. The economic burden of UI has been assessed in multiple studies and shown to be substantial, increasing significantly as the population ages. The total annual service costs in the UK have been estimated at over £230 million in 2005, with a more up-to-date figure of the NHS spending around £80 million per year on incontinence products alone in 2018 [5,6]. The psychosocial impact of UI to a woman includes feelings of shame, low self-esteem, depression, social withdrawal, concerns over sexuality and strained personal relationships [7]. These factors alone can have considerable costs outside of just NHS costs. The NHS is highlighting the importance of this area of medicine with the policy paper, 'Women's Health Strategy for England', produced in 2022.

Initial Assessment

The vast majority of patients will fall into three categories of UI and therefore the aim of the initial clinical assessment is to classify the woman's UI as either:

- stress UI
- mixed UI (MUI)
- urgency UI/OAB.

The National Institute for Health and Care Excellence (NICE) recommends starting initial treatment on this basis. For women with mixed UI, the advice is to direct treatment towards the most predominant symptom [8] (Table 20.1).

Table 20.1 Main symptoms of the different types of UI in women

Stress urinary incontinence	Urge urinary incontinence/OAB
• Urinary leakage on: . Coughing . Exercising . Sneezing . Lifting heavy weights	• Frequency • Urgency • Urge incontinence • Nocturia
Worse when bladder full	Urgency is the main symptoms of OAB
Mixed urinary incontinence can have a mixture of symptoms	

Co-existing Conditions

It is very important to take a comprehensive medical history when diagnosing patients with UI. Co-existing conditions and medications need to be optimised as a priority to aid UI symptom control, as many routine medications can alter bladder function or create fluid shifts, such as diuretics.

Predisposing Conditions

- Poorly controlled diabetes significantly increases urine output.
- Respiratory conditions causing chronic cough symptoms predispose patients to pelvic organ prolapse (POP) and UI symptoms.
- Neurological conditions such as multiple sclerosis, Parkinson's disease, cerebrovascular accident and Alzheimer's diseases are important to note as they can affect nerve stimulation to the bladder, leading to a 'neurogenic bladder' (bladder dysfunction secondary to a neurological disease) as well as causing mobility issues [9].
- Recurrent urinary tract infections (UTIs) are also important to note as this may significantly worsen any UI symptoms.
- Bowel symptoms, including constipation, can weaken pelvic floor muscles and predispose a patient to UI and POP [10,11].
- Lifestyle choices such as alcohol, caffeine, artificial sweeteners, fizzy drinks, fluid intake and smoking tend to worsen UI symptoms.
- Occupations involving heavy lifting can also worsen stress UI symptoms.

Past Medical History

Obstetric and gynaecological risk factors for UI include:

- parity
- mode of delivery (assisted vaginal deliveries, i.e. forceps)
- gynaecological procedures, in particular vaginal hysterectomy
- menopausal status
- any previous urological investigations, surgery and nocturnal enuresis as a child (associated with detrusor overactivity) are also very important to note [10].

Quality-of-Life Assessment

In order to gain a detailed insight of the psychosocial burden associated with a patient's UI, it is vital to ask what restrictions the symptoms put on the patient's daily functions and how they cope with these, such as only shopping in areas with readily accessible toilets.

QoL questionnaires are a useful adjunct in assessing the impact that incontinence and bladder dysfunction have on a woman's life. NICE recommends using a validated urinary incontinence-specific symptom and quality-of-life questionnaire when therapies are being evaluated [8]. ICIQ-UI short form has only four questions and is a good screening tool (Figure 20.1).

Bladder Diaries

These are a method of quantification of urinary frequency, diurnal variations, nocturia, voided volumes, functional bladder capacity, severity of incontinence episodes and fluid input/output [10]. NICE recommends the use of bladder diaries for a minimum of three days spanning over work and leisure days in the initial assessment of women with UI [8].

These diaries enhance the clinical assessment regarding excessive fluid consumption, normal consumption at inappropriate times (e.g. bedtime) or an excessive intake of alcohol or caffeinated drinks. An example of a bladder diary is shown in Table 20.2.

Table 20.2 Bladder diary example. Reproduced with permission from Your Pelvic Floor (https://www.yourpelvicfloor.org/conditions/bladder-diary-2/) [13].

DATE	DRINKS		URINE		LEAKAGE		
Time	**Type**	**How much**	**Volume of Urine (mls)**	**How Urgent 0-3 3 = most urgent**	**Leakage with Urgency**	**Leakage with Activities**	**Pad Change**
0200	-	-	150mls	2	Y	-	-
0700	Mug coffee	250 mls	250 mls	-	-	-	-
0800	-	-	60mls	-	-	□ cough	P
0900	Cup orange juice	200mls	-	-	-	□ sneeze	-
1000	-	-	100mls	-	-	-	-
1200	2 mugs coffee	500 mls	-	-	-	-	-
1400	-	-	300mls	3	Y	-	-
1530	Cup of tea	200mls	-	-	-	□ jogging	P
1600	-	100mls	-	-	-	-	-
1800	Cup of tea	200mls	-	-	-	-	-
1900	-	-	100mls	-	3	Y	-
2000	Glass of beer	200mls	20mls	-	-	-	-
2030	Glass of wine	50mls	-	-	-	□ cough	-
2200	-	-	-	-	-	-	P
2300	-	-	150mls	-	-	-	-

ICIQ-UI Short Form

Initial number

CONFIDENTIAL

DAY MONTH YEAR
Today's date

Many people leak urine some of the time. We are trying to find out how many people leak urine, and how much this bothers them. We would be grateful if you could answer the following questions, thinking about how you have been, on average, over the PAST FOUR WEEKS.

1 **Please write in your date of birth:** DAY MONTH YEAR

2 **Are you** *(tick one)*: Female ☐ Male ☐

3 **How often do you leak urine?** *(Tick one box)*

never ☐	0
about once a week or less often ☐	1
two or three times a week ☐	2
about once a day ☐	3
several times a day ☐	4
all the time ☐	5

4 **We would like to know how much urine <u>you think</u> leaks.**
How much urine do you <u>usually</u> leak (whether you wear protection or not)?
(Tick one box)

none ☐	0
a small amount ☐	2
a moderate amount ☐	4
a large amount ☐	6

5 **Overall, how much does leaking urine interfere with your everyday life?**
Please ring a number between 0 (not at all) and 10 (a great deal)

0 1 2 3 4 5 6 7 8 9 **10**
not at all — a great deal

ICIQ score: sum scores 3+4+5 ☐☐

6 **When does urine leak?** *(Please tick all that apply to you)*

- never – urine does not leak ☐
- leaks before you can get to the toilet ☐
- leaks when you cough or sneeze ☐
- leaks when you are asleep ☐
- leaks when you are physically active/exercising ☐
- leaks when you have finished urinating and are dressed ☐
- leaks for no obvious reason ☐
- leaks all the time ☐

Thank you very much for answering these questions.

Figure 20.1 ICIQ-UI SF quality-of-life assessment tool. Reproduced with permission from Avery et al. (2004) [12].

Physical Examination

A physical examination is required in the assessment of a woman presenting with UI. This assists the diagnosis and management of UI, excludes other related conditions and should routinely include the following.

- BMI.
- Abdominal and pelvic examination is necessary to assess for masses, a palpable bladder, atrophic vaginitis and POP. A cough stress test should be performed to see if demonstrable SUI is present.
- Digital assessment of pelvic floor contractions before commencement of supervised pelvic floor muscle training for the treatment of SUI/MUI is recommended by NICE [8]. The strength of the contraction is graded from no contraction to strong contraction and its duration [Table 20.3].
- If there are symptoms that suggest a neurological cause, it is important to perform a screening neurological exam with emphasis on the sacral roots S2–4 (main innervation of muscarinic receptors of the bladder).
- Deep tendon reflexes (Achilles – S1).
- Abduction and dorsiflexion of toes (S3).
- Sensory innervation at:
  - sole and lateral aspect of foot (S1)
  - perineum (S3)
  - perianal area (S4) [11].
- Assessment of cognitive impairment of women may be required.

Investigations

Urinalysis

Urinalysis in patients with UI is important to detect the presence of blood, protein, leucocytes or nitrites. Symptoms of urinary urgency overlap with those of UTI. The presence of a UTI will worsen irritative bladder symptoms and give false outcomes on any urodynamic investigations.

Women with symptoms of a urinary tract infection with or without a positive (nitrites or leucocyte present) urine dipstick should have a mid-stream urine (MSU) sent for culture and consider empirical treatment.

If a woman is asymptomatic, but has a positive dipstick for leucocytes/nitrites, she should also have an MSU sent but await culture results before treatment [8].

Table 20.3 Modified Oxford grading scale for pelvic floor muscles [9]

Grade	Definition
0	No contraction
1	Flicker of contraction
2	Weak muscle activity
3	Moderate muscle contraction
4	Good muscle contraction
5	Strong muscle contraction

Postvoid Residuals

Postvoid residual (PVR) is the volume of urine remaining in the bladder following micturition. It should be sought in women with symptoms suggestive of voiding dysfunction (e.g. straining, incomplete bladder emptying) or recurrent UTI to assess if the patient is fully emptying the bladder.

Bladder scanning is recommended as a first-line measurement of PVR in view of acceptability and lower incidence of adverse events [8].

Ultrasound

Ultrasound assessment is not routinely recommended for the assessment of women with UI except for PVR measurements or ruling out pelvic masses in obese patients [8].

Cystoscopy

Cystoscopy (direct visualisation of bladder and urethra) is not recommended for the initial assessment of women with UI alone [8].

Urodynamics

Urodynamics aims to demonstrate an abnormality of urine storage or voiding via a combination of tests. It is more useful and accurate for diagnosis of lower urinary tract dysfunction than just symptoms alone [10] and also for selecting the most appropriate intervention to the underlying pathology.

- *Uroflowmetry* measures flow of urine over time. It aids diagnosis of voiding difficulties.
- *Cystometry* measures the pressure–volume relationship of the bladder (intravesical pressure) during filling and voiding. The

Box 20.1 Referral Guidelines for Women with Urinary Incontinence

When to refer a UI patient [8]

Consider referral to a specialist service for:

- persisting bladder or urethral pain
- palpable bladder on bimanual or abdominal examination
- clinically benign pelvic masses
- associated faecal incontinence
- suspected neurological disease
- symptoms of voiding difficulty
- suspected urogenital fistula
- previous continence surgery
- previous pelvic cancer surgery
- previous pelvic radiation therapy
- for patients with suspected cancer symptoms, follow suspected cancer referral pathway to appropriate department, e.g. gynaecology, urology or colorectal.

bladder is filled through a catheter with saline and the woman indicates her first and maximal desires to void. During the filling phase, tests to provoke the bladder for SUI and DO are performed.

Detrusor overactivity (DO) is diagnosed if there are spontaneous or provoked detrusor contractions.

A diagnosis of urodynamic stress incontinence (USI) is confirmed if leakage on coughing occurs, in the absence of detrusor contractions.

NICE recommends that multichannel filling and voiding cystometry are not performed before primary surgery if SUI or stress-predominant MUI is diagnosed based on a detailed clinical history and demonstrated SUI at examination [8].

NICE recommends the use of preoperative urodynamics in cases of SUI that have any of the following:

- urge-predominant MUI or UI in which the type is unclear
- symptoms suggestive of voiding dysfunction
- anterior or apical prolapse
- a history of previous surgery for SUI [8].

In women with overactive bladder symptoms not responding to pharmacological management, offer urodynamics to determine whether detrusor overactivity is causing her overactive bladder symptoms.

Case Scenario 20.2

On examination by her GP, Jane was found to have vaginal atrophy and a first-degree uterine descent with a moderate anterior vaginal wall prolapse. Cough test showed no leak and pelvic floor muscle tone was assessed as moderate (3/5 on the Oxford scale).

Jane's urine dipstick was negative.

Guidelines for referral to secondary care are shown in Box 20.1.

Treatment Options for UI

Management of a patient with UI depends on the underlying diagnosis, with treatment options including conservative, medical and surgical methods.

Conservative and anti-muscarinic drug treatments will most commonly be offered within a primary and community care setting. If these treatments are unsuccessful, the next option for women would involve a surgical option or second-line agent and therefore most women would need to be referred from primary care to receive these interventions.

Conservative Management of UI

Conservative management steps should be used as a first-line approach to treating any patient with UI.

Lifestyle Advice

- NICE advice a trial of caffeine reduction in women with OAB as caffeine increases the irritability of the bladder. Alcohol should also be reduced or avoided [8].
- Modification of high and low fluid intakes to aim for 1–1.5 litres per day will lessen the severity of OAB symptoms.
- Weight loss should be advised to a BMI less than 30. Many hospitals will not operate on patients until BMI is < 35.
- Medication review is advised as various drugs such as diuretics and antipsychotics affect bladder function.
- Dietary advice to prevent constipation if needed.
- Smoking cessation advice to reduce the risk of a chronic cough and urgency episodes.

Physical Therapy and Interventions

Pelvic floor muscle training (PFMT) results in an increase in tone and strength of the pelvic floor muscles and an increased conscious awareness of the muscle groups.

NICE recommends PFMT as a first-line treatment for women with stress or mixed UI. The duration of exercises should be at least eight contractions (working up to an ideal duration of 10 seconds), three times a day for a minimum of three months. If benefit is found these exercises should be continued. PFMT requires high levels of motivation and education and is ideally performed under clinical supervision.

Women who are experiencing difficulty in performing PFMT may benefit from biofeedback or electrical stimulation, although NICE do not recommend this as a routine part of PFMT [8]. There are now mobile applications available to prompt patients to remember to do regular pelvic floor exercises. An example is the 'Squeezy App' which won the national continence care aware in 2015/16.

Vaginal cones act as a form of biofeedback by producing graded resistance levels applied to the pelvic floor muscles. These help to increase muscle strength and endurance of the pelvic floor muscles. A Cochrane review concluded that cones are better than no treatment, although not better than PFMT alone [14].

Electrical stimulation uses short pulses of current from a probe placed transvaginally. For DO, electrical stimulation inhibits detrusor contractions by the sensory feedback it produces. For SUI, it directly stimulates the pelvic floor muscles. NICE found that study results were inconsistent and therefore electrical stimulation is not routinely recommended except in women who have either extremely weak contractions or are unable to produce a muscle contraction [4].

Behavioural Therapy

Bladder drill (retraining) is a behavioural modification used for OAB that involves timed voiding at incremental intervals (15–30 mins). The drill re-educates the bladder into holding increasing volumes of urine for longer periods of time, ultimately up to a desired interval of three to four hours [10].

Bladder training should be used for a minimum of six weeks as first-line treatment for urgency or mixed UI. If a woman does not achieve satisfactory benefit from bladder training programmes, NICE recommend combining OAB drugs with bladder training, especially if frequency is a predominant symptom [8].

Hypnotherapy is used in cases where there are underlying psychological factors exacerbating OAB. Unfortunately, relapse rates are high.

Acupuncture increases the level of encephalins in the cerebrospinal fluid (CSF), which are thought to inhibit detrusor contractions. Studies have shown symptomatic improvement, but usually short-lasting effects.

Alternative Physical Interventions

These include bladder catheterisation, absorbent products and toileting aids.

NICE only recommend these as a coping strategy pending definitive treatment, as an adjunct to ongoing therapy or as a long-term management of UI, only after treatment options have been explored.

Bladder catheterisation (self-catheterisation or indwelling) may be required in patients who suffer with persistent urinary retention causing incontinence, recurrent UTIs or those who have intractable incontinence and are not fit for other treatments.

Vaginal devices can be used (e.g. Contrelle pessary); however, NICE only recommend their use on an occasional basis, for example to prevent leakage during physical exercise.

Case Scenario 20.3

Jane's main complaints come initially from her stress UI symptoms so her initial management should target these, including lifestyle advice (weight loss, smoking cessation, caffeine reduction) and referral to the community-based continence team for PFMT. Alongside PFMT, the specialist team should also commence bladder retraining and the GP start vaginal oestrogen in view of her frequency symptoms and vaginal atrophy found on examination.

As a result of these conservative measures, Jane reports an improvement in her symptoms and reduction in incontinence episodes to three times a week. However, she is still using sanitary pads daily and reports increasing awareness of urgency symptoms.

Pharmacological Treatment for UUI/OAB

Most women with DO will require drug therapy (Table 20.4). Before commencing any treatment, NICE recommends discussing with women:

- likelihood of success
- associated common adverse effects. Some adverse effects of anticholinergic medicines such as dry mouth and constipation may indicate that the medicine is starting to work
- duration of treatment needed to see full effects (four weeks usually)
- the long-term effects of anticholinergic medicines for OAB on cognitive function are uncertain [8].

Before starting an anticholinergic medication for OAB, it is important for the prescriber to consider the following:

- co-existing conditions such as poor bladder emptying, cognitive impairment and dementia
- assessing the total anticholinergic burden (ACB) on a patient including all their current medications. An ACB score of 3 or more may increase the risk of cognitive impairment, falls and mortality in older adults (> 50–65 years). You can work out the ACB score via online calculators such as www.acbcalc.com
- risk of adverse effects including cognitive function.

NICE recommends prescribing the lowest recommended dose and acquisition cost when starting a new OAB medication and then altering according to side effects or efficacy. When the first medication for OAB does not work or is not well tolerated, offer another medication with a low acquisition cost.

Follow-up after starting medication is important. It is recommended to assess treatment affect at four weeks after starting medication and if no benefit is seen to stop the medication and reassess.

If a patient is stable on long-term UI or OAB drug therapy, she should be reviewed annually if under 75 years old or every 6 months if over 75 [8].

Mirabegron is a recommended OAB medication for patients who have contraindications to anticholinergics or no clinical improvement on anticholinergics or if they have unacceptable side effects. It is recommended to have blood pressure checked a week after commencing mirabegron and it should not be commenced in patients with uncontrolled high blood pressure.

Alternative Pharmacological Agents for UUI/OAB

Desmopressin or DDAVP is a long-acting synthetic analogue of vasopressin inhibiting diuresis and is effective in patients with nocturnal polyuria. However, it should be avoided in those with cystic fibrosis or over 65 years old with cardiovascular disease. The main side effects are hyponatraemia and fluid retention (Table 20.3).

Genitourinary Syndrome of Menopause (GSM)

GSM is a hypoestrogenic condition causing a collection of vulvovaginal symptoms including vaginal pain, dyspareunia, vaginal dryness, itching, sexual dysfunction and urinary symptoms including urinary frequency, urgency, incontinence, haematuria and recurrent UTI. Signs of this include atrophic changes to the vagina [15]. This highlights the importance of vaginal oestrogens in maintaining healthy lower genital and urinary tract tissues. NICE recommend the use of intravaginal oestrogens in postmenopausal women with OAB and vaginal atrophy. Systemic hormone replacement confers no extra benefit [8].

Table 20.4 Pharmacological options for OAB/UUI [8]

Drug Anticholinergics	Dosage	Dose titration	Benefits	Side effects
Solifenacin	5–10 mg once daily	Increase after 4 weeks if needed	Extended release Titration of dose Long half-life – offering 24-hour control of bladder smooth muscle tone	Side effects well tolerated[a]
Tolterodine (immediate release)	1–2 mg twice daily	Increase after 4 weeks if needed	High selectivity for bladder receptors thus less side effects Does not cross blood–brain barrier – fewer central nervous system effects[b] Dose can be titrated	Better tolerability than oxybutynin[a]
Oxybutynin (immediate release)	2.5 mg once daily to 5 mg 3 times daily	Gradual increase	Immediate effect, can be used on a PRN basis Targets urgency and urge incontinence Low cost	Marked anti-cholinergic side effects[a,b] High discontinuation rate Not advised for frail older women
Darifenacin (once daily)	7.5–15 mg once daily	After 2 weeks, reassess and increase dose if needed	High selectivity for bladder receptors thus fewer side effects No significant central nervous system effects[b] Extended release Titration of dose	-
OxybutyninXL (extended release)	5–15 mg once daily	Increase after 4 weeks if needed	Extended release Can reduce side-effect profile	Better tolerability than oxybutynin immediate release[a,b]
Oxybutynin patches	3.9 mg/24 hours applied twice weekly	Nil	Extended release Avoids hepatic first pass	Better tolerability than oxybutynin immediate release[a,b] Skin irritation
Tolterodine (extended release)	4 mg once daily	-	Extended release	Better tolerability than oxybutynin[a,b]
Trospium (immediate release)	20 mg twice daily	-	Potent blocking action on detrusor contraction No central nervous system effects[b] – useful in treating elderly patients	Side effects[a]
Trospium (extended release)	60 mg once daily	-	-	-

Table 20.4 (cont.)

Drug Anticholinergics	Dosage	Dose titration	Benefits	Side effects
Fesoterodine	4–8 mg once daily	Increase after 4 weeks if needed	Extended release Dose titration	Better tolerability than oxybutynin[a,b]
Propiverine	15 mg once daily to 3 times daily	Increase after 4 weeks if needed	Anti-muscarinic and calcium-channel blocking actions Improvement in frequency symptoms – useful in OAB dry Extended release	Side effects[a]
Beta- 3-Adrenergic Agonist				
Mirabegron	50 mg once daily	25 mg in renal or hepatic impairment	β–3-adrenoreceptor causing bladder relaxation Similar clinical effectiveness to anti-muscarinics Can be used when anti-muscarinic drugs are contraindicated, clinically ineffective or have unacceptable side effects	Hypertension, headache, painful micturition/UTI, tachycardia and bowel dysfunction
Third line				
Intravesica IBotulinumtoxin A	Botox 100–200 IU Dysport 250 IU	-	See text	-

[a] Common anticholinergic side effects: dry mouth, blurred vision, tachycardia, constipation, dyspepsia.

[b] Central nervous system side effects: disorientation, hallucinations, convulsions, cognitive impairment.

Contraindications: untreated narrow angle glaucoma, myasthenia gravis, bladder retention, bowel obstruction, severe ulcerative colitis.

Case Scenario 20.4

Jane was commenced on solifenacin 10 mg once a day but could not tolerate the problematic side effects. Jane switched to mirabegron 50 mg once a day and continued her vaginal oestrogens with good improvement in her symptoms.

Twelve months after initial presentation, the patient reported her OAB symptoms to be well controlled and significant weight loss to a BMI of 32, but her stress UI had returned. At this point Jane's GP referred her for secondary care assessment which included urodynamic investigation, which confirmed mixed UI (stress UI and detrusor overactivity).

Pharmacological Treatment for Stress Urinary Incontinence

Duloxetine is the only drug therapy licensed for moderate to severe SUI. Duloxetine is a serotonin and noradrenaline reuptake inhibitor, which acts to increase pudendal nerve activity and ultimately increases urethral sphincter contraction and closure pressure.

A short-term study [16] suggests that the use of duloxetine is associated with a reduction in leakage episodes and improved quality of life in women with SUI or MUI, but it causes a high rate of gastrointestinal side effects (mainly nausea and vomiting), leading to a high rate of treatment discontinuation. Starting at a 20 mg BD dose for two weeks and increasing to 40 mg BD after that can reduce the incidence of side effects.

NICE recommends that duloxetine should only be offered as second-line therapy in women wishing to avoid surgery [8].

Surgical Management Options for Urinary Incontinence

Overactive Bladder/Detrusor Overactivity

Botulinum toxin A blocks the release of acetylcholine and can relax the overactive detrusor muscle when injected directly into it. It is important for patients to understand it is a treatment, not a cure, and that the injection would need to be repeated every 6–12 months. In most hospital units it can be performed in the outpatient setting, not just under general anaesthetic.

For patients considering intravesical botox injections, urodynamics must be performed first and the patients case discussed at a local multidisciplinary team meeting. NICE suggests offering bladder wall botulinum toxin A injections:

- in women with proven detrusor overactivity which has not responded to conservative or drug therapy
- in women with symptoms of OAB but urodynamics does not demonstrate DO if symptoms have not responded to conservative or drug therapy.

All women need to understand the risks and benefits of botox before its administration and must be counselled and able to perform intermittent self-catheterisation (5–20% risk of urinary retention). The British Society of Urogynaecology (BSUG) quotes symptom improvement in 70% of patients. There is also evidence that long-term use does not cause bladder damage [17].

Percutaneous sacral nerve stimulation (PTNS) uses implantable electrical stimulation of the sacral (S3) reflex pathway to inhibit the reflex behaviour of the bladder and reduce detrusor overactivity. NICE recommends these treatments should only be offered to women if their OAB symptoms have not responded to conservative management, including drugs, or are unable to perform intermittent self-catheterisation. Prior to having PTNS, patients need discussion at a local or regional multidisciplinary team meeting. Success rates are 55–65% for symptomatic improvement [8].

Adverse effects are pain at implant site, leg pain, disturbed bowel function, urinary retention, anal pain and skin irritation at implant site. It is also important to be aware it is very labour intensive, with patients having to attend weekly for 12 weeks and then often they will need monthly top-ups depending on their symptoms.

Stress Urinary Incontinence

The once popular transvaginal tape is now not recommended after the high-vigilance restrictions put in place in 2018 by NHS England and NHS Improvement. NICE [8] recommends women read the decision aid on surgery for SUI to promote informed patient choice and decision-making. Prior to committing to a surgical intervention, patients need to be aware of:

- benefits and risks of all surgical options and if they are available locally
- uncertainties about long-term complications for all procedures including mesh procedures
- different anaesthetic, length of stay, surgical incisions and post-op recovery needed for each procedure
- any social or psychological factors that may impact on a woman's decision-making.

If the patient fails non-surgical management, then the surgical procedures offered are:

- colposuspension – open, laparoscopic or robotic
- autologous rectus fascial slings
- retropubic mid-urethral mesh slings (less popular and unavailable until a mesh registrar has been created).

If the above procedures are not acceptable to the patient, then you should consider offering *intramural urethral bulking agents*. Bulking agents, such as Bulkamid®, are injected in the urethral submucosa at the bladder neck. This is thought to improve SUI symptoms by increasing resting tone and pressure of the sphincter.

Patients should be seen by six months post-op to review their symptoms post-SUI surgery.

Case Scenario 20.6

Jane was discussed at a multidisciplinary team meeting about her symptoms and urodynamic findings. She opted for surgical intervention with an autologous fascial sling after counselling and review of the NICE operative SUI decision aid. She continued with her anti-muscarinic therapy for treatment of her OAB symptoms. Her three-month postoperative check reported excellent results and Jane's quality of life had significantly improved.

Conclusions

Female UI is a chronic, debilitating symptom that a GP will encounter frequently in their practice. The psychological impact of the condition is far-reaching and clinicians should take an empathic and caring approach to the management of UI.

The aim is for a patient-centred treatment bundle, which educates and empowers women to self-care in adjunct to additional conservative, pharmacological and surgical treatments. Ensuring all conservative and appropriate first-line pharmacological treatments have been undertaken allows swifter action in secondary care and that the right patients are being referred for more invasive interventions.

It is also important to engage multidisciplinary expertise using community-based continence teams and secondary care professionals in a stepwise approach.

References

[1] A. A. Ford, L. Rogerson, J. D. Cody and J. Ogah, 'Mid-urethral sling operations for stress urinary incontinence in women', *Cochrane Database Syst Rev.*, vol. 7, CD006375, 2015.

[2] J. Cooper, M. Annappa and A. Quigley, 'Prevalence of female urinary incontinence and its impact on quality of life in a cluster population in the United Kingdom (UK): A community survey', *Prim Health Care Res Dev*, vol. 16, no. 4, pp. 377–382, 2015.

[3] C. D. D'Ancona, B. T. Haylen, M. Oelke et al., 'An International Continence Society (ICS) report on the terminology for adult male lower urinary tract and pelvic floor symptoms and dysfunction', *Neurourol Urodyn*, vol. 38, no. 2, pp. 433–477, 2019.

[4] B. T. Haylen, D. de Ridder, R. M. Freeman et al., 'An International Urogynecological Association (IUGA)/International Continence Society (ICS) joint report on the terminology for female pelvic floor dysfunction', *Neurourol Urodyn*, vol. 29, pp. 4–20, 2010.

[5] S. Papanicolaou, M. Pons, C. Hampel et al., 'Medical resource utilisation and cost of care for women seeking treatment for urinary incontinence in an outpatient setting: Examples from three countries participating in the PURE study', *Maturitas*, vol. 52(Suppl. 2), pp. S35–S47, 2005.

[6] NHS England, 'Excellence in continence care'. 2018. Accessed: 14 Nov. 2025. [Online]. Available: www.england.nhs.uk/wp-content/uploads/2018/07/excellence-in-continence-care.pdf.

[7] P. Nicolson, Z. Kopp, C. R. Chapple and C. Kelleher, '"It's just the worry about not being able to control it!": A qualitative study of living with overactive bladder', *Br J Health Psychol*, vol. 13(Pt 2), pp. 343–359, 2008.

[8] National Institute for Health and Care Excellence, 'Urinary incontinence and pelvic organ prolapse in women: Management'. 2019. Accessed: 14 Nov. 2025. [Online]. Available: www.nice.org.uk/guidance/ng123.

[9] A. Tamilselvi and A. Rane, *Principles and Practice of Urogynaecology*. Springer, 2015.

[10] M. Parsons and L. Cardozo, *Female Urinary Incontinence in Practice*. The Royal Society of Medicine Press, 2004.

[11] I. Sarris, S. Bewley and S. Agnihotri, 'The pelvic floor and continence'. In Gardiner, M. (ed.), *Training in Obstetrics and Gynaecology: The Essential Curriculum*, Oxford University Press, 2009, pp. 380–390.

[12] K. Avery, J. Donovan, T. Peters, C. Shaw, M. Gotoh and P. Abrams, 'ICIQ: A brief and robust measure for evaluating the symptoms and impact of urinary incontinence', *Neurourol Urodynam*, vol. 23, no. 4, pp. 322–330, 2004. (ICIQ modules can be requested through the ICIQ website, www.iciq.net, and are free for clinical and academic use.)

[13] Your Pelvic Floor, 'Bladder diary'. 2024. Accessed: 14 Nov. 2025. [Online]. Available: www.yourpelvicfloor.org/conditions/bladder-diary-2/#Sample%20Diary.

[14] G. Herbison and N. Dean, 'Weighted vaginal cones for urinary incontinence', *Cochrane Database Syst Rev*, vol. 7, CD002114, 2013.

[15] C. Phillips, T. Hillard, S. Salvatore, L. Cardozo and P. Toozs-Hobson (on behalf of the Royal College of Obstetricians and Gynaecologists), 'Laser treatment for genitourinary syndrome of menopause', *BJOG*, vol. 129, pp. e89–e94, 2022.

[16] P. A. Norton, N. R. Zinner, I. Yalcin and R. C. Bump, 'Duloxetine versus placebo in the treatment of stress urinary incontinence', *Am J Obstet Gynecol*, vol. 187, no. 1, pp. 40–48, 2002.

[17] BSUG, 'Botox injections to treat overactive bladder'. 2019. Accessed: 14 Nov. 2025. [Online]. Available: https://bsug.org.uk/budcms/includes/kcfinder/upload/files/Botox-BSUG-Dec-2019.pdf.

Chapter 21

Managing Cystitis in Primary Care

Catriona Anderson

Key Points

- Cystitis is inflammation of the bladder and can have several causes, but most commonly is due to a urinary tract infection (UTI)/bacteriuria.
- Antibiotics should be considered for patients presenting with two or more classical cystitis symptoms once other causes are eliminated.
- Urine dipsticks are unreliable in up to 50% of cases.
- A standard MSU culture may not detect a UTI.
- Antibiotic or urinary antiseptic prophylaxis can be considered for patients with recurrent UTI.
- Bladder pain syndrome (BPS)/interstitial cystitis (IC) is a poorly understood condition, often misdiagnosed, and causes significant morbidity with limited treatment options.

Cystitis is inflammation of the bladder; it usually affects the mucosa but can involve the muscle layer. Although cystitis most commonly occurs due to infection, it can occur through non-infective causes including tumours and reactions to drugs/chemicals (e.g. chemotherapy or ketamine), as well as immunological, radiotherapy or traumatic irritation (e.g. catheter trauma, post-surgery or post-partum). As the most common cause is infection, of which 90% are due to *E. coli* bacteria, laypeople often use the terms cystitis and urinary tract infection interchangeably which can lead to confusion in the diagnosis.

Urinary Tract Infection

UTIs are a significant cause of morbidity in females of all ages, children and older men. UTIs are the commonest bacterial infection in women; however, there is a paucity of good-quality data regarding their true incidence. Serious sequalae include frequent recurrences, pyelonephritis, sepsis, renal damage, pre-term birth and issues associated with antibiotic use such as gastrointestinal side effects. Because of the high prevalence of UTI, there are large associated socioeconomic consequences as well as widespread impact on the quality of life [1].

Typical symptoms of a UTI include dysuria, frequency, urgency and lower abdominal pain. Risk factors to acquiring a UTI include sexual activity, poor fluid intake, constipation, bladder instrumentation, anatomical anomalies and indeed non-infective cystitis can increase susceptibility to a true UTI. A revision of the National Institute for Health and Care Excellence (NICE) guidance released in February 2023 stated 'women who present with two or more symptoms should not require a dipstick test' to receive treatment [2]. This is a welcome addition to the guidelines which is helping to clear confusion over misuse of urinary dipsticks which are known to give negative results in up to 50% of cases of acute UTI. Hopefully using this guideline will result in more cases receiving prompt treatment, preventing further complications developing if infections are left untreated [3].

The number of false-negative dipsticks and false-negative standard cultures is considerably higher in patients with recurrent UTIs, leading to false reassurance and increases the risk of a worsening condition. There is also evidence that enhanced rather than standard culture techniques will give a more comprehensive analysis resulting in better clinical outcomes [4].

NICE states 'empirical antibiotics can be considered depending on the severity of the symptoms, risk of developing complications and previous infections and antibiotic use'. Non-pregnant adult women should be counselled about self-care measures such as fluids and simple analgesia with a backup prescription for a three-day course of first-line antibiotic such as Nitrofurantoin or Trimethoprim; of course, local guidelines, culture results and the patient's antibiotic history should also be considered when selecting the antibiotic. Pivmecillinam and Fosfomycin are considered second-line choices. Longer courses of antibiotics (usually seven days) are advocated for pregnant women and complicated infections; attention to national and local guidelines is advised when selecting which type [5].

An 'uncomplicated infection' can be described as an infection of the bladder caused by typical pathogens in individuals with a normal urinary tract and kidney function and no predisposing co-morbidities (such as immunosuppression or poorly controlled diabetes). The definition excludes UTIs with an increased likelihood of complications such as persistent infection, treatment failure and recurrent infection. It also excludes cases where there are symptoms of pyelonephritis, such as fever or flank pain [6].

Recurrent UTI

UTI is a common infection with a high degree of recurrence. Recurrent UTI is medically defined as 2 or more episodes in 6 months or 3 in 12 months [6]. Three episodes in 12 months is usually regarded as the standard definition because 2 episodes within 6 months may simply represent a relapse of the initial infection.

More than 53% of women over the age of 55 experience a recurrence within one year of an infection, whereas approximately 36% of younger women will experience a recurrence within the year [7]. Urinary symptoms are noted to be most common in menopausal and postmenopausal women [26]; 8–11% of postmenopausal women report persistently recurrent UTIs and, across all ages, approximately 3% of women [8].

Although generally not life-threatening, the impact of recurrent UTIs on quality of life, healthcare and socioeconomic costs should not be underestimated. Some women suffer such frequently recurrent UTIs that their symptoms can be regarded as chronic and, in common with other chronic diseases, report associated high levels of anxiety and depression [9].

There is currently no medical definition for a chronic UTI, although key opinion leaders acknowledge that the phenomenon exists, underpinned by recent research discoveries [10]. The original research by Hultgren et al. demonstrated that bacteria could embed within uroepithelial cells lining the bladder, forming small reservoirs of infecting bacteria which seed repeated infections and most likely underpin chronic symptoms of cystitis (see Figure 21.1) [7]. Indeed, a SNOMED CT (Systemized Nomenclature of Medicine – Clinical Terms) code for chronic UTI exists and it is anticipated that a medical definition will be available in the near future.

Interestingly, there is now evidence to support the theory that certain genetic polymorphisms render some people more susceptible to bacterial infection with respect to vaginal and bladder mucosal receptor expression. This may be observed in the family history with patients describing a family tendency to recurrent UTIs [11].

Treatment

For patients meeting the diagnostic criteria for recurrent UTI, a prophylactic course of low-dose antibiotics can be given. A narrow-spectrum antibiotic should be the first choice, given to adults over the age 16, after behavioural and self-care measures have failed to reduce infections [4]. A large Cochrane database meta-analysis showed antibiotics confer a 79% risk reduction for recurrence while on prophylaxis, which falls to 18% risk reduction for recurrence upon completing the prophylactic treatment [12].

NICE recommend six-monthly reviews of antibiotic prophylaxis to assess for adverse effects and to consider the risk of resistance with long-term use. An alternative option is methenamine hippurate, a urinary antiseptic which has been in use for many decades but decreased in use when antibiotic prophylaxis took over, mainly due to lack of trial evidence. This was addressed when the *BMJ* published the ALTAR study in March 2022 demonstrating non-inferiority of this urinary antiseptic in comparison to first-line antibiotic prophylaxis in this intention-to-treat, head-to-head trial.

The Role of Oestrogen

It is known that oestrogen deficiency can contribute to urogenital atrophy exhibiting vaginal and/or urinary symptoms and an increased risk of recurrent UTI. Hormone receptors have been found in vaginal, urethral, bladder and pelvic floor tissues and are known to play a vital role in maintaining health in these areas [14].

Reduced oestrogen levels lead to decreased glycogen and thinning of vaginal epithelium, resulting in loss of a both healthy microbiome and

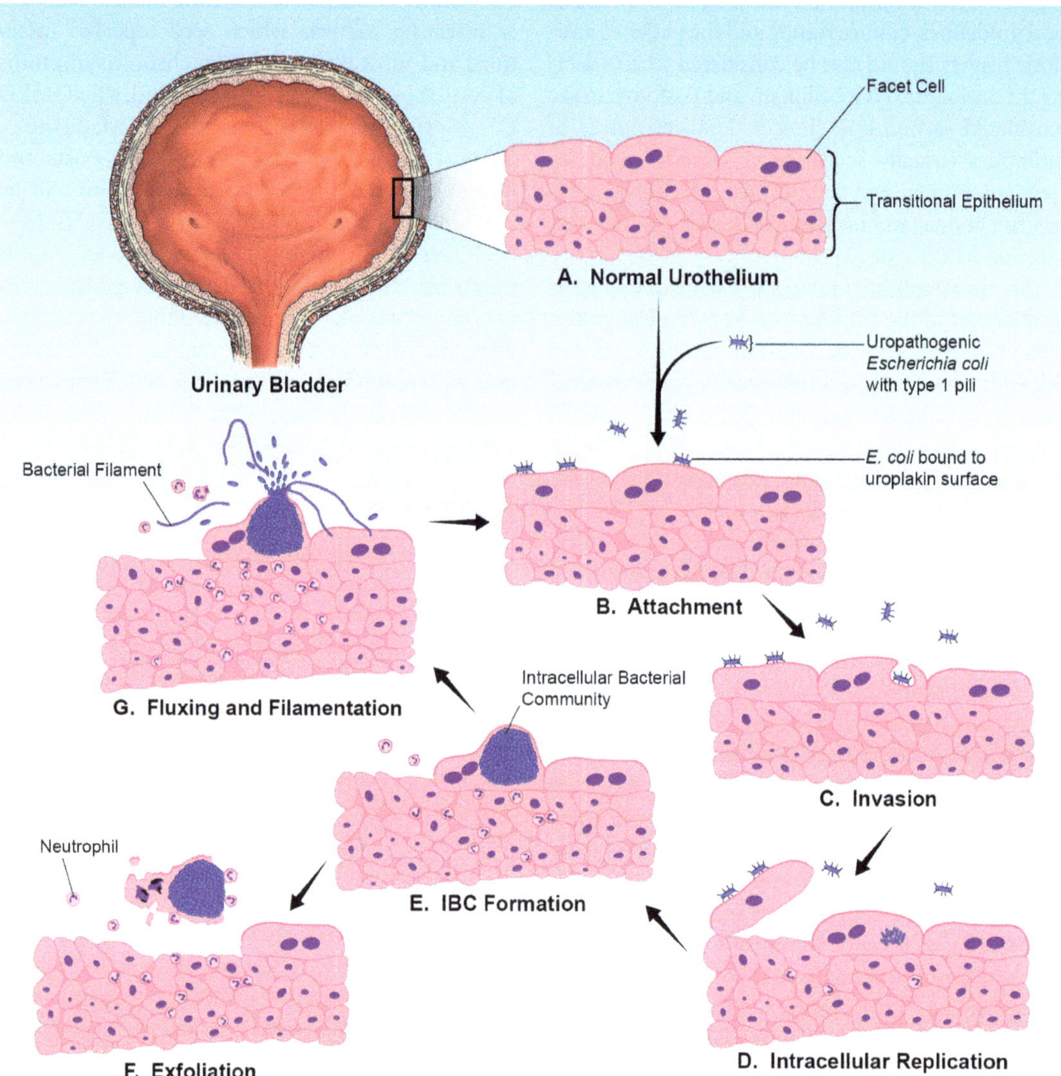

Figure 21.1 Uropathogenic *Escherichia coli* (UPEC) bind to, invade and replicate within the murine bladder urothelium to form intracellular bacterial communities (IBCs) observed in murine cystitis model [27].

vaginal acidity, with subsequent colonisation of uropathogens such as *E. coli* bacteria [15]. Once a vaginal reservoir of uropathogens has been established, the risk of transfer to the urethra is high, potentially leading to recurrent UTIs.

Randomised controlled trials in the 1990s demonstrated that intravaginal oestrogen treatment significantly decreased the incidence of UTI and reduced vaginal pH without adverse events. It was also claimed that systemic oral oestrogen hormone replacement therapy (HRT) was not effective in reducing recurrent UTIs and may cause unwanted side effects [16,17]. However, the data came from old trial evidence and systemic HRT preparations have since improved. It would be advantageous to repeat a trial using modern systemic preparations across a larger study population to establish if there is any benefit to be gained from systemic HRT in addition to local topical oestrogen.

Looking at its mode of action, oestrogen has been shown to stimulate secretion of antimicrobial peptides in both bladder and vaginal cells which contribute to innate defence mechanisms [18]. It has been well demonstrated that for postmenopausal women the most significant risk factor in recurrent urinary symptoms/recurrent

UTIs is oestrogen deficiency [19]. NICE guidelines state that topical vaginal oestrogen reduces the risk of recurrent UTIs in postmenopausal women compared to placebo and recommends the use of topical oestrogen. This is based on evidence cited in a systematic review in 2018 [20].

There are several options for topical hormone replacement ranging from low-dose estriol cream, pessaries or gel to the more potent oestradiol pessaries. An alternative is dehydroepiandrosterone (DHEA), a steroid prohormone in the biosynthetic pathway of oestradiol and testosterone. DHEA provides an acceptable and effective alternative for women whose symptoms do not improve with vaginal oestrogen, or simply as an alternative. Vaginal metabolism of DHEA leads to activation of oestrogen and testosterone receptors in the three layers of the vaginal wall without activating any response in the endometrium [21,22].

Interstitial Cystitis/Bladder Pain Syndrome

With refractory cystitis symptoms a further diagnosis to consider is interstitial cystitis (IC), also known as bladder pain syndrome (BPS). It is a poorly understood condition of unknown aetiology and diagnostic uncertainty with a paucity of effective treatments.

IC/BPS generally presents with lower urinary tract symptoms which meet with the description of cystitis, namely urinary frequency, nocturia, urgency and lower abdominal pain which is relieved on urination. Typically, this sensation is felt in the supra-pubic area, but it can be referred to areas located in the pelvis including the urethra, vagina, labia, inguinal area, perineum, lower abdomen and back. A diagnostic criterion for IC/BPS is the absence of infection underpinning the cystitis; however, it is said that up to 50% of patients will have a previous history of UTI. It is important to elicit a comprehensive medical history, including past pelvic surgery or radiation, medications that can cause cystitis (non-steroidal anti-inflammatory drugs, cyclophosphamide and ketamine), fibromyalgia, depression, sexual dysfunction, autoimmune diseases, allergies and other gynaecological conditions (vulvodynia, endometriosis, dyspareunia). The past medical history is important for diagnosis but also because many conditions may coexist. Frequency of micturition is by far the most common symptom, presenting in 92% of sufferers [23]. A diagnosis of IC/BPS is one of exclusion, but are we using accurate means to exclude other causes of this life-altering disease?

The lack of more accurate testing methods, together with a paucity of up-to-date evidence examining the validity of current quantitative threshold criteria for diagnosing UTI across the Western world, is known to result in gross underestimation of the true numbers of cystitis-like symptoms caused by bacteria.

A Belgian study in 2017 looked at 220 women with typical cystitis symptoms but negative standard culture. Urine samples were processed via more detailed extended culture and qPCR molecular analysis. In the symptomatic group, 80.9% of the urine cultures were positive for any uropathogens and 95.9% (211/220) were *E. coli* qPCR-positive. For the control group, healthy students, cultures for *E. coli* and *E. coli* qPCR were positive in 10.5% (9/86) and 11.6% (10/86), respectively. The authors concluded that almost all women with typical urinary complaints and a negative culture will have an infection with *E. coli* [24].

So, we must ask ourselves, are we failing to diagnose UTI effectively in some cases, relegating patients to a diagnosis of unknown aetiology and thereby failing to treat their infection due to our poor diagnostic methodology? Should we re-examine our approach in chronic cystitis? IC and BPS may well exist, but many urologists, urogynaecologists and GPs interested in this area think the real numbers of BPS/IC are very much lower than the numbers currently suggest. Studies examining quality of life among IC/BPS-affected patients reveal that females with IC had an overall lower quality of life than patients with end-stage renal failure [25]. So, is this another devastating condition suffered predominantly by women which has not attracted enough research and funding? See Table 21.1 for differential diagnoses for these patients.

Diagnosis and Treatment of IC/BPS

Diagnosis is one of exclusion but is largely based on history of urinary frequency and pain when the bladder is full. Cystoscopic appearances may be helpful in diagnosis; a biopsy will likely demonstrate chronic inflammatory change but is also important for ruling out neoplasm.

Table 21.1 Relevant diseases that may be confused with IC/BPS [28,29]

Disease	History details that can help exclude or diagnose
Endometriosis	Pain worse during menses or few days prior
Non-infectious cystitis	History of radiation, non-steroidal anti-inflammatory drugs, cyclophosphamide and/or ketamine use
Vulvar disorders	Pain occurs only during voiding, when urine contacts vulva and/or during painful sexual intercourse
Overactive bladder	Good response to anti-muscarinics, patient voids to avoid incontinence (vs. to relieve pain); no significant perceived bladder pain
Pudendal nerve entrapment	Worse with sitting, positional dependency suggests a neurogenic or musculoskeletal process
pelvic floor disorders	Trigger point, fascial or muscle pain, spasm on palpation

Treatments for this condition include: lifestyle and dietary modification; analgesia; neuromodulating medications including amitriptyline; intravesical treatments including dimethyl sulfoxide (DMSO), hyaluronic acid, chondroitin sulfate and lidocaine; implantable neurostimulation devices; cystoscopy and hydrodistension; and in some refractory cases surgery may even be offered following referral to a tertiary centre and multidisciplinary team review.

Conclusion

Lower urinary tract symptoms are one of the commonest presentations in primary care and most cases of cystitis will be caused by a bacterial infection. A negative dipstick and even a negative culture do not rule out the possibility that the patient's symptoms are caused by infection. A useful revision to the NICE guidelines in 2023 advises treating suspected UTI based on two or more typical symptoms. Patients with recurrent UTI should be offered prophylactic treatment and more complex cases should be referred into secondary care for further investigation and expert opinion. Recurrent and chronic cystitis can have a huge detrimental effect on a woman's physical, psychological health and overall wellbeing. Signposting the worst-affected patients to support organisations (see below) may be a useful step in helping to provide holistic care and reduce patient anxiety associated with this potentially life-altering condition.

Bladder & Bowel UK: www.bbuk.org.uk.

Bladder Health UK: www.bladderhealthuk.org.

Chronic Urinary Tract Infection Campaign: https://cutic.co.uk.

References

[1] B. Foxman, 'Epidemiology of urinary tract infections: Incidence, morbidity, and economic costs', *Am J Med*, vol. **113** (Suppl. 1A), pp. 5S–13S, 2002, http://doi.org/10.1016/s0002-9343(02)01054-9.

[2] NICE, 'Quality statements: Urinary tract infections in adults – Quality standards'. Accessed: 18 Nov. 2025. [Online]. Available: www.nice.org.uk/guidance/qs90/chapter/Quality-statements.

[3] S. Nys, T. van Merode, A. I. Bartelds and E. E. Stobberingh, 'Urinary tract infections in general practice patients: Diagnostic tests versus bacteriological culture', *J Antimicrob Chemother*, vol. **57**, no. 5, pp. 955–958, 2006, http://doi.org/10.1093/jac/dkl082.

[4] T. K. Price, T. Dune, E. E. Hilt et al., 'The clinical urine culture: Enhanced techniques improve detection of clinically relevant microorganisms', *J Clin Microbiol*, vol. **54**, no. 5, pp. 1216–1222, 2016, http://doi.org/10.1128/JCM.00044-16.

[5] NICE, 'Recommendations: Urinary tract infection (lower) – Antimicrobial prescribing guidance'. 2018. Accessed: 18 Nov. 2025. [Online]. Available: www.nice.org.uk/guidance/ng109/chapter/Recommendations#treatment-for-women-with-lower-uti.

[6] G. Bonkat, R. Pickard, R. Bartoletti et al., *EAU Guidelines on Urological Infections*. European Assoc Urology, 2018.

[7] C. M. Mitchell and L. E. Waetjen, 'Genitourinary changes with aging', *Obstet Gynecol Clin North Am*, vol. **45**, no. 4, pp. 737–750, 2018, http://doi.org/10.1016/j.ogc.2018.07.010.

[8] A. R. Brumbaugh and H. L. Mobley, 'Preventing urinary tract infection: Progress toward an effective Escherichia coli vaccine', *Expert Rev Vaccines*, vol. **11**, no. 6, pp. 663–676, 2012, http://doi.org/10.1586/erv.12.36.

[9] R. Ikäheimo, A. Siitonen, T. Heiskanen et al., 'Recurrence of urinary tract infection in a primary care setting: Analysis of a 1-year follow-up of 179 women', *Clin Infect Dis*, vol. **22**, no. 1, pp. 91–99, 1996, http://doi.org/10.1093/clinids/22.1.91.

[10] N. J. De Nisco, M. Neugent, J. Mull et al. 'Direct detection of tissue-resident bacteria and chronic inflammation in the bladder wall of postmenopausal women with recurrent urinary tract infection', *J Mol Biol*, vol. **431**, no. 21, pp. 4368–4379, 2019, http://doi.org/10.1016/j.jmb.2019.04.008.

[11] A. S. M. Ali, C. Mowbray, M. Lanz et al. 'Targeting deficiencies in the TLR5 mediated vaginal response to treat female recurrent urinary tract infection', *Sci Rep*, vol. **8**, no. 7(1), 11039, 2017, http://doi.org/10.1038/s41598-017-10445-4.

[12] X. Albert, I. Huertas, I. I. Pereiró, J. Sanfélix, V. Gosalbes and C. Perrota, 'Antibiotics for preventing recurrent urinary tract infection in non-pregnant women', *Cochrane Database Syst Rev*, vol. **3**, 2004, http://doi.org/10.1002/14651858.CD001209.pub2.

[13] C. Harding, H. Mossop, T. Homer et al., 'Alternative to prophylactic antibiotics for the treatment of recurrent urinary tract infections in women: Multicentre, open label, randomised, non-inferiority trial', *BMJ*, vol. **376**, 2022, http://doi.org/10.1136/bmj-2021-0068229.

[14] D. Robinson, P. Toozs-Hobson and L. Cardozo, 'The effect of hormones on the lower urinary tract', *Menopause Int*, vol. **19**, no. 4, pp. 155–162, 2013, http://doi.org/10.1177/1754045313511398.

[15] K. Gupta and W. E. Stamm, 'Pathogenesis and management of recurrent urinary tract infections in women', *World J Urol*, vol. **17**, no. 6, pp. 415–420, 1999, http://doi.org/10.1007/s003450050168.

[16] R. Raz and W. E. Stamm, 'A controlled trial of intravaginal estriol in postmenopausal women with recurrent urinary tract infections', *N Engl J Med*, vol. **329**, no. 11, pp. 753–756, 1993, http://doi.org/10.1056/NEJM199309093291102.

[17] J. Barclay, R. Veeratterapillay, C. Harding, 'Non-antibiotic options for recurrent urinary tract infections in women', *BMJ*, 23 Nov., j5193, 2017.

[18] V. Taneja, 'Sex hormones determine immune response', *Front Immunol*, vol. **9**, 1931, 2018, http://doi.org/10.3389/fimmu.2018.01931.

[19] I. Medina-Estrada, N. Alva-Murillo, J. E. López-Meza and A. Ochoa-Zarzosa, 'Immunomodulatory effects of 17β-estradiol on epithelial cells during bacterial infections', *J Immunol Res*, vol. 2018, 6098961, 2018, http://doi.org/10.1155/2018/6098961.

[20] V. Antoniou and B. K. Somani, 'Topical and oral oestrogen for recurrent urinary tract infection-evidence-based review of literature, treatment recommendations, and correlation with the European Association of Urology guidelines on urological infections', *Eur Urol Focus*, vol. **8**, no. 6, pp. 1768–1774, 2022, http://doi.org/10.1016/j.euf.2022.05.006.

[21] F. Labrie, D. F. Archer, W. Koltun et al. (VVA Prasterone Research Group), 'Efficacy of intravaginal dehydroepiandrosterone (DHEA) on moderate to severe dyspareunia and vaginal dryness, symptoms of vulvovaginal atrophy, and of the genitourinary syndrome of menopause', *Menopause*, vol. **23**, no. 3, pp. 243–256, 2016, http://doi.org/10.1097/GME.0000000000000571.

[22] I. Naumova and C. Castelo-Branco, 'Current treatment options for postmenopausal vaginal atrophy', *Int J Womens Health*, vol. **10**, pp. 387–395, 2018, http://doi.org/10.2147/IJWH.S158913.

[23] S. H. Berry, M. N. Elliott, M. Suttorp et al., 'Prevalence of symptoms of bladder pain syndrome/interstitial cystitis among adult females in the United States', *J Urol*, vol. **186**, no. 2, pp. 540–544, 2011, http://doi.org/10.1016/j.juro.2011.03.132.

[24] S. Heytens, A. De Sutter, L. Coorevits et al., 'Women with symptoms of a urinary tract infection but a negative urine culture: PCR-based quantification of Escherichia coli suggests infection in most cases', *Clin Microbiol Infect*, vol. **23**, no. 9, pp. 647–652, 2017, http://doi.org/10.1016/j.cmi.2017.04.004.

[25] Y. L. Michael, I. Kawachi, M. J. Stampfer, G. A. Colditz and G. C. Curhan, 'Quality of life among women with interstitial cystitis', *J Urol*, vol. **164**, no. 2, pp. 423–427, 2000.

[26] J. Anger, U. Lee, A. L. Ackerman et al., 'Recurrent uncomplicated urinary tract infections in women: AUA/CUA/SUFU Guideline', *J Urol*, vol. **202**, no. 2, pp. 282–289, 2019, http://doi.org/10.1097/JU.0000000000000296.

[27] D. A. Rosen, T. M. Hooton, W. E. Stamm, P. A. Humphrey and S. J. Hultgren, 'Detection of intracellular bacterial communities in human urinary tract infection', *PLoS Med*, vol. **4**, no. 12, 2007.

[28] A. Cox, N. Golda, G. Nadeau et al., 'CUA guideline: Diagnosis and treatment of interstitial cystitis/bladder pain syndrome', *Can Urol Assoc J*, vol. **10**, no. 5–6, 2016, http://doi.org/10.5489/cuaj.3786.

[29] D. G. Tincello and A. C. Walker, 'Interstitial cystitis in the UK: Results of a questionnaire survey of members of the Interstitial Cystitis Support Group', *Eur J Obstet Gynecol Reprod Biol*, vol. **118**, no. 1, pp. 91–95, 2005, http://doi.org/10.1016/j.ejogrb.2004.06.012.

Chapter 22

The Management of Ovarian Cysts in Primary Care

Aamena Salar

Key Points

- Almost all ovarian cysts in premenopausal women are benign.
- A transvaginal (TV) scan is far superior to a transabdominal scan.
- Care with the nomenclature used with patients helps to manage anxiety.
- The CA 125 assay is of little value in premenopausal women but should be used in all postmenopausal women.
- Risk assessment tools are more useful in postmenopausal women and will simplify management.
- In premenopausal women:
  - a simple cyst, measuring less than 50 mm in diameter, requires no follow-up
  - a larger simple cyst (50–70 mm) requires annual follow-up, and those greater than 70 mm are more likely to cause problems and should be referred.
- In postmenopausal women, where the risk of a malignancy is greater:
  - simple unilateral, unilocular ovarian cysts of less than 50 mm with a normal CA 125 can be managed conservatively; 50% of these will resolve spontaneously within three months
  - cysts of 20–50 mm should be rescanned every four months for one year, with repeat CA 125 assays every four months for one year
  - women with concerning features on ultrasound or raised CA 125 should be referred to the gynaecological oncologist.
- A widespread screening programme is not thought to be cost-effective.

Case Scenario 22.1: Alice

Alice, aged 47, attends the morning surgery. She is distressed. She presented with right iliac fossa pain one month ago, and some irregularities of her periods. She takes the progesterone-only pill as contraception. An ultrasound scan was requested, and this was performed yesterday. The report of the abdominal scan has not yet arrived, but on accessing the online report, it would appear that she has a right-sided loculated thin-walled simple ovarian cyst measuring 48 mm in its maximal diameter. The septum is thin. Her endometrial thickness is 10 mm and appropriate for the time in her menstrual cycle. Her aunt had ovarian cancer at the age of 72 and she wants to know what is going to happen next.

Definition

An ovarian cyst is a fluid-containing structure arising from the ovary measuring more than 30 mm in diameter. An ovarian follicle is an integral part of the ovary and should not exceed 30 mm in diameter.

Introduction

Ovarian cysts are extremely common, and up to 10% of women will have an operation during their life for investigation of an ovarian mass [1,2]. Most ovarian cysts are incidental findings on ultrasound scans performed for non-specific reasons such as irregular or heavy menstrual bleeding, pain or bloating. Of healthy postmenopausal women, 21% may have an ovarian cyst [3].

The risk of malignancy in a unilocular ovarian cyst in a premenopausal woman is very low at 0.1% [1], but the finding of solid and cystic elements on the ultrasound scan increases the risk of malignancy up to 17%. The risk of malignancy increases with cyst size, patient age and menopausal status.

The 2011 National Institute for Health and Care Excellence (NICE) guidelines [4] suggest that non-specific symptoms, such as persistent abdominal distension, satiety, bloating, pain, difficulty eating and urinary symptoms occurring regularly, particularly in the postmenopausal woman, should raise the index of suspicion of malignancy. Further investigations are warranted, with the recommendation that a vaginal examination is undertaken, and then the appropriateness of a serum CA 125 and transvaginal ultrasound considered. Care should be taken in menopausal women with a family or personal history of ovarian or breast malignancies.

Case Scenario 22.2: Alice

Alice is aged 47 and has regular menses. If her ovarian cyst is simple, she has approximately a 1:1000 risk of malignancy.

Physiology of the Menstrual Cycle

During the first half, or follicular phase, of the menstrual cycle, follicle-stimulating hormone (FSH) is released to stimulate follicular growth of both the endometrium and the ovaries. One of the ovarian follicles grows, and by about day 7, a dominant follicle will be established, usually in just one ovary. This follicle continues to grow, but any other stimulated follicles start to degenerate. The developing follicle produces oestrogen, and this has several effects. Firstly, it encourages the thickening of the endometrium, but secondly, at a certain level, the oestrogen also has a negative effect on the FSH production, ensuring that only one follicle matures. Thirdly, the rising oestrogen triggers the release of luteinising hormone (LH) from the pituitary gland over a 24-hour period (the LH surge), which is the stimulus for the follicle to release the ovum. The release of the ovum, or ovulation, generally occurs 36 hours after the LH surge.

The second half, or proliferative phase, of the menstrual cycle sees the remains of the dominant follicle (or corpus luteum as it is now called) producing oestrogen. This is driven by the LH. If fertilisation has not occurred, then the corpus luteum regresses, and levels of both hormones fall. The falling progesterone level is associated with the shedding of the endometrium, and menstruation begins.

Physiology of Ovarian Cysts

With the complex relationships between FSH, LH, oestrogen and progesterone, and the production of a dominant follicle with every menstrual cycle, it is not difficult to understand why, in some women, ovulation and the subsequent disintegration of the corpus luteum does not occur. Several dominant follicles may appear without one single follicle dominating. Why some premenopausal women appear to be regular cyst formers, and why it occurs at all in postmenopausal women, remains a mystery. There is no doubt, however, that the use of the correct terminology can alleviate anxiety. Women generally consider a 'cyst' to be pathological but a 'follicle' to be physiological, so care with the nomenclature at the outset of the diagnosis can pave the way for less stressful management. In gynaecological terms, a 'follicle' is anything up to 30 mm in diameter, but 'cyst' is anything larger than this.

Case Scenario 22.3: Alice

So, what do we do with Alice? She wants to know if she has cancer.

Assessment of Patients with Ovarian Cysts

Initially, a thorough history should be taken, and particular attention should be paid to her risk factors, protective factors, menopausal status and symptoms.

Risk factors include personal or family history of breast, uterine, colonic or ovarian cancer, including the hereditary cancer syndromes (BRCA gene mutation or Lynch syndrome).

Protective factors include a previous pregnancy and breastfeeding, which confer a 50% reduction in risk. It is thought that current use of the combined oral contraceptive pill also confers protection, but use of hormone replacement therapy (HRT) can increase the risk [5].

Symptoms of concern include persistent abdominal bloating, feeling full and/or loss of appetite, pelvic or abdominal pain and increased urinary urgency and/or frequency, particularly if they occur more than 12 times each month. Other worrying symptoms would be unexplained weight loss, fatigue or changes in bowel habit. It is rare for women to develop irritable bowel syndrome over the age of 50, so symptoms suggestive of this should trigger the exclusion of ovarian pathology. These are, of course, very common symptoms in primary care, making it easy to overlook the diagnosis of ovarian malignancy.

Clinical examination should include an assessment for a pelvic or abdominal mass, ascites, abdominal pain and lymphadenopathy.

The Vaginal Examination

If a cyst has already been diagnosed on ultrasound scan, then a pelvic examination will not offer much additional information. An assessment of mass tenderness, mobility, nodularity and the presence or absence of ascites or lymphadenopathy may aid the diagnosis. The vaginal examination is known to have poor sensitivity in the detection of ovarian masses (between 15% and 51%) [6].

What Sort of Scan Is Best?

It is now widely accepted that a transvaginal ultrasound scan is considered the gold standard and is preferable to an abdominal ultrasound scan, because the better resolution gives much clearer images (Figure 22.1). This is particularly true for women with a high body mass index (BMI), simply because the TV transducer starts imaging much closer to the pelvic organs, with less chance of artefactual deterioration of the scanned images. Women may be initially concerned at the appearance of the TV probe, which can look quite intimidating, but anecdotal evidence would suggest that women prefer the TV scan to the discomfort associated with the pressure being applied to the abdomen in the presence of a full bladder. The TV probe has a scanning depth of 5–10 cm whereas the abdominal transducer has a scanning depth of 10–15 cm. Certainly the TV scan is essential when looking for small pelvic changes, such as a tiny intrauterine gestation sac, or a possible ectopic pregnancy. However, the abdominal transducer may be preferred in some groups of women:

- those who have never experienced sexual intercourse
- those with such a large pelvic mass that 10 cm is an inadequate scanning depth to visualise the mass fully
- those with an axial uterus (as opposed to anteverted or retroverted), which can be more difficult to visualise with the TV probe, particularly in the larger woman.

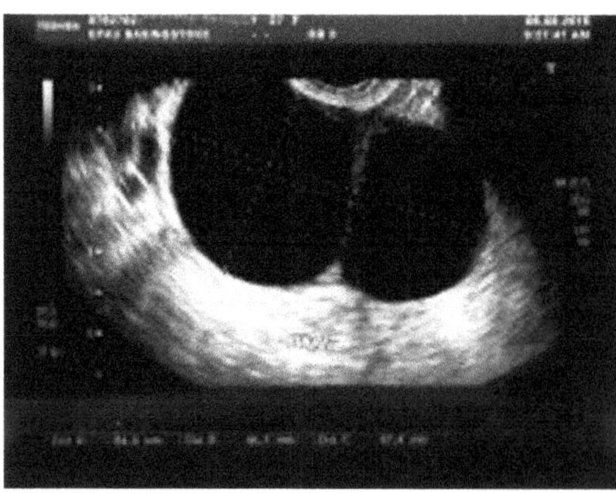

Figure 22.1 Bilocular ovarian cyst on TV scan.

The use of colour doppler has not really helped scanning diagnostic accuracy but may help in the more detailed assessment of a complex mass and is favoured by some specialists. Unless the cyst is large (greater than 10 cm in diameter), the use of CT or MRI scanning often adds little to the diagnostic process, but may help in the assessment of complex lesions, lymphadenopathy or metastases.

How Does a Clinician Assess an Ovarian Cyst on Scanning?

The system most widely used in the assessment of ovarian cysts is that of 'pattern recognition' of specific ultrasound findings [7,8]. Pattern recognition assesses the appearance of the cyst on ultrasound and classifies the findings into benign (B-rules) and malignant (M-rules). The sonographer essentially considers:

- size
- wall thickness
- whether it is unilocular or multilocular
- the thickness of the division between the locules
- the presence or absence of solid components
- the presence of acoustic shadowing
- the presence of ascites
- bilateral lesions
- blood flow.

This allows the clinician to assign an objective numerical score to the ultrasound report. A small, thin-walled unilocular cyst with no solid components would be described as simple and of low concern. Unsurprisingly, the expertise of the sonographer is extremely important in this assessment.

Case Scenario 22.4: Alice

Alice will be best assessed with a transvaginal scan undertaken by an experienced sonographer. The scan she had done was an abdominal scan, with consequent images, and it may be that she needs to be re-referred for a second transvaginal scan, because in Alice's case the cyst is not truly 'simple'.

Which Are the Best Serum Markers to Use, and How Are They Interpreted?

The serum CA 125 glycoprotein antigen serum marker is currently considered the best serum marker available. However, it can be affected by many conditions seen in the premenopausal woman, such as menstruation, fibroids, adenomyosis and endometriosis. It is raised in only 50% of early epithelial carcinomas. A raised result should be treated with caution and considered only in addition to the ultrasonographic findings. It does not need to be assayed in all premenopausal women [1], and indeed, some consider it useless in these women [8].

The Royal College of Obstetricians and Gynaecologists (RCOG) therefore states that:

- a serum CA 125 is not necessary when a clear ultrasonographic diagnosis of a simple ovarian cyst has been made
- if a serum CA 125 is slightly raised, but less than 200 u/mL, further investigations may be necessary to exclude/treat the common differential diagnoses
- when a CA 125 level is raised, serial monitoring (after four to six weeks) may be helpful, as rapidly rising levels are more likely to be associated with malignancy
- if a CA 125 level is greater than 200 u/mL, discussion should take place with a gynaecological oncologist for further evaluation.

Lactate dehydrogenase (LDH), alpha fetoprotein (aFP) and human chorionic gonadotropin (hCG) should also be measured in all women under the age of 40 years with a complex ovarian mass, because of the possibility of germ-cell tumours. Human epididymis protein4 (HE4) is a tumour marker currently undergoing evaluation, and may prove superior to CA 125.

The Risk of Malignancy Index

The risk of malignancy index (RMI) is a risk assessment tool, used by hospital gynaecologists, first developed in 1991 by Sassone [9]. Used in the assessment of complex cysts, it is most useful in postmenopausal women. The RCOG suggests that it should only be employed if ovarian carcinoma is suspected in a premenopausal woman but used every time for a postmenopausal woman. Sassone [9] suggested:

$$\text{RMI} = \text{U} \times \text{M} \times \text{CA125}$$

where U = ultrasound score and M = 3 for all postmenopausal women, but M = 1 for premenopausal women multiplied by the absolute value of the CA 125. Postmenopausal status is considered to be the absence of periods for 12 months, or women over 50 years of age who have had a hysterectomy. Anything above 250 was deemed to be at high risk of malignancy. This index, set at this level, has a sensitivity of 70% and a specificity of 90% [10].

- RMI < 25, the risk of cancer is < 3%.
- RMI > 25, but < 250, risk of cancer 20%.
- RMI > 250, risk of cancer 75%.

Many other models have been produced in an attempt to improve upon the RMI, but the original 1991 model remains the best and most widely used.

So, What Is the Best Diagnostic Tool for Ovarian Cancer?

ROCkeTS (2024) is a multicentre, prospective diagnostic accuracy study aimed to identify the best diagnostic test for ovarian cancer in symptomatic patients, through head-to-head comparisons of risk-prediction models, in the postmenopausal cohort. The study concluded that ultrasound using International Ovarian Tumour Analysis (IOTA) group ultrasound rules for ovarian masses had a higher sensitivity than RMI at 250. The recommendation was that IOTA should be considered as the new standard-of-care diagnostic in ovarian cancer for postmenopausal patients.

Ovarian Cysts in Premenopausal Women

The chance of sinister pathology in premenopausal women is very low. The overall incidence of a symptomatic ovarian cyst in a premenopausal woman being malignant is approximately 1:1000, increasing to 3:1000 by the age of 50. Differentiation between benign and malignant ovarian masses in the premenopausal women can be difficult, as the CA 125 serum marker is not very helpful. The markers, AFP, hCG, and LDH [11], may be of use with a complex cyst.

A functional or simple ovarian cyst is a thin-walled cyst without any internal structures seen on the ultrasound scan and measuring less than 50 mm in their maximum diameter. The Society of Radiologists in Ultrasound concluded that asymptomatic simple cysts 30–50 mm in diameter do not require further imaging or follow-up as these usually resolve over two to three menstrual cycles [12]. Test of resolution is not required. A cyst greater than 50 mm is more likely to incur an ovarian accident, including torsion, rupture or haemorrhage.

Case Scenario 22.5: Alice

Alice has some concerning features on her ultrasound scan. The cyst is described as loculated, 40 mm in diameter, thin-walled and the septum between the locules is described as being thin. As her cyst is loculated, Alice requires a serum CA 125 performing. However, assuming she is premenopausal, her RMI will remain low.

Management of Ovarian Cysts in Premenopausal Women

The RCOG states that:

- as most women with small (less than 50 mm diameter) simple ovarian cysts are likely to be physiological, and will almost always resolve within three menstrual cycles, these women do not require follow-up and can be managed conservatively
- those with slightly larger simple unilocular ovarian cysts (50–70 mm in diameter) should have annual ultrasound follow-up
- those with symptomatic or larger simple cysts (> 70 mm) should be considered for further imaging or surgical intervention.

Alice's thin-walled 48 mm ovarian cyst with two locules and a family history of ovarian carcinoma may cause continuing concern. With this ultrasound appearance, however, her CA 125 and RMI will almost certainly be low. However, her family history may persuade you to rescan in three to four months' time, specifically requesting a transvaginal scan, for reassurance.

Asymptomatic cysts that persist or increase in size are unlikely to be functional and may warrant surgical management. Mature cystic teratomas (dermoid cysts) will grow over time, increasing the risk of pain and ovarian accidents. These cysts have a characteristic ultrasound appearance and would not be described as 'simple', so the guidelines would suggest CA 125 and referral. An evidence-based consensus regarding the upper limit of size that would indicate surgical management does not exist, but most studies would suggest an arbitrary maximum diameter of 50–60 mm.

Case Scenario 22.6: Alice

Alice accepts that you have considered her clinical condition and ultrasound findings carefully and you have agreed with her that, in view of her family history but low CA 125, she should be rescanned in three to four months.

However, after 10 weeks, Alice re-presents to you with right iliac fossa pain of sudden onset 6 hours previously. She has been vomiting with the pain. Her bowels remain normal. She assures you that she has continued to take the contraceptive pill on a regular basis with no missed pills. Clinical examination reveals that she is apyrexial, her pulse is 85 b/min and she has significant abdominal pain, but no guarding or rebound. Her bowel sounds are normal. A pregnancy test is negative, and her urine is clear on dipstick testing.

What Can Go Wrong with Ovarian Cysts?

Rupture

Women who present acutely with lower abdominal pain, and a collapsed cyst on ultrasound with free fluid in the pouch of Douglas, may have a ruptured ovarian cyst. An ectopic pregnancy needs to be excluded by ensuring a pregnancy test is negative. Uncomplicated cyst ruptures can be managed at home with analgesia and advice, as symptoms usually resolve within 24–72 hours. However, some patients develop a haemoperitoneum, and management in a hospital may be required. Occasionally, a laparoscopy may be indicated.

Torsion

If an ovary twists partially or completely on its pedicle of supporting ligaments, it may cut off its blood supply. The patient might present with sudden onset lower abdominal pain, vomiting and possibly a palpable, tender adnexal mass. The diagnosis is usually made clinically, but a USS will contribute to the diagnosis and could show a reduced ovarian blood flow on doppler and maybe the presence of free fluid in the pouch of Douglas. Benign cysts greater than 50 mm, and particularly dermoid cysts, are at the greatest risk of torsion.

Laparoscopy is usually required to de-tort and conserve the ovary, but oophorectomy may take place if the ovary is not viable.

Pregnant Women with Ovarian Cysts

Women are scanned more frequently in pregnancy and incidental ovarian cysts are commonly found; 50% resolve spontaneously during the pregnancy. These may be related to a persistent corpus luteum of early pregnancy. With expectant management, the reported rate of complications is < 2% [13]. A cyst seen on an eight-week dating scan will be reviewed regularly at routine antenatal scans. Intervention will be required if there is a suspicion of malignancy, if there is a complication, such as torsion, or if the size is so large that it is likely to cause obstetric problems. The best time to intervene is after the first trimester, when the miscarriage rate decreases. The risk of cancer in a pregnant woman is less than 1% [14].

The Prevention and Treatment of Ovarian Cysts in Premenopausal Women

A small Cochrane review concluded that the combined oral contraceptive probably did not prevent the formation of new cysts or the resolution of existing cysts [15].

If intervention is required, the consensus is that it should be performed laparoscopically as it is safer, aesthetically more pleasing and more cost-effective. However, with a large mass, with solid components and a possible risk of malignancy, a laparotomy may be considered more appropriate. The aspiration of ovarian cysts, either vaginally or laparoscopically, is associated with high recurrence rates.

Case Scenario 22.6: Alice

Alice was admitted acutely under the gynaecologists and rescanned later that day. Her ovarian cyst had gone, but she had some free fluid in the pouch of Douglas. Her symptoms settled quickly with analgesia and with the reassurance that her scan was normal she was discharged from hospital.

Ovarian Cysts in Postmenopausal Women

Ovarian cysts are less common in postmenopausal women, but many are still found as incidental findings with the increasing use of ultrasound. Up to 21% may have abnormal morphology [2]. The RCOG states that as the risk of malignancy is greater in ovarian cysts in postmenopausal women, a TV ultrasound and a CA 125 assay should be performed in all these women. However, the risk of malignancy in a simple, unilateral, unilocular cyst less than 50 mm in diameter is still less than 1% [16]. A CA 125 of more than 30 u/mL has a sensitivity of 81% and specificity of 75% for the diagnosis of ovarian cancer in older women. The transvaginal ultrasound, in experienced hands, achieves a sensitivity of 89% and specificity of 73%. This result should be used in conjunction with the ultrasound findings and menopausal status. Other markers, such as the carcinoembryonic antigen (CEA) and cancer antigen 19.9, are of uncertain clinical significance.

Management of Ovarian Cysts in Postmenopausal Women

The RCOG states that:

- simple unilateral, unilocular ovarian cysts of less than 50 mm with a normal CA 125 can be managed conservatively; 50% of these will resolve spontaneously within three months
- cysts of 20–50 mm should be rescanned every four months [16,17] for one year, with repeat CA 125 assays every four months for one year [2]
- women with concerning features on ultrasound or raised CA 125 should be referred to the gynaecological oncologist
- any woman who does not meet the criteria for conservative management should be offered surgical management. An oophorectomy is recommended rather than a cystectomy, if a malignancy is suspected, as this allows complete removal of the cyst and the avoidance of any spillage into the

peritoneal cavity. Bilateral oophorectomy may be appropriate, as the contralateral ovary could be affected either now or in the future.

Screening the Population for Ovarian Cancer

For the general population routine screening does not have adequate sensitivity or specificity to be used as a mass screening test but is useful on an individual basis. Screening with the transvaginal ultrasound has a high false-positive rate, as it may be difficult to differentiate between malignant and benign masses. The serum CA 125 is affected by benign conditions and is not always raised. Women with a strong family history of ovarian or breast malignancies should have genetic counselling. Those who carry the BRCA1 mutation have a lifetime risk of ovarian cancer of 60%, and BRCA2 in the region of 40% [18].

Although there is no clear screening tool for ovarian cancer, recent research has emphasised the effectiveness of symptom-triggered testing for ovarian cancer. Kwong et al. [20] demonstrated that one in four women identified with high-grade serous ovarian cancer through the fast-track pathway following symptom-triggered testing was diagnosed with early-stage disease. Symptom-triggered testing may help identify women with a low disease burden, potentially contributing to high complete cytoreduction rates. This highlights the need for raising awareness among women about the symptoms of ovarian cancer. This is particularly including women of ethnic-minority backgrounds as the 2022 report *Achieving Excellence in Ovarian Cancer Care*, published by Target Ovarian Cancer, highlights significant disparities in ovarian cancer diagnosis and treatment across ethnic groups in the UK. It found that 34% of black women are diagnosed through an emergency presentation – the highest rate among ethnic groups – compared to 29% of white women. The report also revealed differences in treatment start times following referral: Asian women wait an average of 74.5 days, black women 73.5 days and white women 68 days [21] (Figure 22.2).

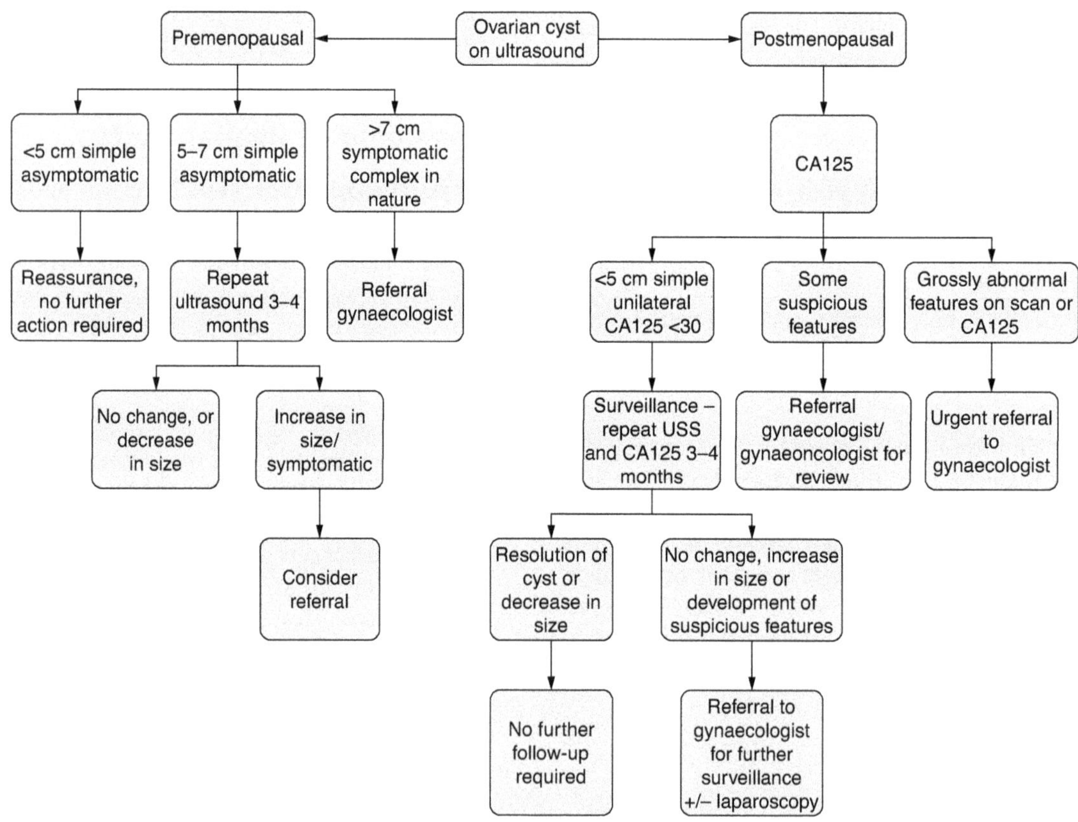

Figure 22.2 Management of ovarian cysts.

Conclusion

The discovery of an ovarian cyst can cause a great deal of anxiety for both patients and doctors. Appropriate risk assessment using the available tools in the correct hands will simplify their management and reduce concern. Using the correct nomenclature early in the diagnosis is important. Greater care is essential for postmenopausal women, particularly given the absence of an available screening programme.

References

[1] Royal College of Obstetricians and Gynaecologists, 'Management of suspected ovarian masses in premenopausal women'. Green-Top Guideline No. 62. RCOG, 2011.

[2] Royal College of Obstetricians and Gynaecologists, 'Ovarian cysts in postmenopausal women'. Green-Top Guideline No. 34. RCOG, 2003.

[3] U. Menon, A. Gentry-Maharaj, R. Hallett et al., 'Sensitivity and specificity of multimodal and ultrasound screening for ovarian cancer, and stage distribution of detected cancers: Results of the prevalence screen of the UK Collaborative Trial of Ovarian Screening (UKCTOCS)', *Lancet Oncol*, vol. **10**, no. 4, pp. 327–340, 2009.

[4] National Institute for Health and Care Excellence (NICE), 'Clinical guidance on ovarian carcinoma guidelines'. CG 122. 2011.

[5] Z. Kmietowicz, 'Short term use of HRT increases the risk of ovarian carcinoma', *BMJ*, vol. **350**, 2015.

[6] L. Padilla, D. Radosevich, M. Milad, 'Accuracy of the pelvic examination in detecting adnexal masses', *Obstet Gynecol*, vol. **96**, no. 4, pp. 593–598, 2000.

[7] D. Timmerman, L. Valentin, T. H. Bourne et al., 'Terms, definitions and measurements to describe the sonographic features of adnexal tumors: A consensus opinion from the International Ovarian Tumour Analysis (IOTA) Group', *Ultrasound Obstet Gynecol*, vol. **16**, no. 5, pp. 500–505, 2000.

[8] D. Timmerman, A. C. Testa, T. Bourne et al., 'Simple ultrasound-based rules for the diagnosis of ovarian cancer', *Ultrasound Obstet Gynecol*, vol. **31**, no. 6, pp. 681–690, 2008.

[9] A. M. Sassone, I. E. Timor-Tritsch, A. Artner, C. Westhoff and W. B. Warren, 'Transvaginal sonographic characterization of ovarian disease: Evaluation of a new scoring system to predict ovarian malignancy', *Obstet Gynecol*, vol. **78**, no. 1, pp. 70–76, 1991.

[10] A. P. Davies, I. Jacobs, R. Woolas, A. Fish and D. Oram, 'The adnexal mass: Benign or malignant? Evaluation of a risk of malignancy index', *Br J Obstet Gynaecol*, vol. **100**, no. 10, pp. 927–931, 1993.

[11] S. Sundar, R. Agarwal, C. Davenport et al., 'Risk-prediction models in postmenopausal patients with symptoms of suspected ovarian cancer in the UK (ROCkeTS): A multicentre, prospective diagnostic accuracy study', *Lancet Oncol*, vol. **25**, no. 10, pp. 1371–1386, 2024.

[12] American College of Obstetrics and Gynecology, 'Management of adnexal masses', *ACOG Bulletin*, vol. **110**, p. 1, 2007.

[13] D. Levine, D. L. Brown, R. F. Andreotti et al., 'Management of asymptomatic ovarian and other adnexal cysts imaged at US: Society of Radiologists in Ultrasound Consensus Conference Statement', *Radiology*, vol. **256**, no. 3, pp. 943–954, 2010.

[14] G. Zanetta, E. Mariani, A. Lissoni et al., 'A prospective study of the role of ultrasound in the management of adnexal masses in pregnancy', *BJOG*, vol. **110**, no. 6, pp. 578–583, 2003.

[15] G. S. Leiserowitz, G. Xing, R. Cress et al., 'Adnexal masses in pregnancy: How often are they malignant?', *Gynecol Oncol*, vol. **101**, no. 2, pp. 315–321, 2006.

[16] D. A. Grimes, L. B. Jones, L. M. Lopez and K. F. Schulz, 'Oral contraceptives for functional ovarian cysts', *Cochrane Database Syst Rev*, vol. **2**, CD006134, 2009.

[17] C. L. Bailey, F. R. Ueland, G. L. Land et al., 'The malignant potential of small cystic ovarian tumors in women over 50 years of age', *Gynecol Oncol*, vol. **69**, no. 1, pp. 3–7, 1998.

[18] J. M. Aubert, C. Rombaut, P. Argacha et al., 'Simple adnexal cysts in postmenopausal women: Conservative management', *Maturitas*, vol. **30**, no. 1, pp. 51–54, 1998.

[19] National Health and Medical Research Council, 'Clinical practice guidelines for the management of women with epithelial ovarian cancer'. CP98. NHMRC, 2004.

[20] F. L. A. Kwong, C. Kristunas, C. Davenport et al., 'Symptom-triggered testing detects early stage and low volume resectable advanced stage ovarian cancer', *Int J Gynecol Cancer*, vol. **36**, 101848, 2024, http://doi.org/10.1136/ijgc-2024-005371.

[21] Target Ovarian Cancer, 'Tackling inequalities in ovarian cancer care'. Accessed: 18 Nov. 2025. [Online]. Available: https://targetovariancancer.org.uk.

Chapter 23

Managing Menopause in Primary Care

Sarah Gray

Key Points

- Menopause is technically the last menstrual period. The term is more generally applied to the phase of midlife when women transition from regular periods to amenorrhoea.
- Oocyte numbers are maximal in the fifth month of gestation and reduce throughout life by the process of apoptosis. Spontaneous menopause is the final phase of this with symptoms attributable to the depletion in numbers and quality of remaining oocytes.
- Menstrual bleeding is driven by the cyclical change of ovarian hormones. Menopause transition is revealed by changes in bleeding patterns as well as symptoms. These arise from insufficiency of ovarian hormones, predominantly oestrogen, which act on many tissues but their effect on the central nervous system predominates in the early phases.
- Individuals vary greatly in their response to these changes and hence the expression of symptoms relating to menopause is not consistent. Symptom assessment relies on the identification of patterns.
- The diagnosis of menopause is clinical. As part of the assessment, clinicians should:
    - assess the health and social background of their patient. Menopause provides the ideal opportunity to discuss lifestyle modification that could affect both symptoms and longer-term health risks
    - offer options for intervention that are appropriate for the individual. Ensure that they understand how they should be used and their relative risks and benefits
    - review three months after initiation of any treatment or any change. Once stable, women should be reviewed annually.
- There is no set duration of intervention except for women with premature ovarian insufficiency (POI) who should be offered hormone replacement at least to the average age of menopause. After this age, an annual review should be continued to

  agree the most appropriate regime at lowest dose that is effective.

National guidance for the diagnosis and management of menopause was published in the UK in 2015 (NICE NG23). Their thorough review of available evidence, plus celebrity endorsement, media prominence and social media, has changed the landscape in the UK significantly. This is not yet mirrored globally.

GPs in the UK have experienced a significant increase in women presenting explicitly to discuss menopause. These patients have more information at the time of presentation than they would have had ten years ago. They want to discuss their difficulties with a confident and knowledgeable clinician. They want help.

This chapter will:

- summarise the physiological changes which occur during menopause transition
- develop clinical confidence in the diagnosis of menopause and provide a framework for risk benefit assessment
- develop an understanding of the options that can be offered in the primary care setting and strategies for explaining their suitability to the patient
- discuss review, problem-solving and troubleshooting.

Background

The term 'menopause' is derived from the Greek language and refers to the very last menstrual bleed that a woman experiences. It is a retrospective diagnosis identified when no bleeding has occurred for one year. This can be obscured if bleeding is suppressed by an intrauterine device, systemic hormone treatments or surgery. Symptoms relating to the reduction in hormone production can begin years before, at or after the last bleed, and a significant minority of women will have none that bother them. Try to understand which symptoms are experienced and the impact that they have on the woman's quality of life.

Physiology

The last bleed generally represents the cessation of cyclical ovarian activity. Women are born with a complement of oocytes which are progressively lost throughout life through programmed cell death (apoptosis). Each cycle involves recruitment and stimulation of one or more oocytes which produce oestrogen as they develop. Oestrogen levels peak at ovulation and then fall away, this becoming more marked with age. It is common for women in their 40s to describe oestrogen deficiency symptoms at the end of their luteal phase which during the early menstrual phase then resolve. These symptoms may begin up to 10 years before the last bleed.

The first change that is usually noticed at the beginning of menopause transition is a shortening of the menstrual cycle. This is attributed to the increasing oocyte resistance to stimulation, resulting in higher levels of follicle-stimulating hormone (FSH) and more rapid progression when response occurs. Fertility services will check FSH early in the cycle as a marker of ovarian response. Persistently raised levels suggest lack of response and are consistent with, but not diagnostic of, the postmenopausal state. Anti-Müllerian hormone (AMH) is used to assess ovarian reserve prior to assisted conception. Neither are recommended to diagnose menopause.

Progressively, oocyte resistance increases and when ovulation fails the woman will experience a longer than usual cycle and miss a period. She may or may not experience symptoms in the interim which resolve with the next period. It is impossible to predict an individual women's experience other than to say that anything could happen.

In the phase of menstrual chaos, it is important to remain alert for potential endometrial disease. Women who are obese, diabetic or have previous polycystic ovarian syndrome are more at risk. Bleeding which is post-coital, persistent, heavy or more than a year after the last period should be investigated.

Early loss of ovarian function can occur spontaneously and is thought to affect 1% of women under the age of 40. If under the age of 30, significant genetic/chromosomal causes should be considered.

Age at menopause can be affected by family history, nutrition, smoking, medication (particularly chemotherapy), radiation, infection, surgery and many other factors. It is particularly important to identify POI to avoid degenerative sequelae – particularly osteoporosis, but also coronary artery disease and loss of cognition. The term premature ovarian insufficiency has replaced ovarian failure as sometimes function will return, often sporadically.

In women, circulating androgen levels are much less than in men but still functionally important. Approximately half is derived from the ovarian stroma. Therefore, surgical removal, radiotherapy, significant vascular disruption or infection affecting the whole ovary can compromise androgens as well as oestrogen with associated symptoms.

Symptoms

Typical symptoms result from sensitivity to the reduction in oestrogen. This sensitivity will vary between women and is an explanation for the difference in experience. Oestrogen is pervasive, with receptors along with their activators/repressors in many tissues and the potential spectrum of deficiency symptoms is broad.

The absence of luteal phase progesterone may be seen as positive if this resolves a previous premenstrual syndrome.

Androgen lack can only be considered after correction of oestrogen deficiency.

Consider the following groups of symptoms.

Centrally Modulated Effects of Oestrogen – Due to Its Effect on the Central Nervous System

- *Flushes and sweats* – these are due to overreactivity of heat-losing mechanisms and are thought to result from a loss of temperature homeostasis (the thermoregulatory centre is located in the hypothalamus). Women will say that they feel as if their thermostat has 'packed up' and this appears to be close to the truth. After extreme sweating some women will feel cold and shiver as the response swings in the opposite direction.

Vasomotor symptoms are often the most recognised menopause-associated complaint. They tend to resolve with time, but this varies greatly. We quote three to seven years as typical, but some women continue to flush through their 60s and into their 70s with a few continuing beyond that.

- Sleep disturbance – although nighttime sweating can disturb sleep, it is now recognised that sleep disturbance is a separate phenomenon which can persist beyond the resolution of flushing. For some women this can be quite disabling.
- Mood change – a proportion of women will experience mood change. This can manifest as low mood, heightened anxiety, loss of confidence and emotional lability with a tendency to cry. Some describe themselves as irritable. Many of these women have had problems earlier in their lives with postnatal depression or premenstrual syndrome. Be alert for reported intolerance to contraceptive hormones as this may also indicate sensitivity.

Some women who previously experienced premenstrual mood change will paradoxically feel better after menopause if intolerance of progesterone had been their main problem rather than lack of oestrogen.

- Concentration and memory problems – these are very difficult to tease out as being menopausal. Life stresses, sleeping difficulties and age-related changes will all have an effect. Word-finding difficulty is commonly recognised and may be linked as there are many oestrogen receptors in the centre for verbal memory. Difficulty concentrating and making decisions are often described by women after early surgical menopause and abrupt loss of ovarian function. There is some research linking this to an increased risk of dementia in later life.

Musculoskeletal Effects of Oestrogen

Oestrogen has many roles in the metabolism of collagen, cartilage and bone. It is well established that bone resorption increases as oestrogen is depleted with a loss of 8–10% of bone mineral density in the first five or so postmenopausal years. Early menopause is a significant risk for subsequent osteoporosis and fracture. Bone loss does not cause symptoms until a fracture occurs. Some women do experience otherwise unexplained aches and pains which resolve with oestrogen replacement. This is poorly characterised but potentially linked to effects on collagen.

Urogenital Effects of Oestrogen

Oestrogen exerts a trophic influence on the tissues of the vagina and lower urinary tract. With depletion comes progressive atrophic change that results in thinning, loss of elasticity and vaginal dryness, which affects almost 50% of women by three years after the last period. There may be itching (often misinterpreted as fungal infection), soreness and difficulty with intercourse, tight clothes or even walking. Urinary symptoms include urgency, frequency, nocturia, cystitis and an increased likelihood of infection. Surveys have shown these symptoms to be under-reported. It is important to determine if and how much of a problem genitourinary symptoms of menopause (GSM) are for the individual as this can significantly affect management decisions.

Testosterone-Deficiency Symptoms

Women who are adequately replaced with oestrogen and yet have a loss of sexual interest that is causing distress may have an associated testosterone deficiency. A thorough biopsychosocial assessment is vital as there are multiple potential contributing factors. If, however, androgen deficiency is significant, then there are likely to be symptoms of myalgia, lethargy and mood change such as anxiety. It is recommended that a testosterone assay is checked to exclude pre-existing high levels prior to any prescription.

Clinical Pathway

Consider the following general practice scenario (Figure 23.1).

Case Scenario 23.1

Linda is 52 years old. She does not come to the surgery often and there is nothing of note in her medical summary. She is concerned as she has always been very calm and organised but recently has become irritable and struggles to cope with previously minor challenges. This is a problem as she teaches at a local secondary school and the youngsters exploit any perceived weakness. She feels that this is worse because she is not sleeping and asks for some sleeping tablets.

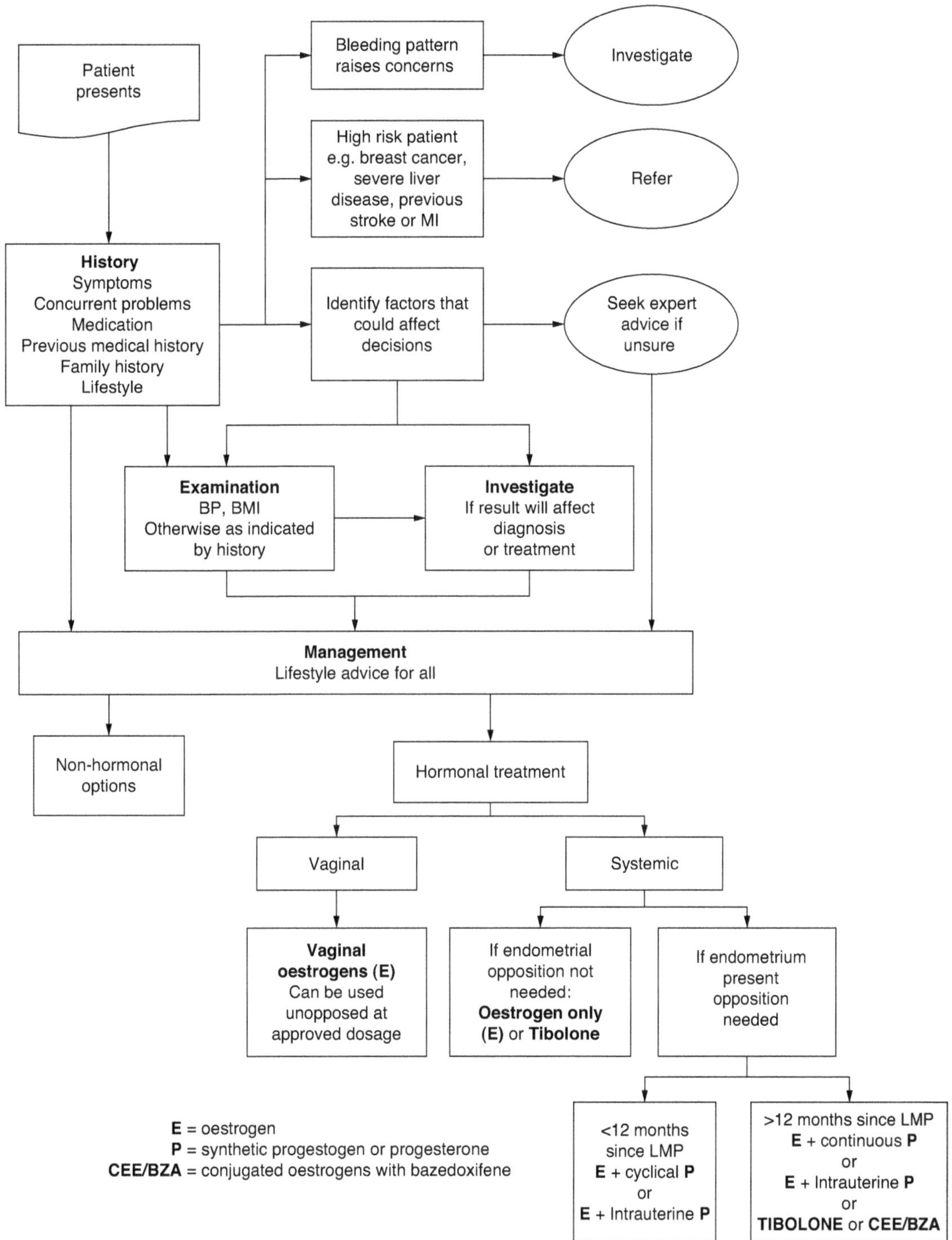

Figure 23.1 Menopause clinical pathway.

Do not simply assume that it is a mental health issue. She is 52 years old, the median age of menopause, so in this context begin by asking about her periods.

She tells you that her last period was six months ago, and the previous one was three months before that.

This is enough information to indicate that she is perimenopausal. It allows you to explore further.

As flushing and sweating are the most common problems, ask about these.

She gets very hot at night and so wet that she has to get out and change her nightclothes most nights. She is then cold and shivery and often finds it difficult to get back to sleep. She has a few daytime flushes but manages by wearing layers of clothes and takes her cardigan on and off.

You now know that she is missing periods, and she is troubled by the most typical menopausal symptoms. At this point you can make a clinical diagnosis; she does not need any biochemical tests.

Linda has come to discuss her sleeping difficulties so return to that issue and ask if her problem is going to sleep or staying asleep. If she is waking, ask if she can tell why and whether it is because of the sweating.

She tells you that going to sleep is not the problem, but that she wakes three or four times in the night starting at 01:30. Sometimes it is because she is hot but mostly, she wakes up and then sweats. It can be difficult to get back to sleep and that is why she is so tired.

This is a typical description of menopause-linked sleep disturbance.

Linda is grateful that you have listened. If you have built sufficient rapport and use appropriate language, it will not be difficult to ask about the next most common issues of menopause – urogenital atrophy and sexual function.

Linda tells you that she does have some vaginal dryness and it is uncomfortable to have sex, but she is really not interested and would rather go to bed with a cup of hot milk and a good book to help her to get to sleep. This is causing some tension at home, which is not helped by her lack of patience and tendency to snap at her husband.

You can appreciate that there are many aspects of her life that are currently difficult and coping is a problem. Reassure her that resignation from work does not need to be considered but you can help. You have no information so far that raises any concerns or requires any physical examination or investigation.

There are a variety of NHS and other organisations providing accredited information and support and the patient can be signposted to these. If she has not already done so, it might be helpful for Linda to read about and consider her options and then return if she wishes to discuss how they might apply to her.

Assessment and Advice

Menopause is a biological process and may offer an opportunistic time to review all health issues including cardiovascular, bone and cancer risk profiles. These are the major causes of mortality and risk reduction should be addressed. Relevant risk assessment tools (QRisk3, FRAX or Qfracture, etc.) can be used to inform your discussion.

There is nearly always an element of lifestyle modification that could help. This might be increasing exercise, stopping smoking/vaping, reduction in weight or moderation in caffeine and alcohol consumption. These changes will optimise ongoing health and may reduce symptoms.

Management Options

Women may choose to manage their difficulties with techniques such as mindfulness, cognitive behavioural therapy (CBT), acupuncture or relaxation therapy. There is established evidence that CBT can help women and is recommended for consideration by the National Institute for Health and Care Excellence (NICE).

There is some evidence that isoflavones (botanicals with some oestrogenic properties) and black cohosh may relieve flushing in the short term, but their safety profile is unclear and longer-term trials have not shown benefit. They are not available on prescription in the UK. Should they wish to try these, women should be advised to choose a quality accredited standardised brand.

Research has shown that other therapeutic options can address some but not all of the symptoms associated with menopause:

- Serotonin reuptake inhibitors (SSRIs) and serotonin and norepinephrine reuptake inhibitors (SNRIs) can ease the symptoms of flushing at lower dosage ranges. They are not as effective as oestrogen and may exacerbate flushing at high dose. The side-effect profile includes loss of sexual interest and anorgasmia, and this should be taken into consideration. They are not licensed in the UK for this indication and are not recommended as a first-line option.
- Gabapentin has been shown to reduce flushing at moderate dose, but is not licensed and not recommended first-line due to its sedative side-effect profile. Oxybutynin has been shown to reduce flushing in some women but is not licensed and has

a significant side-effect profile. A novel range of medicines termed Neurokinin3 (NK3) receptor antagonists are becoming available at the time of writing. These can reduce flushing in women who choose not to or cannot use oestrogen.

- Vaginal moisturisers and lubricants can help vaginal dryness and sexual difficulty and can be recommended. These are available on prescription in the UK.

Hormone Replacement Therapy

Most menopausal symptoms are attributable to oestrogen deficiency. Many systematic reviews have confirmed that hormone replacement therapy (HRT) remains the most effective and holistic therapeutic option where symptoms have sufficient impact to require intervention. It is recommended for women with early loss of ovarian function for bone protection even if symptoms are manageable.

Women should be provided with up-to-date and evidence-based information regarding what is known and what is not known, to allow them to form an opinion about whether this is a course of action they wish to try. The guidance published by NICE (NG23 November 2015 and updated in 2024) can be used as a reference.

Choosing an HRT Regimen

Prescribers are advised to develop a simple and logical list of familiar preparations with which they are familiar (Table 23.1).

Progestogenic Opposition

The role of a progestogen/progesterone in an HRT is to oppose the effect of oestrogen which alone over a sustained period of time increases risks of endometrial hyperplasia and then malignancy. The dose required will vary with the regime, the dose of oestrogen and the background risk of the patient. Figure 23.2 provides an indication.

Choosing an HRT Regimen

Determine:

- Where is she in the menopause transition?
- What symptoms does she complain of?
- What is her main problem?
- What are her concerns?
- What is her risk profile? – Consider
  - lifestyle
  - gynaecological factors
  - cardiovascular factors
  - breast factors
  - musculoskeletal factors
  - metabolic factors
  - mental health.

Consider the example of Linda given earlier.

Decision-Making

This is how the answers Linda gives might work into the options you can offer (Table 23.2).

Decision-Making

1. Consider if vaginal (local) oestrogen alone may be adequate.
2. If a systemic regimen is indicated:
   a. Choose an oestrogen, route of administration and dose.
   b. Add progestin if endometrial tissue is present to suppress proliferation.
      i. Cyclical for predictable bleeding.
      ii. Continuous once postmenopausal.

For Linda, we have no information that would point to the need for a bespoke combination and a ready-formulated first-line cyclical combination would be reasonable. She has had a period within the last year so, is not postmenopausal and would potentially bleed if prescribed a continuous preparation. This could lead to unnecessary anxiety and investigation. Two distinct advantages of a cyclical regimen are that any bleeding should be predictable and that assessment of response to the two different hormones involved is possible.

It is reasonable to offer a fixed-dose oral sequential combination that is easy to use and ensures that both components are taken correctly.

If it is an option, consider starting at the lower end of the effective dose range (e.g. 2 mg oral oestradiol for young women and 1 mg for those at typical menopausal age), and allow three months before reassessment and potential increase.

Table 23.1 A summary of different HRT regimens.

Types	Comment	
Oral oestrogens	-	Easy to take Inexpensive *But:* Potential to interact via first-pass effects in the liver and affect: • thrombotic pathways • concomitant medication • other hormone treatment via SHBG induction • gall bladder physiology Potential for direct gastrointestinal side effects
Conjugated equine oestrogens (CEE)	-	Mixture of oestrogens derived from the urine of pregnant mares. Products used for > 60 years and in many of the trials. Now rarely used
Estradiol valerate (E2Val)	-	Oestradiol that is esterified to ensure absorption
17β-Estradiol (E2)	-	Oestradiol that is micronised to ensure absorption (1 mg~1.2 mg E2Val)
Non-oral oestrogens	-	Minimal gut effects and consequences of hepatic first-pass metabolism (notably effects on clotting and drug interaction) Preferred for women with higher cardiovascular risk profiles, gut absorption difficulty and significant liver disease or drug interaction potential
Gel	17β oestradiol (E2) 0.06% pump provides 0.75 mg/dose 0.1% sachets provide 0.5 mg or 1 mg options	Applied to clean dry skin of upper arm or thigh daily Early peak in serum levels then release from reservoir in fat tissue
Patch	All 17β oestradiol (E2)	Applied to clean dry skin below the waist and changed weekly or twice weekly Some differences in adhesive and dose ranges between brands, but all use matrix technology providing consistent release
Spray	17β oestradiol delivers 1.53mg/spray	Applied to the forearm, 1–3 measures daily
Implant	17β oestradiol (E2) in oily crystalline matrix 25 mg 50 mg	Implanted into fat tissue No licensed product in the UK bit may be available in specialist clinic
Vaginal ring	17β oestradiol (E2) 7.5 mcg/day	Retained for 12 weeks and then replaced Low dose licensed for atrophic vaginitis – not effective for systemic symptoms but can help bladder symptoms – opposition not needed
Vaginal tablets	17β oestradiol (E2)	

	10 mcg	Used daily initially then twice a week (licensed) – more frequent use is out of license but safety data from previous 25 mcg product Low dose – licensed for atrophic vaginitis – not effective for systemic symptoms but can help bladder symptoms – opposition not needed
Vaginal cream	Estriol 0.1%–0.01% Both deliver 500 mcg/dose but excipient different	Used daily initially then twice a week Low dose – licensed for atrophic vaginitis – not effective for systemic symptoms but can help bladder symptoms – opposition not needed
Vaginal gel	Estriol 50 mcg/g in aqueous gel base	Very low dose – can help vaginal dryness
Vaginal pessary	Estriol 30 mcg in an emollient base	Very low dose – can help vaginal dryness
Progestogens	-	Required to prevent hyperplasia and malignant change in endometrial tissue
Testosterone derivatives	Norethisterone	Available in form of progesterone-only contraceptive pills and as a component of many oral proprietary regimens in both continuous and cyclical forms Can be absorbed through skin and used in some combination patches
-	Levonorgestrel and norgestrel	Available in form of progesterone-only pills and as a component of limited number of oral proprietary regimens Can be absorbed through skin and used in some combination patches Delivery via an intrauterine system highly effective with limited systemic impact
-	Dienogest	Available in combined contraception and for use in endometriosis but not specifically licensed for endometrial protection
-	Desogestrel	Available in combined contraception but not specifically licensed for endometrial protection Can provide contraception/cycle blockade
-	Drospirenone	Available in combined contraception but not specifically licensed for endometrial protection Can provide contraception/cycle blockade
Progesterone derivatives	Dydrogesterone	Available in one range of fixed-dose oral combinations
-	Progesterone	Available as: • micronised oral capsules (licensed) • micronised vaginal capsules (unlicensed) • Pessaries/suppositories (unlicensed)
-	Medroxyprogesterone acetate	Available as oral tablets and as a component of limited number of oral proprietary regimens
Mineralocorticoid derivative	Drospirenone	Previously available in one fixed-dose continuous combination Available in combined and progestogen only contraception

Table 23.1 (cont.)

Types	Comment	
Selective oestrogen receptor modulator (SERM)	CEE/Bazedoxifene	New continuous combination using a third-generation SERM to oppose the endometrial effects of 0.45 mg combined equine oestrogen
Testosterone	-	For relief of androgen deficiency symptoms, particularly low libido
Gel	40.5 mg in 2.5 g sachets	Not licensed for women but may be in small doses and specialist practice initiated
-	2% testosterone pump	Not licensed for women but may be used in specialist practice – 10 mg bolus dose used on alternate days to deliver 5 mg/day
Cream	1% testosterone	Produced and licensed in western Australia – unlicensed in the UK – available on private prescription
Implants	100 mg in oily crystalline matrix	Not recommended as dose too high for most women
Gonadomimetic	Tibolone 2.5 mg tablets	Steroidal pro-drug metabolised to active metabolites with oestrogenic, androgenic and progestogenic activity. Limited breast and endometrial activity, not thrombotic Consider for postmenopausal women with low libido

Table 23.2 A review of information relevant to the decision-making process

Information	Relevance
Para 2 with previous postnatal depression	She has previously had a hormone-related effect on mood – to have a mood effect at menopause would not be unusual
Her husband has had a vasectomy 10 years ago Periods previously never caused concerns No intermenstrual or post-coital bleeding	Contraception is not needed (guidance is to continue contraception a year after the last period in women over 50) We have no information about previous hormone intolerance No gynaecological concerns
No personal or family history of breast problems	No raised background risks or anxieties
Mother has had a recent hip fracture age 81 and has thoracic kyphosis	Parental history of hip fracture approximately doubles risk of osteoporosis. Consider using a risk calculator
BP 132/74 BMI 24.5 Not diabetic 10 units alcohol/week and never smoked	In primary care these are usually recorded but check that information is up to date to provide a current cardiovascular risk profile This does not reveal any higher-risk indicators
No other medication	No interaction to be considered

Progestogenic opposition

Perimenopause → Post menopause

52mg levonorgestrel LNG-IUD – effective for 5 years

Sequential use 12–14 days per cycle

Oestrogen dose	Low	Typical	High*
Norethisterone	0.5mg	1mg	1mg
Dydrogesterone	10mg	10mg	20mg
MPA	5mg	10mg	10–20mg
Progesterone	200mg	200mg	300mg

Continuous use

Oestrogen dose	Low	Typical	High*
Norethisterone	0.5mg	1mg	1mg
Dydrogesterone	2.5mg	5mg	10mg
MPA	2.5mg	5mg	10–20mg
Progesterone	100mg	100mg	200mg

*Consider for typical dose but higher risk patient

Figure 23.2 The dose of progestogen needed will vary with the regime, oestrogen and risk profile of the patient.

Agree Follow-Up

Linda may be prescribed three cycles of a low-dose cyclical oral combination containing oestradiol 1 mg with dydrogesterone 10 mg for 14 days. It is important to ensure that the relevant risk and benefit advice is explained and that she should expect it to take six to eight weeks to perceive full benefit. Advise her to monitor when she bleeds and if any unexpected change occurs, note where in the pack she is.

Individualisation and Choice

Many women will have an increased baseline risk of cardiovascular issues – they may be taking medications that interact with oestrogen, have gallstones or other hepatic issues – and for these women the option of oral oestrogen is therefore best avoided. Others will choose non-oral oestrogen to avoid the hepatic effect. Even if they do not have these medical risks, the different options should still be discussed with the patient; they may not want what they perceive to be a 'badge of menopause' or 'gloopy gel'. Some women may struggle with using separate components, leading to chaotic bleeding or even risk hyperplasia. The best regime is tailored to the individual's symptoms and medical history and should be one that she feels comfortable to use.

Counselling

Vaginal Products

Vaginal oestrogen products are highly effective for urogenital atrophy and can be used alone or in conjunction with systemic therapy.

Vaginal oestrogen products used in accordance with the manufacturer's advice have not been shown to affect systemic risks due to the very low dose used. However, patient information leaflets are required to include all cautions as for systemic oestrogen without making this distinction.

Seek expert advice regarding use of any hormone-containing products in women being treated for breast cancer. This includes the low-dose vaginal oestrogen products, though their use may not be precluded. There is evidence indicating no increase in recurrence risk in breast cancer survivors not taking aromatase inhibitors (avoid in women who are).

Vaginal moisturisers and lubricants can be used by all women, including those with breast cancer and women already using oestrogen-containing products.

Cardiovascular Risk

This can be explained in three sections. It is important to evaluate the background risk of the woman in each area to consider the effect of hormone therapy.

- *Coronary artery disease*: For women starting HRT up to 10 years after typical menopause, there is no increase in the risk of coronary artery disease and younger women may be offered protection. There is no increased risk of death. If existing risks are managed, this does not exclude the choice to use HRT.
- *Stroke*: Oral oestrogen is associated with a small increase in stroke risk, but this is not significant for up to 10 years after typical menopause. Most women at this age have a low baseline risk. Standard doses of non-oral oestrogens have not shown an increase in stroke risk and are preferred if the patient has a higher risk profile.
- *Venous thromboembolism*: Oral oestrogens have been shown to increase risk of deep vein thrombosis (DVT) and pulmonary embolism (PE). This is further influenced by the progestogen component. Dydrogesterone appears to offer least additional risk. Standard doses of non-oral oestrogens have not shown this effect and are preferred if the patient has a higher risk profile.

Breast Disease

Benign breast disease may remain uncomfortable if taking HRT, but this is not a risk for malignant transformation.

HRT is believed to act as a growth promoter of pre-existing breast cancer and its effect is slowly lost after stopping. Oestrogen alone is associated with a small increase in breast cancer diagnosis. Combined regimes are associated with a further increase in cancer diagnosis after three to five years of exposure. The size of this effect is, however, still small and of similar magnitude to that associated with regular alcohol consumption or having a body mass index (BMI) of 30. In women under 50, the effect of HRT is similar to that of cyclical ovarian hormones. Older women have a greater background risk as incidence increases with age and hence the numbers of additional diagnoses due to the effect of HRT will be higher.

Musculoskeletal Problems

The risk of fracture is reduced while taking HRT. This effect increases with time. While some effect is lost after stopping, a difference can persist for many years. There is some evidence that HRT may improve muscle mass and strength.

Diabetes

HRT does not adversely affect blood sugar control or increase the risk of a diagnosis of type 2 diabetes.

Dementia

We do not know enough about the effects of HRT on dementia to be able to advise.

Review and Modification

Encourage your patient to return before the end of three months for review.
Consider:

- relief of original symptoms
- onset of new symptoms (and when this happens)
- bleeding
- any change in risk profile.

Problem-Solving Suggestions

- Persistence/reappearance of flushing:
  - increase oestrogen dose
  - consider change to non-oral regime
- Breast tenderness:
  - often settles in four to six weeks
  - reduce oestrogen and increase very slowly
  - try a non-oral oestrogen
  - change progestogen class or consider 52 mg LNG-IUD
  - consider tibolone
- Premenstrual syndrome:
  - increase oestrogen
  - change class of progestogen
  - change route of progestogen – consider 52 mg LNG-IUD
- Bleeding too early in cyclical regime:
  - increase progestogen dose
  - change progestogen class
  - consider previous bleeding schedule
- Bleeding after starting a continuous combined regime:
  - allow three to six months to settle initially
  - REDUCE oestrogen
  - increase progestogen
  - consider 52 mg LNG-IUD
  - try Tibolone
  - revert to cyclical regime
- Unscheduled bleeding with any regime:
  - may reflect endogenous hormone release but should be investigated if previously settled for the last six months – it may be a sign of structural or histological abnormality
  - this is not the same as true postmenopausal bleeding as although HRT may increase the likelihood of bleeding, the risk of an underlying malignancy is lower than in women not taking HRT. The starting point for investigation is usually transvaginal ultrasound.

Stopping

There is little evidence regarding the best way to stop HRT but most experts would recommend reducing gradually. If symptoms return, then these have not been deferred, merely masked, and it may be that an informed decision is made to continue for longer at the lowest effective dose.

Further Reading

- NICE, 'Menopause: Diagnosis and management'. NG23. November 2015, updated December 2019. Accessed: 19 Nov. 2025. [Online]. Available: www.nice.org.uk/guidance/ng23.
- H. Boardman, L. Hartley, A. Eisinga et al., 'Hormone therapy for preventing cardiovascular disease in post-menopausal women', *Cochrane Database Syst Rev*, vol. 10, no. 3, CD002229, 2015. Accessed: 19 Nov. 2025. [Online]. Available: www.ncbi.nlm.nih.gov/pmc/articles/PMC10183715.
- College of Sexual and Reproductive Healthcare. FSRH Clinical Guideline: Contraception for Women Aged over 40 Years. London: College of Sexual and Reproductive Healthcare; August 2017 (amended July 2023). Available: www.cosrh.org/Public/Documents/fsrh-guidance-contraception-for-women-aged-over-40-years-2017.aspx.
- Qfracture, '10 year fracture risk'. Accessed: 19 Nov. 2025. [Online]. Available: www.qfracture.org.
- FRAX, '10 year fracture risk and guide to intervention'. Accessed: 19 Nov. 2025. [Online]. Available: https://frax.shef.ac.uk/FRAX.
- QRisk3, 'Cardiovascular risk calculator'. Accessed: 19 Nov. 2025. [Online]. Available: www.qrisk.org.
- The International Menopause Society. Accessed: 19 Nov. 2025. [Online]. Available: www.imsociety.org.
- The European Menopause and Andropause Society. Accessed: 19 Nov. 2025. [Online]. Available: https://emas-online.org.
- The British Menopause Society. Accessed: 19 Nov. 2025. [Online]. Available: www.thebms.org.uk.

Chapter

24 Vulval Dermatoses in Primary Care

Kate London and Sue Towers

Key Points

- Women with generalised skin conditions such as eczema or psoriasis should be proactively asked about vulval symptoms; many women don't mention these symptoms, due to embarrassment, or because they do not think that the problems are linked.
- The principles of management of a vulval skin problem are the same as many skin conditions; irritant avoidance, repair of skin barrier function (with the use of emollients) and reduction of inflammation.
- Emollients require regular use; decanting into a small, easy-to-carry pot is useful for frequent application.
- Using controlled amounts of high- or mid-potency steroid ointments is important to reduce inflammation and the consequences of persistent vulval scratching once a diagnosis has been made.
- Always make a diagnosis before treating with ultra-potent or potent topical steroids as they will mask the signs and may make it impossible to make the diagnosis later.
- Women may need support and understanding to choose the preparation of emollient or steroid that they find most comfortable.
- Women with vulval problems are often embarrassed and feel stigmatised. They may experience emotional distress, needing careful assessment and possible referral for psychological support.
- Signposting to useful resources may help women understand the importance of self-management and improve adherence to treatment.
- Women with lichen planus and lichen sclerosus should be aware of the increased risk of vulval intraepithelial neoplasia or carcinoma. This may present as an unresolving vulval lump, ulceration or change in skin appearance and requires an urgent review. This risk is decreased by long-term maintenance with regular emollient and a twice-weekly topical steroid.
- Prescribe topical oestrogen in adult women who are likely to be hypo-oestrogenic (post-partum, breastfeeding, peri- and post-menopausal).

Introduction

Vulval skin conditions may not be revealed to health professionals due to several factors, including:

- embarrassment
- not knowing who to talk to
- physical pain
- fear of being stigmatised
- previous misdiagnoses or treatment failure.

The 2015 British Association of Dermatology (BAD) Vulval Health Survey revealed that one in five women had experienced thoughts of self-harm because of their vulval condition [1].

Comments recorded include:

> 'I feel broken, hopeless and often at times less of a woman'
>
> 'disgusted with my own body'
>
> 'like a freak'
>
> 'going out was difficult and I couldn't talk to anyone about my symptoms in detail'

Treatment of vulval conditions, though often not curative, can make a significant difference to quality of life and alleviate distress.

History-Taking

A good history is paramount in establishing diagnosis and management. Stopping the patient from doing some things can be just as important as active treatment.

Important points include:

- Symptoms: including itching, dryness, dysuria, burning or pain.

- No symptoms, but a partner or health professional has noticed a change in the skin appearance, or discolouration of the vulva.
- Other areas affected, such as scalp, elbows, knees, hands, nails or mouth.
- Duration – this may also tell you about her perception of the cause. This could be a clue, such as a topical allergen, or a misconception (e.g. a food allergy), or not feeling clean, leading to excessive washing after an uncomfortable sexual experience.
- Aggravating and relieving factors, previous treatment success or failure.
- Urinary and bowel symptoms (e.g. incontinence or frequency) and measures to cope with these, such as use of pads or deodorisers.
- Personal or family history of dermatological conditions.
- Medical history such as diabetes, autoimmune conditions or thyroid disease.
- Washing/grooming habits such as use of soap, sponges, hair removal, douches, clothing, frequency of washing. What are her cultural habits after toileting?
- Gynaecological, obstetric and smear history including sexual history, any dyspareunia and any abnormal smears.
- Hobbies which might aggravate a vulval problem, such as wearing tight clothes for exercising, cycling or horse-riding.
- Social history, including smoking; this increases the risk of diagnosis and recurrence of vulval intraepithelial neoplasia and squamous cell carcinoma and also makes human papillomavirus (HPV) elimination less likely.

Examination

As the vulva consists of a mixture of keratinised epithelium, modified epithelium and mucous membrane, it is important to check the whole skin surface, including the oral mucosa, as particular sites may provide clues to help with diagnosis.

The scalp, elbows and knees may reveal typical rough scaly plaques and the natal cleft/axilla may show red, shiny and well-demarcated areas. These findings suggest psoriasis [2].

Nail changes can be suggestive of eczema [3], psoriasis [2] or lichen planus [4].

Examination of the skin of the wrists, lower back and ankles may reveal the shiny flat-topped purplish papules of lichen planus [4]. Additional findings may include eroded areas on the buccal mucosa (lacy appearance) or gingivitis. Examine the perianal skin by asking the woman to lie in the left lateral position.

Vulval examination may reveal the following:

- Erythema which may be diffuse or well demarcated and may involve or spare the flexural creases. It may be dusky, bright red or orange red.
- Lichenification, suggestive of chronic scratching.
- Specific or generalised pigmentation or depigmentation.

On parting the labia majora you may see depigmentation suggesting vitiligo [5], or pallor suggestive of lichen sclerosus.

Architectural change can include the following:

- Loss of the labia minora, fusion of the clitoral hood or midline fusion, which may be secondary to disease or female genital mutilation (FGM). There is a mandatory duty in England and Wales to report FGM in anyone aged under 18 [6].
- Scarring secondary to ulceration or trauma.
- Redness or erosion at the introitus.

Differential Diagnosis

Possibilities include:

- eczema – atopic, irritant or seborrhoeic
- psoriasis
- intertrigo (may be flexural psoriasis or tinea) [7]
- vitiligo
- lichen sclerosus [8]
- lichen planus.

Management

In medicine it is unusual for 'always' and 'never' to apply; however, in the management of vulval conditions this isn't the case:

- *Always* stop irritants (Box 24.1).
- *Always* restore the skin barrier function.
- Suppress inflammatory response where indicated.

Box 24.1 Irritants

Any topical cream or ointment can be an irritant. Common irritants include:

- Soaps, shower gels, sponge, loofah, flannel (cosmetic soaps and shower gels are all detergents – like washing-up liquid!).
- 'Feminine washes'.
- Wipes.
- Cosmetic bath additives, bath oils, foams and bombs.
- Excessive frequency/duration of washing (even water alone dries the skin).
- Vigorous drying.
- Topical anti-itching remedies (can be contact allergens).

Box 24.2 Choosing an Emollient

- Creams work better than bath emollients as soap substitutes and are often more comfortable and acceptable to patients.
- Emollients work in different ways. Some are occlusive (prevent water loss from skin); some draw water up into the stratum corneum (humectant); some do both.
- Creams need preservatives which can themselves be irritant, ointments less so.
- Ointments generally come in pots or tubs rather than pump dispensers. Advise the patient to use a spoon or spatula to remove ointment from the pot; this avoids contaminant from fingers, as ointment is a perfect growing medium for bacteria.
- The 'emollient ladder' (Box 24.3) may help with emollient choice.

Irritant Avoidance

Patients may not associate use of soaps and shower gels with symptoms and are often not aware of how these can damage the barrier function of the skin. This problem occurs particularly in pre-pubertal children and postmenopausal women and in those with a dermatological problem of the vulva, where the skin barrier is intrinsically weakened. It is important to be very specific in understanding washing/hygiene procedures for each patient.

> 'What exactly do you use to wash with?' 'How long do you bath/shower/wash for?'
>
> 'How often do you shower or bath?' 'Then what do you do?'

Avoidance of tight-fitting clothes of synthetic material should also be avoided, if possible, such as tight layers of Lycra, thongs and so on [9].

Restoring Barrier Function

Having identified potential causes of damage to the skin's barrier function, the patient needs a regime to restore it.

Emollients restore barrier function by improving the water-resistant lipid lamellae encasing the corneocytes (bricks). The corneocytes are held together by corneodesmosomes (cement), which depend on a balance of proteases to remain intact.

This important barrier function can be destroyed by environmental factors, such as soap and other detergents, which enhance protease activity. This causes the corneodesmosomes to break and inhibits lipid lamellae synthesis and subsequent 'brick' shrinkage. This allows increased water loss from the skin and increased ingress of irritants and allergens, producing a vicious cycle of skin barrier breakdown.

An emollient should be used as a soap substitute but it will not foam up as it is not a detergent. Skin will be clean, even if it does not feel as clean as with soap, because the natural barrier has been left intact.

Clear instructions should be given on using emollients as a soap substitute. Place at least a 50p size amount in the palm of the hand/fingers (Box 24.2) and apply to the vulva and perianal area, then rinse off. After bathing, 'pat' the vulva dry with a soft towel (avoid rubbing and irritating the skin). Then apply emollient again directly to the vulva and perianal area and leave it on. Emollients can be used liberally (in contrast to topical steroid) and should be applied several times a day, also putting some on the toilet paper to wipe with, therefore removing traces of irritant urine, or after toileting and washing as in some cultures, leaving an emollient-protective film on the vulva.

The best emollient is the one that the patient prefers. Advice about emollient choice is in Box 24.2.

Correct emollient use is essential for the management of vulval disease. Emollient bath additives can be used in addition, but not instead of emollients.

Box 24.3 Emollient Choices

Ointments (very greasy) occlusive

- Hydromol® ointment
- Cetraben® ointment
- Aproderm® ointment
- Liquid paraffin 50% in white soft paraffin ointment
- QV ointment®

Greasy creams and gels (all below humectant and occlusive)

- Cetraben® cream
- Aproderm® cream
- Doublebase® Gel (does not contain cetyl alcohol)
- Aveeno® cream
- Hydromol® Cream
- Dexeryl® Cream (does not contain cetyl alcohol)
- Dermol® cream (do not use for more than 2 weeks as it can become an irritant)

Sprays (useful in people who have difficulty applying or find touch very painful)

- Emollin®
- Dermamist®

Urea-containing creams (sting more)

- Aquadrate®
- Eucerin®
- Balneum Plus®
- Hydromol Intensive®

Lotions (not moisturising enough for dry skin)

- Aveeno® lotion
- Dermol 500® (can be irritant, do not use long term)

An important exception to the 'emollient rule' is that aqueous cream should not be left on the skin. It contains sodium lauryl sulfate which can change skin pH and may aggravate the condition.

Suppression of Inflammation

Suppression of any inflammatory process is likely to require a topical steroid regularly or intermittently.

Steroid and emollient application should be separated by about 15–30 minutes. Patients often ask whether to use their emollient or steroid first. The authors of this chapter would suggest emollient first, but dermatologists can disagree on this; the most important point is that both are used, never just topical steroid alone.

Cream or ointment formulations of most steroids are available; the steroid ladder (Box 24.4) can clarify the preparations in order of potency. The potency required will depend on the condition and the patient. Ointment is usually preferred to cream, as this contains fewer preservatives and stabilisers and is therefore less likely to cause contact allergy.

The Fingertip Unit (FTU) [10] guides the quantity of topical steroid to use. One FTU is the length of cream squeezed from a tube which spreads from the distal fold on the index finger to the tip (about 0.5 g). One FTU treats an area equivalent to both palms. Generally for the vulva and perianal area we use one FTU per treatment application. Prescribing a 30 g tube can enable the prescriber and patient to monitor the quantity used and decreases the likelihood of side effects from overuse. Always use the topical steroid in the morning; close-fitting clothing such as underwear will prevent transfer onto the inner thighs, causing atrophic changes such as striae.

Do not start treatment with a potent or ultra-potent topical steroid if you are unable to make the diagnosis; this will make it very difficult to make a diagnosis later. If you cannot make the diagnosis, refer to a specialist vulval clinic, start the patient on an emollient and consider a weak topical steroid if necessary.

For women who may have low levels of vaginal oestrogen, vulval symptoms will improve more if vaginal oestrogen is given. This includes women who are perimenopausal or menopausal and those who are post-partum, particularly if breastfeeding.

Who to Refer

- Diagnostic uncertainty.
- Those with unusual presentations: 'it just doesn't look right'.
- Failure to respond to treatment, having checked adherence.
- Persistent lesions such as thickened white or red patches, ulceration, red or pigmented

Box 24.4 Example of a Steroid Ladder

Potency	Active ingredient	Brand name example
Very potent	Clobetasol propionate 0.05%	Dermovate®
Potent	Betamethasone (as valerate) 0.1%	Betnovate®
	Mometasone furoate 0.1%	Elocon®
	Fluocinolone acetonide 0.025%	Synalar®
	Hydrocortisone butyrate 0.1%	Locoid®
Moderate potency	Clobetasone butyrate 0.05%	Eumovate®
	Betamethasone (as valerate) 0.025%	Betnovate RD®
	Clobetasone butyrate with nystatin and oxytetracycline (cream only)	Trimovate®
	Fluocinolone acetonide 0.00625%	Synalar 1 in 4®
Mild potency	Hydrocortisone 1%	Hc45®
	Hydrocortisone 1% + clotrimazole 1%	Canesten HC®
	Hydrocortisone 1% + miconazole nitrate 2%	Daktacort®
	Hydrocortisone 0.5% + nystatin 100,000 u/gm + chlorhexidine 1%	Nystaform HC®

patches. Refer on the suspected cancer pathway if there is an unexplained vulval lump, ulceration or bleeding [11].

Case Studies

Case Scenario 24.1

Hayley, 27, comes to surgery angry and upset because of her psoriasis. She feels 'fobbed off' with creams which don't work and that she hasn't 'been clear' for many years. You elicit that Hayley has plaque psoriasis affecting her elbows and knees, but also genital problems, which is embarrassing; sex is uncomfortable and condoms make her sore.

Hayley is unlikely to disclose genital problems unless specifically asked. She has been too embarrassed to talk about this previously and did not know whether it was linked to her psoriasis, although she suspects that it might be.

Surveys suggest that up to two-thirds of those with psoriasis may have genital involvement which has a significant effect on quality of life, sexual health and relationships. Many are too embarrassed to tell their healthcare professional [12]. Most people with genital psoriasis also have symptoms elsewhere, but it may be the only area affected in up to 5% of those with psoriasis [13].

Hayley hasn't used any treatment in the genital area as she is 'frightened' and does not know what she can use. She also finds the itching embarrassing if she needs to scratch in public.

On examination, Hayley has classic changes of psoriasis on the other typical sites and the redness in the vulva and groins is well demarcated and shiny, with splitting in the groins and natal cleft. The vagina is not involved, and the labial structures look normal. Unlike other affected body sites, the genital area and flexures are not generally scaly due to the hydrating effect of the skin folds.

Hayley is currently washing with water alone. She uses Dovobet® on her elbows and knees, but nothing in the genital area.

Management

Hayley should use an emollient to wash and moisturise; you show her how to use this as a soap substitute as well as a leave-on emollient, explaining why this is important.

For management of the psoriatic inflammation, a moderately potent or potent topical steroid ointment should be applied once daily in the morning. Clobetasone or mometasone are suitable; a vitamin D analogue such as tacalcitol or calcitriol at night could be added. Calcipotriol is too much of an irritant for the vulva.

Initially, she should use both the steroid and vitamin D analogue, in addition to the emollient, then decrease the steroid to alternate days, then two to three times a week. Continue daily use of vitamin D analogue and emollient long-term, noting the maximum weekly doses of vitamin D emollient which should be clear in the packaging.

Using condoms may have aggravated the psoriasis due to a Koebner effect from trauma, therefore advice about use of a suitable water-based lubricant may help. She should also use another method of contraception, partly because condoms alone have a high typical failure rate, and also because oil-based preparations may damage condoms.

Case Scenario 24.2

Rita, 58, comes to see you. She has 'thrush again' and would like some more clotrimazole and hydrocortisone cream, which seemed to help last time.

You see she has been treated for 'thrush' without examination on three occasions in the past eight months.

Taking a history, you find that she does not have a discharge; clotrimazole with hydrocortisone eases the symptoms a little while she is using it, but the vulval irritation returns when she finishes the treatment. She is very careful about keeping clean but has stopped using soap as it seemed to make the 'thrush' worse; she uses an over-the-counter genital detergent cream instead. Her last period was about eight years ago, and she did not have much trouble with menopausal symptoms.

Rita is embarrassed about being examined, but this is essential as the problem is recurring and examination findings will help determine the diagnosis management.

Vaginal candidiasis is uncommon in postmenopausal women, although the risk is higher in those with co-morbidities such as diabetes or immunosuppression and in those who use tamoxifen or hormone replacement therapy [14]. Postmenopausal women (and premenopausal women with immunosuppression) with candidiasis may be more likely to have a non-albicans species cultured [15].

On examination, there is some redness of the vulva and the clitoris cannot be seen; the labia minora have almost disappeared bilaterally and there is pallor and whiteness consistent with lichen sclerosus. The pallor extends around the perianal area and there is some thickening from scratching.

Management

Review anything that may be irritating the problem, by making sure that she stops using any soaps or detergents that could be reducing or damaging skin barrier function, including the one that she is buying over the counter.

It is important that she understands that her problem is lichen sclerosus, not thrush. There are good information leaflets on the BAD and British Society for the Study of Vulval Disease (BSSVD) websites.

Advise about avoidance of soaps and irritants and start Rita on a regimen to restore skin barrier function by using an emollient as a soap substitute and to leave on.

Lichen sclerosus requires an ultra-potent topical steroid such as clobetasol propionate, or a potent topical steroid ointment such as mometasone. She should use this daily for up to four weeks until itching is controlled, followed by a weaning-down period, for example alternate day use, followed by lifelong maintenance, once or twice a week. She should use the FTU as a guide to the amount of steroid cream needed. On the perianal area she is better using mometasone ointment, as clobetasol propionate can cause atrophic changes. As she is postmenopausal, a vaginal oestrogen will also help to improve symptoms.

A review appointment should be made for three or four weeks after treatment is started to assess adherence and response. Advise her that it is essential to control the condition to prevent inflammation from damaging the vulval structures. Damage from lichen sclerosus can progress without itching, hence maintenance treatment is important, as well as control of symptoms.

There is a small increased risk of vulval intraepithelial neoplasia (VIN) and squamous cell carcinoma with lichen sclerosus. Adherence to treatment may be improved if she is aware that she has a 5% risk of vulval carcinoma, which is reduced if the lichen sclerosus is well controlled. If she notices any changes to the vulval skin which do not resolve, such as white patches, lumps or ulceration, she needs an urgent medical review; it would be sensible to give that advice in writing. Otherwise, once her symptoms are controlled, annual examination by a healthcare professional experienced in vulval examination is advised [9]. Any patch which looks different from the vulva surrounding it should prompt referral, on the suspected cancer pathway if the clinician is concerned about malignancy.

Case Scenario 24.3

Mary is 74. She walks awkwardly into your clinic room and sits down carefully. She is clearly in discomfort and on questioning informs you that for the past four months she has been very sore and itchy 'down there'; the soreness is 'unbearable'. She has used clotrimazole and various barrier creams, with no effect.

Mary's medical history includes ischaemic heart disease and Bowen's disease of the lower leg.

She is washing with water alone now and cannot bear any intimate contact with her husband due to the soreness of her vulva; this is putting a strain on her marriage.

She agrees to examination reluctantly, as she knows it will be painful. Examination reveals a well-defined, red, angry erosion at the introitus, which extends into the vagina, and some resorption of the right labia minora. This is consistent with lichen planus. It is important to check the oral mucosa, as oral lichen planus is present in around half of those with lichen planus. It can also affect the vagina, lacrimal ducts, external auditory canal, oesophagus and urethra [4,16].

Management

The treatment for lichen planus is similar to that of lichen sclerosus; irritant avoidance, emollient use and potent or ultra-potent topical steroids. Vaginal lichen planus may present as a profuse irritant watery discharge. Topical steroids can be introduced using a FTU of clobetasol propionate or mometasone on a dilator and inserting into the vagina three times weekly. This will decrease vaginal scarring and stenosis. As she is postmenopausal, intravaginal oestrogen will improve her symptoms.

Case Scenario 24.4

Sam, 60, comes to see you because of itching and soreness 'down below'. This has been going on for a couple of years and is getting worse. She is fed up, tearful and at the end of her tether. She has been treated with fluconazole and clotrimazole, but this only improves things briefly.

You notice that she has well-controlled type 2 diabetes and that she has been on canagliflozin for five years. She tells you that the itching started when she was treated twice with antibiotics for a urinary tract infection and then a chest infection; it has not gone away since.

She washes with soap and has no history of skin problems.

Examination shows marked redness over the mons pubis, labia majora, labia minora and the inner thighs. It is well demarcated and slightly scaly; it looks very sore and 'angry'. There is also some oedema of the labia majora and minora.

A swab shows *Candida*.

Management

The most appropriate treatment is to stop the canagliflozin and change to an alternative anti-diabetic medication, stop her using soap and use an emollient to wash and moisturise. Give fluconazole 150 mg every 72 hours and then weekly for up to six months. Arrange to review her in about three weeks.

On review, she feels a lot better but there is still some itching and soreness. On examination, the redness and oedema have decreased but she still has a well-demarcated scaly erythema. The SGLT 2 inhibitor has provoked a psoriasiform dermatitis. This needs emollients, a vitamin D analogue and a moderate topical steroid, which can be gradually decreased over a few weeks.

This is a relatively new problem that has been seen since the introduction of SGLT 2 inhibitors for diabetes; it can occur at any stage of SGLT2 inhibitor treatment. Control is difficult while the drugs is continued, as it will increase urinary excretion of glucose, giving favourable conditions for genital thrush.

Conclusion

Vulval conditions cause embarrassment, debilitating physical symptoms and emotional upset. In most cases, relatively simple irritant avoidance and restoration of barrier function will make life much more comfortable. It is important that women can feel able to talk about their bodies without fear of stigmatisation.

Lichen sclerosus can be over-diagnosed; however, the SWIFT model (Soreness, Whiteness, Urinary Incontinence, Fissures, Clitoral hood Thickening) improves the accuracy of diagnosis in premenarchal girls [17].

Examination of women who complain of vulval symptoms is important, particularly if the problem is recurrent. Women who have a chronic skin disease, such as psoriasis and eczema, may not report the symptoms unless specifically asked and if they admit to or present with vulval problems, examination is essential.

The principles of irritant avoidance and restoration of barrier function are applicable across a wide range of vulval conditions, similar to the advice necessary to improve other skin conditions routinely managed in primary care.

The BSSVD [18] is an excellent resource for professionals and patients wanting to know more about vulval conditions. Patient information leaflets can be found on their website, as well as on the BAD website [19]. Other useful resources include the Primary Care Dermatology Society (PCDS) [2,4,5,7,8], International Society for the Study of Vulvovaginal Disease (ISSVD) [20] and Dermnet [13].

References

[1] S. Arnold, S. Fernando, S. Rees S. Living with vulval lichen sclerosus: a qualitative interview study. *Br J Dermatol.* vol **187**, no 6, pp. 909–918, 2022.

[2] Primary Care Dermatology Society, 'Psoriasis'. Dec. 2023. Accessed: 26 Feb. 2024. [Online]. Available: https://www.pcds.org.uk/patient-info-leaflets/psoriasis.

[3] B. Y. Chung, Y. W. Choi, H. O. Kim et al., 'Nail dystrophy in patients with atopic dermatitis and its association with disease severity', *Ann Dermatol*, vol. **31**, no. 2, pp. 121–126, 2019.

[4] Primary Care Dermatology Society, 'Lichen planus'. Dec. 2023. Accessed: 26 Feb. 2024. [Online]. Available: www.pcds.org.uk/clinical-guidance/lichen-planus.

[5] Primary Care Dermatology Society, 'Vitiligo'. May 2022. Accessed: 26 Feb. 2024. [Online]. Available: www.pcds.org.uk/clinical-guidance/vitiligo.

[6] Home Office and Department for Education, 'Mandatory reporting of female genital mutilation – procedural information'. Jan. 2020. Accessed: 26 Feb. 2024. [Online]. Available: www.gov.uk/government/publications/mandatory-reporting-of-female-genital-mutilation-procedural-information.

[7] Primary Care Dermatology Society, 'Intertrigo'. Apr. 2023. Accessed: 26 Feb. 2024. [Online]. Available: www.pcds.org.uk/clinical-guidance/intertrigo.

[8] Primary Care Dermatology Society, 'Lichen sclerosus'. Oct. 2023. Accessed: 26 Feb. 2024. [Online]. Available: www.pcds.org.uk/clinical-guidance/lichen-sclerosis.

[9] NHS, 'Lichen sclerosus'. Oct. 2021. Accessed: 26 Feb. 2024. [Online]. Available: www.nhs.uk/conditions/lichen-sclerosus.

[10] NHS, 'Topical corticosteroids'. May 2023. Accessed: 26 Feb. 2024. [Online]. Available: https://www.nhs.uk/medicines/steroids/.

[11] NICE, 'NG12. Suspected cancer: Recognition and referral'. Oct. 2023. Accessed: 26 Feb. 2024. [Online]. Available: www.nice.org.uk/guidance/ng12.

[12] J. C. Cather, C. Ryan, K. Meeuwis et al., 'Patients' perspectives on the impact of genital psoriasis: A qualitative study', *Dermatol Ther*, vol. **7**, pp. 447–461, 2017.

[13] DermNet, 'Genital psoriasis'. Jun. 2014. Accessed: 26 Feb. 2024. [Online]. Available: https://dermnetnz.org/topics/genital-psoriasis.

[14] M. Becker and R. Sobel, 'Vulvovaginal candidiasis in postmenopausal women', *Curr Infect Dis Rep*, vol. **25**, pp. 61–66, 2023.

[15] A. Farr, I. Effendy, B. Frey Tirri et al., 'Guideline: Vulvovaginal candidosis (AWMF 015/072, level S2 k)', *Mycoses*, vol. **64**, no. 6, pp. 583–602, 2021.

[16] R. Gall and I. N. Navarro-Fernandez, 'Lichen planus erosive form'. StatPearls Publishing, 2024.

[17] M. Wang, M. Wininger and A. Vash-Margita, 'The SWIFT model for lichen sclerosus among premenarchal girls', *J Low Genit Tract Dis*, vol. **26**, no. 1, pp. 46–52, 2022.

[18] British Society for the Study of Vulval Disease, 'Patient information leaflets'. Accessed: 26 Feb. 2024. [Online]. Available: https://bssvd.org/practitioner-portal/external-resources.

[19] British Association of Dermatologists, 'Vulval skincare'. May 2023. Accessed: 26 Feb. 2024. [Online]. Available: www.bad.org.uk/pils/vulval-skincare.

[20] International Society for the Study of Vulvovaginal Disease. Accessed: 26 Feb. 2024. [Online]. Available: www.issvd.org.

Chapter 25

Management of the Patient with Pelvic Organ Prolapse in Primary Care

Christian Phillips

Key Points

- A prolapse is a protrusion of any pelvic organ or structure beyond its normal anatomical position. These are graded from first to fourth degree, depending on severity.
- Damage to the major supports of the vagina (endopelvic fascia, ligaments and levator ani muscle) leads to prolapse.
- Childbirth is the major risk factor for the development of prolapse.
- Patients with prolapse present with a variety of symptoms depending on the compartment affected.
- Patients should only be referred for treatment of prolapse if their symptoms are bothersome. Asymptomatic prolapse can be left untreated.
- Patients with anterior compartment prolapse often have urinary symptoms and should be questioned for this.
- Patients with posterior compartment prolapse often have concomitant bowel symptoms and need to be questioned for this.
- Diagnosis is made on clinical examination, usually with the patient in a left lateral position using a Sims' speculum.
- Women opting for conservative management including lifestyle changes, pelvic floor exercises or a pessary can be managed successfully in primary care with regular review.
- Surgery should only be considered after all risk factors have been considered and the patient has completed her family.

Introduction

Pelvic organ prolapse (POP) is a common condition that presents regularly in primary care. Many women with a prolapse will be asymptomatic and can be reassured. They should be provided with general advice about risk avoidance and pelvic floor exercises. However, those with symptoms need a methodical history and examination to help determine the type and stage of prolapse and the management options most suitable for her.

Case Scenario 25.1

Andrea is a 33-year-old woman who attends your general practice clinic to discuss her prolapse. The prolapse was noted by the practice nurse when Andrea attended for a cervical smear. She works as a healthcare worker in a nursing home, smokes 20 cigarettes a day and has a body mass index (BMI) of 36. She has had two vaginal deliveries in the past with children aged five and seven years. She had forceps delivery with an episiotomy and a normal vaginal delivery but sustained a second-degree tear which was sutured by the midwife. She is divorced but has recently acquired a new partner with whom she co-habits. Andrea is worried and concerned about her prolapse and wants your advice about having something done about it. She has heard that her friend has had a 'sling procedure' and she was wondering whether she should have the same.

What Are the Structures That Support the Pelvic Organs?

Let us first consider the mechanisms of support for the pelvic organs. The pelvic organs comprise:

- the urethra and bladder in the anterior compartment
- the uterus and vaginal vault in the apical compartment
- the small bowel, peritoneum and rectum in the posterior compartment.

The pelvic organs are supported by three mechanisms [1]:

- the endopelvic fascia with its condensations forming the uterosacral and cardinal ligaments
- the levator ani with its intact nerve supply
- the posterior angulation of the vagina when the woman is standing.

Fascia

The endopelvic fascia is formed of connective tissue with occasional smooth muscle that envelopes the pelvic organs. They form condensations of fascia inserted into the top of the vagina (paracolpium) and cervix/uterus (parametrium). These form the uterosacral ligaments posteriorly, the transverse (cardinal) ligaments laterally and the thin pubocervical ligaments anteriorly.

DeLancey describes three levels of pelvic organ support (Figure 25.1). The condensations of fascia that insert into the cervix and upper vagina are the 'Level 1' supports. Tears or avulsion in the Level 1 support causes uterine prolapse or if the uterus is absent, vault prolapse. The vagina, with bladder anteriorly and rectum posteriorly, is enclosed in connective tissue/endopelvic fascia. These form sheet-like structures to partition the vagina from the bladder and the rectum. These are the 'Level 2' supports. Tears in these structures can cause a cystocele or rectocele. The 'Level 3' supports form the sphincter complex and suburethral hammock anteriorly and the perineal body posteriorly [2].

Muscle

The levator ani muscles form a diaphragm for the pelvic organs to sit upon. Integrity between the connective tissue of the endopelvic fascia and its connections to the levator ani ensure that the pelvic organs are suspended within the pelvis. Denervation or direct injury to the muscle at the levator ani or avulsion/tears of the endopelvic cause lack of continuity between the levator ani and the connective tissue and the pelvic organs. This will result in prolapse.

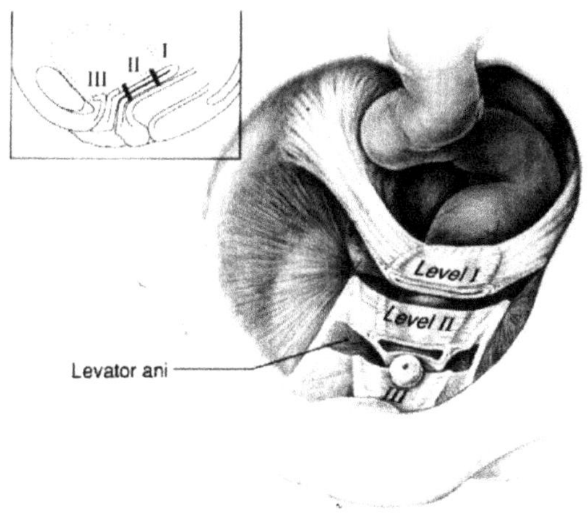

Figure 25.1 Levels of support for pelvic organs.

What Are the Risk Factors That Andrea Has for Pelvic Organ Prolapse?

The primary mechanism in the aetiology of POP is obstetric injury and childbirth [3]. Andrea has had a forceps delivery and a spontaneous vaginal delivery. At both deliveries she sustained either an episiotomy or a tear. Parturition through the birth canal can cause injury both in the form of tears in the pelvic fascia, but also injury to the pudendal nerve which innervates the levator ani or direct injury to the levator muscles themselves and their attachments to the pelvic sidewall [4].

Andrea has had two children in the past, but it is noted from the history that she has started a new relationship, and she may wish to have further children with her new partner. This needs to be considered when counselling her. Certainly, any surgical correction (which will be discussed later) needs to be deferred until her family is complete. Furthermore, on counselling her about subsequent pregnancies there is sometimes the temptation to open the discussion about elective caesarean section with the aim of trying to prevent further obstetric injury and prolapse. There is, however, no evidence that caesarean section reduces the risk of a prolapse or urinary incontinence [5].

In this case, although she already has a degree of pelvic floor injury resulting in prolapse, a caesarean section will not prevent deterioration of this and on balance is likely to have a greater morbidity than a further vaginal delivery. The advice should therefore be to aim for a vaginal delivery unless there is an obstetric reason to plan otherwise. The patient could receive conservative therapy for the prolapse until her family is complete and then surgical correction may be considered if she so wishes [5].

Other causes for the development of prolapse are those that predispose to prolonged or sustained periods of raised intra-abdominal pressure. In this case, Andrea has a high BMI, smokes and has an occupation that may involve lifting patients. It is important to also ask if she suffers with constipation. All these factors predispose her to having sustained periods of straining, which increases intra-abdominal pressure, forcing the pelvic organs down into the vagina. These risk factors should all be addressed before any form of surgical treatment is considered.

Other risk factors for the development of prolapse include collagen/connective tissue disorders [6]. The most severe forms of this include Ehlers–Danlos syndrome. Ageing is the other major risk factor [7] as atrophic tissues can be associated with prolapse. There is no evidence in the postmenopausal patient that hormone replacement therapy (HRT) would reduce or reverse the development of a sustained prolapse. However, HRT (especially in the form of topical administration) can be useful as an adjunct to surgery or pessary usage. This will be discussed later.

What Should You Look for When Assessing This Patient?

History

As discussed previously, prolapse can affect all three compartments of the pelvis (anterior, apical and posterior). As such, prolapse from each compartment can cause symptoms from the organs that are present in that compartment. Anteriorly sits the urethra and bladder and patients with a cystocele or a urethrocele can present with urinary symptoms, including stress incontinence, urinary frequency and nocturia, urinary urgency and poor voiding (in advanced prolapse). Posterior compartment involvement suggests injury to the supporting structures of the rectum and small bowel. Patients can present with obstructive defecation, incomplete evacuation of the bowel requiring digitation and perineal splinting, and occasionally concomitant faecal urgency or incontinence. Non-specific symptoms of prolapse include vaginal bulge (often worse at the end of the day or on straining), pelvic aching (which may extend down to both thighs), backache and dyspareunia. A careful detailed history is necessary to elicit which compartments may be affected before going on to clinical examination.

What Other Salient Features in Andreas's History Would You Want to Elicit?

The most important thing to ascertain from Andrea is whether the prolapse does indeed bother her in day-to-day life. In other words, does it negatively impact her quality of life? If the prolapse has been noted by the practice nurse and is an incidental finding and completely asymptomatic with little effect on her day-to-day living, the advice should always be to leave things well alone until it does become bothersome. Often, reassurance that a prolapse is not dangerous is all that is needed. Lifestyle advice, including maintaining a healthy BMI, regular exercise and avoiding smoking, should still be given. Patients can sometimes be concerned that it may get worse in the future and would therefore like to have it corrected now while they are still young. The advice from the surgeon should always be only to undergo surgery when the prolapse becomes an issue, as age is seldom a cause not to operate.

Clinical Examination

It is first worth looking on clinical examination for risk factors to the development of prolapse including high BMI, co-morbidities such as chronic obstructive pulmonary disease (COPD) or asthma or any scars to the perineum caused by obstetric injury. An abdomino-pelvic examination should be performed to exclude any pelvic masses with the patient lying supine. Then, in the left lateral position, the vagina is inspected using a Sims' speculum (Figure 25.2). This is inserted initially retracting the posterior vaginal wall to inspect the anterior compartment and apex. The speculum is then slowly withdrawn back out through the introitus, to see if any ensuing enterocele or rectocele falls into the vagina behind the lip of the retracted speculum. Urinalysis should also be performed as routine to exclude haematuria or urinary tract infection.

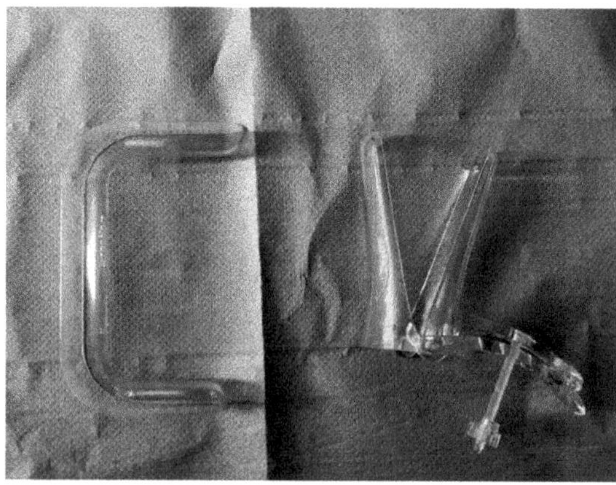

Figure 25.2 Sims' and Cusco's speculum. Sims' is used with the patient in the left lateral position and enables inspection of each compartment for prolapse.

Any obvious pelvic mass or haematuria should be referred to the appropriate rapid access clinic at the hospital, and any urinary tract infection treated. Signs of atrophy should be noted and treated with topical oestrogens if felt appropriate and symptomatic.

Classification of Pelvic Organ Prolapse

As explained earlier, prolapses can be classified into the appropriate compartment:

- anterior compartment – urethra, bladder
- apical – uterus, vaginal vault (if uterus is absent)
- posterior compartment – small bowel, rectum.

The prolapse derives its nomenclature from the affected organ (Table 25.1).

The prolapse can further be graded by severity. This can be done in two ways. Commonly clinicians in primary care and gynaecology use the Baden–Walker classification:

- Stage 1 – prolapse has descended to halfway to the hymen (> 1 cm above the hymen).
- Stage 2 – the prolapse has descended to the hymen (within +/−1 cm of the hymen).
- Stage 3 – the prolapse has descended past the hymen (> 1 cm below the hymen).
- Stage 4 – prolapse is at maximum descent (eversion of the lower genital tract is complete).

Clinicians in secondary care may sometimes refer to the POPQ (pelvic organ prolapse quantification) grading. This involves taking quantitative measurements of six vaginal points representing anterior, apical and posterior vaginal prolapse in centimetres relative to the hymen [8].

Investigation

Very little in the way of investigation is needed for a patient with POP. Once abdominopelvic examination has excluded any pelvic masses and urine dipstick analysis is negative, investigations are dependent on the patient's symptoms and can be geared accordingly. If the patient has a retroverted uterus or is obese, then pelvic masses can be difficult to feel on bimanual examination and a pelvic ultrasound scan may be necessary. Urodynamics are not necessarily routine but are warranted if surgery is being considered. Patients with concomitant bowel symptoms that are refractive to stool softeners may need referral to a coloproctologist or combined pelvic floor clinic (if available) for clinical assessment. Those with symptoms of obstructed defaecation may need proctography (conventional or MRI) to look for an intussusception, as well as rectocoele or enterocele. If they have faecal urgency or incontinence, then endoanal ultrasound may be necessary to assess anal sphincter integrity. Anal manometry is occasionally indicated to assess sphincter function.

Table 25.1 Classification of prolapse

Compartment	Structure	Prolapse
Anterior	Urethra Bladder	Urethrocoele Cystocoele
Apex	Uterus Vault	Uterine prolapse Vault prolapse
Posterior	Small Bowel Omentum Rectum	Enterocoele Enterocoele Rectocoele

What Are the Treatment Options for Prolapse?

Conservative Therapies

Conservative treatments are centred round reducing or preventing predisposing factors for the development or worsening of prolapse. These include weight loss in the obese patient, treatment of chronic cough or constipation and also smoking cessation. It is important to take a good, detailed history of the patient's bowel habit as often concomitant constipation and straining exist. Review of the patient's Bristol stool score can help to educate the patient on what a normal stool consistency should be [9]. The use of stool softeners such as Laxido, Fybogel or Movicol are all helpful in aiming to increase the water content of the stool and thus reducing its hardness. If obstructive defecation and incomplete emptying persist despite optimising the patient's stool consistency, one may consider referral to a combined pelvic floor clinic. Here patients can be assessed with a proctogram or even magnetic resonance proctography to rule out concomitant intussusception which may co-exist with the vaginal prolapse.

Studies have shown that pelvic floor exercises may be helpful in the treatment of prolapse, especially in stage 1 and stage 2, and so referral to pelvic floor physiotherapy should be made for these patients [10,11,16].

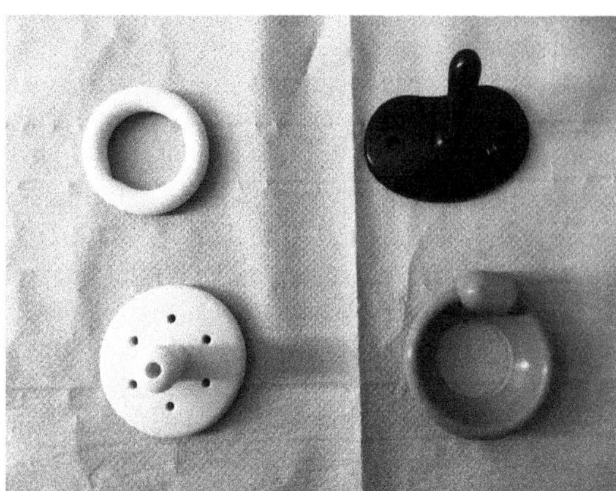

Figure 25.3 Common types of pessaries used in clinical practice. Top left: ring, top right: shelf, bottom left: Gellhorn, bottom right: hinged ring.

Pessaries are one of the most common forms of conservative therapy with a high (70–90%) level of patient satisfaction [12,13]. These are inserted into the vagina and require replacement every three to six months, depending on the type of pessaries used. Silicone ring pessaries can be changed every six months, while shelf pessaries have a greater chance of causing ulceration and incarceration, and need changing every three months. The size and shape necessary vary on type of prolapse and the patient's wishes. The use of pessaries can cause vaginal ulceration and infection, and therefore the vagina should be carefully inspected at the time of replacement or insertion. Topical oestrogens in the form of pessaries or creams may be beneficial in reducing vaginal ulceration. The main indications for pessary treatment are:

- the patient wishes to avoid surgical intervention
- the patient is medically unfit to undergo surgery
- symptomatic relief while waiting for surgery
- the patient has not completed their family or is currently pregnant or in the early post-partum period/breastfeeding
- as a therapeutic test to ascertain whether correction of the prolapse will improve the patient's symptoms before considering surgery.

The commonest pessaries used in the past have been ring and shelf pessaries. There is now a greater variety such as the Gellhorn, cube pessaries and the hinged ring pessary, which the patient can take out and insert by themselves (Figure 25.3).

Surgical Therapies

The aim of surgery is to restore normal anatomy, as well as normal function. There are a variety of vaginal and abdominal operations designed to correct prolapse. Although one would not expect a GP to counsel a patient fully about the variety of surgical procedures, a knowledge of the surgery is essential to discuss with the patient prior to referral and also to help manage any postoperative problems [16].

Anterior Compartment Surgery

Anterior repair (colporrhaphy) is the most commonly performed surgical procedure. An anterior vaginal wall incision is made and the defect in the endopelvic fascia underlying the bladder is isolated and closed, usually with interrupted absorbable sutures. With the bladder position restored, any redundant vaginal epithelium is removed and the lesion closed.

Posterior Compartment Surgery

Posterior colporrhaphy is performed in the instance of a rectocele. A similar incision is made to an anterior colporrhaphy, but on the posterior vaginal wall. The fascial defect is closed, preventing the rectum herniating into the vagina. Once the anatomy of the rectum is restored, any redundant epithelium is excised and the incision closed.

Repair of an enterocele involves excision of the peritoneal sac containing the small bowel and then approximating the peritoneum and/or the uterosacral ligaments at the same time. This is often performed with concomitant posterior colporrhaphy.

Apical Compartment Prolapse

The commonest procedure for uterine prolapse is vaginal hysterectomy. This is one of the oldest major operations with the references dating back to Hypocrites in the fifth century BC. The operation involves incising the vaginal epithelium around the cervix and then entering the peritoneal cavity between the bladder and the uterus and the rectum and the uterus. The major blood vessels are then ligated and the uterus removed through the vagina. The vault is then closed and supported by sutures into the uterosacral-cardinal ligament complex.

Uterine-Preserving Surgery for Uterine Prolapse

The uterus can be preserved if the patient so wishes. Ideally, surgery should not be contemplated until the patient has completed their family; however, there have been case reports of successful pregnancies following uterine-preserving prolapse surgery. The uterus can be suspended to a variety of structures, including the anterior longitudinal ligament overlying the sacrum (sacro-hysteropexy with mesh) or to the sacrospinous ligament (vaginal sacrospinous hysteropexy).

Manchester Repair

This procedure is seldom performed. It involves accessing the uterus vaginally, shortening the cervix and then using the uterosacral and cardinal ligament complex to support the uterus. This has gone out of vogue due to problems with cervical stenosis or cervical incompetence and risk of miscarriage.

Le Fort's Colpocleisis

This operation is used in very frail patients who are unfit for major surgery. It involves partial closure of the vagina by suturing the anterior and posterior vaginal walls together, thus preventing the uterus from falling through the vaginal opening.

Vault Prolapse

After a hysterectomy, failure of support to the vaginal vault can occur in a proportion of patients. In this situation the vault needs to be attached back within the pelvis either to the anterior longitudinal ligament that overlies the sacrum (open/laparoscopic sacrocolpopexy with mesh) or to the sacrospinous ligament (vaginal sacrospinous fixation).

Mesh Procedures

The use of mesh to treat prolapse of the uterus or vaginal vault has declined significantly since a report by the Food and Drug Administration (FDA) in 2009 recommended caution in its usage. This was due to the recognised risk of mesh erosion or exposure leading to pain, vaginal discharge or infection, or dyspareunia [14]. National Institute for Health and Care Excellence (NICE) guidance recommends patients should be counselled about the possible short- and long-term risks of synthetic mesh. In 2018 the use of vaginal mesh was banned in the UK and can only be confined to abdominal placed mesh (sacrohysteropexy/sacrocolpopexy) [15].

Patients may find decision aids for surgical treatments options of prolapse, including information on mesh, on the British Society of Urogynaecology website: www.bsug.org.uk [16].

Conclusion

Prolapse is a common condition that presents regularly in primary care. Treatment is only necessary if the patient has bothersome symptoms; asymptomatic prolapse requires reassurance alone. Pessaries and physiotherapy can be provided in the community if the patient wishes. Although the mainstay of treatment is surgery, referral for surgery should only be considered if the patient is symptomatic, has completed their family and wishes surgical intervention.

References

[1] V. Bonney, 'The principles that should underlie all operations for prolapse', *BJOG*, vol. **1**, no. 5, pp. 669–683, 1934.

[2] J. DeLancey, 'Anatomy and biomechanics of genital prolapse', *Clin Obstet Gynecol*, vol. **36**, no. 4, pp. 897–909, 1993.

[3] A. H. MacLennan, A. W. Taylor, D. H. Wilson and D. Wilson, 'The prevalence of pelvic floor disorders and their relationship to gender, age, parity and mode of delivery', *BJOG*, vol. **107**, no. 12, pp. 1460–1470, 2000.

[4] J. Mant, R. Painter and M. Vessey, 'Epidemiology of genital prolapse: Observations from the Oxford Family Planning Association Study', *Br J Obstet Gynaecol*, vol. **104**, no. 5, pp. 579–585, 1997.

[5] H. P. Dietz and J. M. Simpson, 'Levator trauma is associated with pelvic organ prolapse', *BJOG*, vol. **115**, no. 8, pp. 979–984, 2008.

[6] I. Malfouz, F. Asali and C. Phillips, 'The management of urogynaecological problems in pregnancy and early postpartum', *Obstet Gynaecol*, vol. **14**, no. 3, pp. 154–158, 2012.

[7] C. H. Phillips, F. Anthony, C. Benyon and A. K. Monga, 'Collagen metabolism in the uterosacral ligaments and vaginal skin of women with uterine prolapse', *BJOG*, vol. **113**, no. 1, pp. 39–46, 2006.

[8] C. Persu, C. R. Chapple, V. Cauni, S. Gutue and P. Geavlete, 'Pelvic Organ Prolapse Quantification System (POP–Q): A new era in pelvic prolapse staging', *J Med Life*, vol. **4**, no. 1, 75, 2011.

[9] I. McCallum, S. Ong and M. Mercer-Jones, 'Chronic constipation in adults', *BMJ*, vol. **338**, b831, 2009.

[10] S. Hagen, D. Stark, C. Maher and E. Adams, 'Conservative management of pelvic organ prolapse in women', *Cochrane Database Syst Rev*, vol. **2**, CD003882, 2004.

[11] S. Hagen, D. Stark, C. Glazener et al., 'A multicentre randomised controlled trial of a pelvic floor muscle training intervention for women with pelvic organ prolapse'. *41st Annual Meeting of the International Continence Society, 29 August–2 September 2011*, Abstract 000129.

[12] B. H. Lamers, B. M. Broekman and A. L. Milani, 'Pessary treatment for pelvic organ prolapse and health-related quality of life: A review', *Int Urogynecol J*, vol. **22**, pp. 637–644, 2011.

[13] C. Bugge, E. J. Adams, D. Gopinath and F. Reid, 'Pessaries (mechanical devices) for pelvic organ prolapse in women', *Cochrane Database Syst Rev*, vol. **2**, CD004010, 2013.

[14] US Food and Drug Administration, 'FDA safety communication: Update on serious complications associated with transvaginal placement of surgical mesh for pelvic organ prolapse'. 2011. Accessed: 1 May 2024. [Online]. Available: www.fda.gov/MedicalDevices/Safety/AlertsandNotices/ucm262435.htm.

[15] National Institute for Health and Care Excellence, 'Surgical repair of vaginal wall prolapse using mesh'. Accessed: 1 May 2024. [Online]. Available: www.nice.org.uk/guidance/ipg267.

[16] National Institute for Health and Care Excellence, 'Urinary incontinence and pelvic organ prolapse in women: Management'. 2019. Accessed: 1 May 2024. [Online]. Available: www.nice.org.uk/guidance/ng123.

Chapter 26

Ovarian Cancer

A Primary Care Perspective

Ken S. Metcalf

Key Points

- Ninety per cent of ovarian cancers arise from the epithelium.
- Ovarian cancer presents late – only 30% are diagnosed in an early stage when the prognosis is better.
- There is no screening process with an acceptable risk/benefit profile.
- The presenting symptom with the greatest positive predictive value (PPV) is abdominal distension – the PPV is over 5% if this is associated with appetite loss.
- CA 125, clinical examination and ultrasound (USS) are important in the assessment of suspected ovarian cancer, as is calculating the risk of malignancy index (RMI). Advances in USS assessment are likely to be of greater importance in the immediate future.
- CA 125 over 200 in a premenopausal, and over 65 in a postmenopausal woman, would give a high RMI and alone act as a red flag.
- The commonest hereditary syndrome is the breast ovarian cancer syndrome associated with BRCA 1 and 2. Lynch syndrome (hereditary nonpolyposis colorectal cancer) is another.
- Laparoscopic bilateral salipingo-oopherectromy (BSO) is a safe and effective strategy for women identified as at increased personal risk.
- Use of the oral contraceptive pill (OCP) confers considerable risk reduction for ovarian cancer.

The term ovarian cancer tends to represent the group of tumours arising from the ovarian surface epithelium (epithelial ovarian cancer or EOC). EOC is by far the commonest malignant tumour of the ovary and represents over 90% of all ovarian tumours.

One in 52 women will be diagnosed with ovarian cancer during their lifetime. Around 7,500 women are diagnosed with ovarian cancer in the UK each year, making it the sixth most common cancer, representing 4% of all new cancer cases in women. Among gynaecological cancers, ovarian cancer has the highest mortality, with over 4,000 deaths per year, accounting for 5% of all cancer deaths in women.

Ovarian cancer incidence is strongly related to age, with the highest incidence rates being in older women. In the UK in 2016–2018, more than a quarter of new cases (28%) were in females aged 75 and over [1].

Analysis of ovarian cancer mortality rates throughout the UK shows very little variation between health boundaries, and European age-standardised mortality rates do not differ significantly to those in the UK.

For patients where the stage was recorded at diagnosis, 57% were advanced disease (stage III or IV, indicating tumour spread beyond the pelvis). The one-year relative survival rate for early-stage disease (stages I or II – tumours confined to pelvis) is good (88.6–98.1%) in comparison to late-stage disease (51.5–71.3%) [1,2]. As such, a major goal in improving outcomes from this disease would be to stage shift diagnosis and increase the proportion of early-stage tumours detected.

Early Diagnosis

Currently, only 30% of patients are diagnosed with early-stage disease. Early symptom recognition and screening are two key areas that could lead to early-stage shift.

Symptoms

Symptoms associated with ovarian cancer are also common in non-malignant conditions. One estimate suggested that as many as 95% of women attending primary care have a symptom potentially representing ovarian cancer [3].

Hamilton et al. [4] looked at the PPV of symptoms for ovarian cancer; that is, the chance that a woman with a specific symptom has ovarian cancer. This large case-control study involved a retrospective review of case records in 39 general practices to identify all (212) women aged > 40 diagnosed with ovarian cancer in 2000–2007. Of these, 32% were stages I and II, 45% stage III and 23% stage IV. Their medical records were examined in the year prior to diagnosis and the PPV was calculated for seven key symptoms: abdominal distension 2.5%, loss of appetite 0.6%, abdominal pain 0.3%, increased urinary frequency 0.2%, abdominal bloating 0.3% and rectal bleeding 0.2%. Abdominal distension in combination with any other of the key symptoms increased the PPV, particularly with loss of appetite where the PPV was > 5%.

The small PPVs identified in this study reflect both the common nature of such symptoms and the low incidence of ovarian cancer, but it seems that persisting abdominal distension (in contrast to bloating, which is an intermittent symptom) should be a red flag symptom and lead to urgent further investigation. Whether early symptom recognition will lead to a stage shift diagnosis remains unproven, but it is noteworthy that in this study 34% of the early-stage cancers and 35% of late-stage cancers presented with abdominal distension within a year of diagnosis, in comparison to 0.6% of controls. One might hypothesise that a fraction of the late-stage disease patients may have progressed from an earlier stage during the course of the year.

NICE

The National Institute for Health and Care Excellence (NICE) guidelines [5] recommend that in women (especially if over the age of 50) with suspicious symptoms for ovarian cancer, a clinical examination should be performed along with a serum CA 125. An elevation in CA 125 over 35 IU/mL or the presence of a pelvic mass should lead to a pelvic ultrasound assessment. For women who have a CA 125 of 35 IU/mL or greater, but normal pelvic ultrasound, NICE recommends careful assessment for other clinical causes of symptoms and investigation if appropriate. If no cause is found the woman should be advised to return to the GP if symptoms become more frequent and/or persistent.

Adopting the NICE guideline measures meant that many women were reassured on the basis of a normal CA 125 result. However, it has long been known that patients with early-stage ovarian cancers often have normal CA 125 levels [6]. More recent data from the United Kingdom Collaborative Trial of Ovarian Cancer Screening (UKCTOCS) has shown serial CA 125 estimation to be important and that velocity change, even within the normal reference range, can confer high risk when interpreted using their risk of ovarian cancer algorithm (ROCA) [7]. These data indicate that a new paradigm will need to be defined to ensure maximum reassurance is provided.

Screening Tests

Employing a general-population screening test to detect ovarian cancer at an early stage remains the subject of ongoing global research, but to date a successful screening strategy has not been found.

A major concern in screening is to establish a successful balance between sensitivity (the ability to detect the problem when present) and specificity (the ability to not detect a problem when absent) of the screening test. Sensitivity reflects the false-negative rate and a high level of sensitivity will indicate a low false-negative rate. Specificity reflects the false-positive rate and a high level of specificity reflects a low false-positive rate. An ideal test has very high sensitivity and specificity. In terms of cancer screening, it is clearly important to have the highest sensitivity possible to ensure the tumour is detected and not missed by the test. A very high specificity will also reduce the likelihood of a false-positive result. This is particularly important as the consequences of a positive result often include invasive tests or surgery, both of which have significant complication risks in terms of morbidity and even mortality.

Even with very good test performance (high specificity), the low background prevalence of ovarian cancer means that the number of unnecessary interventions can be unacceptable. Assuming the prevalence for ovarian cancer of 1:2500 women and a test specificity as high as 99.6% (i.e. 0.4 false-positive cases in every 100 tests), there would be 10 false positives per case detected – an unacceptable ratio.

There is a wide range of commercially available biomarker blood tests for ovarian cancer. While these are of significant value in secondary care triage for known pelvic pathology, none has demonstrated a high enough sensitivity and specificity to be recommended and at this time patients should be discouraged from using commercially available screening kits.

Current screening strategies are most focused on combinations of transvaginal ultrasound scanning and CA 125 testing. Two large studies have looked at this, but in different ways.

The Prostate, Lung, Colorectal and Ovarian (PLCO) multicentre American trial [8] looked at annual screening with ultrasound and CA 125. It failed to show any reduction in mortality and in those women with false-positive results, 15% sustained a major complication from the subsequent surgical intervention.

In 2001, the UKCTOCS trial commenced and recruited more than 200,000 women aged between 50 and 64 who were randomly assigned to one of three groups – control, annual ultrasound or annual CA 125 test. In the latter group, instead of relying on the absolute value of the CA 125 level, the result was utilised as part of the ROCA test (see earlier). Early published data showed an increase in the number of ovarian cancers diagnosed at an early stage with screening, but the latest published results have not shown any confirmed impact on overall mortality from this trial in either screening arm [9]. The early results suggest that approximately 15 ovarian cancer deaths could be prevented for every 10,000 women who attend for screening that involves annual blood tests between 7 and 11 years, but longer-term follow-up is required to confirm this. In the UKCTOCS study, for every three women having surgery for presumed ovarian cancer (based on their blood test), two of them turned out not to have cancer. This represents a lot of unnecessary surgery for the screened population. Notwithstanding the undoubted psychological effects of false-positive results, major complications occurred in 3% of women having surgery. It is still unclear whether the risk/benefit ratio is in favour of screening in this way.

Results Assessment and Secondary Care Referral Patterns

Where investigations indicate an abnormality, correct interpretation is vital in both counselling the patient and determining the most appropriate route for secondary care referral. In many cases the results will indicate a greater likelihood of benign abnormality. In such cases expectant management may be appropriate or referral on a non-urgent pathway for a general gynaecological opinion and management. For others at greater risk, urgent referral to a specialist gynaecological oncology multidisciplinary team is essential, as there is strong data to indicate better outcomes for women with gynaecological malignancies, particularly ovarian cancer, where treatment is undertaken in specialised centres [10].

In a postmenopausal woman, an abnormal CA 125 level or the presence of a pelvic mass on ultrasound should lead to urgent referral for a secondary care opinion, usually as a cancer two-week wait referral. This approach is also appropriate for the premenopausal patient where CA 125 level is greater than 200 IU/mL or the ultrasound report indicates suspicion of malignancy. For other premenopausal cases where the CA 125 level is raised but < 200 IU/mL and where the ultrasound report indicates a cystic adnexal mass with minimal complexity, there may be a dilemma faced by the referring clinician in terms of the urgency and/or best place for secondary care referral. In such circumstances it may be helpful to consider the calculation made by secondary care specialists for overall risk of malignancy, the RMI [11].

The RMI assessment involves calculating the product of the formula:

Age score × CA 125 score × Ultrasound score

Commonly, an RMI calculation of > 200 would be taken as conferring a significant enough risk of malignancy to merit urgent and specialist referral. The age score relates to menopausal status (score 1 for premenopausal, 3 for postmenopausal). The CA 125 score is the absolute level of CA 125 in IU/mL. The ultrasound score is either 1 or 3, where 3 would be an ultrasound report indicating more than one of five possible features on scan (multilocularity, bilaterality, presence of solid components within cyst, presence of pelvic fluid/ascites, presence of possible abdominal implants).

It is noteworthy that a CA 125 level of 200 in a premenopausal patient or 65 in a postmenopausal patient will result in a high risk RMI calculation even where the ultrasound findings are not particularly suspicious (i.e. score 1). It is useful to keep these two CA 125 levels in mind as red flags.

Advances in ultrasound technology and operator-dependent skills are leading to much greater accuracy with risk prediction using ultrasound alone. The International Ovarian Tumour Analysis (IOTA) Study algorithms show a better sensitivity and specificity for cancer prediction than RMI in both pre- and postmenopausal women [12]. The ultrasound variables which IOTA has shown to be required are within the capacity of non-expert ultrasonographers and will undoubtedly soon become represented widely in mainstream ultrasound reporting. This will help guide referral from primary care level, leading to the most appropriate level of triage and choice of surgical specialist at secondary and tertiary care level.

Identifying High-Risk Women

The recognition of women at significantly increased risk of developing ovarian cancer and referral for preventative surgery is an important component in any strategy to improve ovarian cancer outcomes.

The strongest known risk factor is a family history of the disease, which is present in 10–15% of women with ovarian cancer. Women with a single family member affected with ovarian cancer have a 4–5% lifetime risk (general-population risk 1.4%). With two affected relatives the risk is 7%. In some circumstances a definite hereditary ovarian cancer syndrome is identified and such women have a lifetime risk as high as 50%.

The commonest hereditary syndrome is the breast ovarian cancer syndrome, accounting for over 90% of hereditary ovarian cancers. This syndrome is associated with mutations in the BRCA1 or 2 genes and confers high risk for both ovarian and breast cancer. Risk-reducing strategies therefore take account of both ovarian and breast cancer. BRCA1 mutations increase risk significantly for both cancers from age 35, so it is important that risk-reducing measures are implemented early for both. For BRCA2 mutations, breast cancer risk is significantly increased from age 35, whereas ovarian cancer risk appears to only be significantly increased from age 45. This leaves the opportunity to delay ovarian cancer risk-reducing measures for BRCA2 cases if desired.

Lynch syndrome, also known as hereditary nonpolyposis colorectal cancer (HNPCC), is the other common hereditary ovarian cancer syndrome. This syndrome is associated with mutation of the MLH1, MSH2, MSH6 and PMS2 genes. Affected patients have high risk to develop colon, endometrial and ovarian cancers, so risk-reduction strategies must consider all sites.

Where a patient is identified as having a family history of ovarian, breast, colon or endometrial cancer, it will be helpful to refer for a formal genetics consultation. In many circumstances this will be initially conducted by genetic counsellors and where high risk is suspected, a more accurate risk stratification calculation is done with potential genetic testing.

Risk-Reducing Surgery

Even in high-risk women who have a known familial or genetically increased risk for ovarian cancer, annual screening has no impact on mortality. Further study is underway to establish if more frequent screening intervals might confer greater advantage. Until such time, risk-reducing surgery remains the only way to reduce mortality from ovarian/fallopian tube cancers for these women [13].

BSO in women who carry the BRCA1 or BRCA2 mutations will considerably reduce the lifetime risk for ovarian, tubal or peritoneal cancers, although not eliminate it completely (residual risk approximately 0.1%). BSO in these women reduces their breast cancer risk by 50% also [14]. Women that undergo risk-reducing BSO, compared to those that do not, have an associated lower all-cause mortality (10% vs. 3%), breast cancer-specific mortality (6% vs. 2%) and ovarian cancer-specific mortality (3% vs. 0.4%) [15].

The vast majority of risk-reducing surgeries will be laparoscopic. This approach is associated with little morbidity and is usually performed as day case surgery. In practice, most women are concerned about timing of surgery, whether to have a concurrent hysterectomy and the hormonal implications of the intervention.

In BRCA1 carriers the risk for both breast and ovarian cancer starts to rise significantly from age 35 and general consensus would be that risk-reducing surgery to both breasts and ovaries should be considered after this age, as soon as childbearing is complete. For BRCA2 carriers, while increased breast cancer risk still occurs early, as for BRCA1, the ovarian cancer increased risk occurs later (significantly from age 45). These women may choose to delay risk-reducing BSO, but they would not then get the benefit of breast cancer risk reduction from earlier BSO.

A minimum surgical intervention for risk reduction is BSO in isolation. The fallopian tubes should be removed in addition to the ovaries as it is now recognised that many ovarian cancers first arise in the fallopian tubes [16]. In some cases there are convincing concurrent gynaecological indications for total hysterectomy also. The presence of a significant increase in endometrial cancer risk with Lynch syndrome (HNPCC) is a compelling indication. Women on tamoxifen therapy may also choose to eliminate the small associated increased endometrial cancer risk with concomitant hysterectomy. Concerns raised in relation to the increased risk of breast cancer in combined hormone replacement therapy (HRT) users compared with oestrogen only users [17] are a strong stimulus for many women choosing hysterectomy as part of their risk-reducing surgery as subsequent HRT may then be oestrogen only.

The inclusion of hysterectomy as part of the surgical strategy obviously increases the scale of the surgical intervention and potential risk in comparison to BSO alone, but many women will be suitable candidates for a total laparoscopic approach (TLH), which has clear benefits in terms of perioperative morbidity and time to recovery.

For those women having risk-reducing surgery with a preceding history of breast cancer, oestrogen replacement therapy would be inadvisable as some data suggests an increase in recurrence risk. Nevertheless, where intractable menopausal symptoms arise, decision-making will need to be individualised. For others, available data suggests that HRT may be given to women up to the age of 50 with no loss of benefit in terms of breast cancer risk reduction [18]. This guidance appears to be reasonable for BRCA1 carriers also, where only 3.9% of breast cancers are oestrogen-receptor positive. A slightly greater anxiety may be required for BRCA2 carriers where incident breast cancers are more often oestrogen-receptor positive [19].

Non-Surgical Risk-Reduction Strategies

Screening may be offered to women who decline risk-reducing surgery. In this setting a six-month /yearly screening interval should be considered. This should start from age 35 (or 5 years earlier than the youngest age of ovarian cancer diagnosis in the family).

It has long been known that use of the OCP is associated with a significant reduction in risk of ovarian cancer. This effect increases with duration of use. The odds ratio for ovarian cancer incidence in ever-users compared to never-users is 0.73. With more than 10 years' OCP use, lifetime incidence of ovarian cancer is reduced by 50% [20].

In BRCA mutation carriers, OCP use has a significantly protective effect for ovarian cancer (odds ratio 0.58) and, while the association with breast cancer showed a suggestion of increased risk, this was not significant [21].

Summary

EOC remains a major health problem with poor overall outcomes. Strategies for early diagnosis have so far proven disappointing and shown negligible impact on overall mortality. However, continued recognition of the risk reduction conferred by OCP use and identification of those high-risk women who will benefit from risk-reducing surgery are clear goals from a primary care and public health perspective.

References

[1] Cancer Research UK, 'Ovarian cancer statistics'. Accessed: 19 Nov. 2025. [Online]. Available: www.cancerresearchuk.org/health-professional/cancer-statistics/statistics-by-cancer-type/ovarian-cancer.

[2] S. McPhail, S. Johnson, D. Greenberg et al., 'Stage diagnosis and early mortality from cancer in England', *Br J Cancer*, vol. **112**, S108–S115, 2015.

[3] B. Goff, L. Mandel, C. Melancon, H. Muntz, 'Frequency of symptoms of ovarian cancer in women presenting to primary care clinics', *JAMA*, vol. **291**, no. 22, pp. 2705–2712, 2004.

[4] W. Hamilton, T. Peters, C. Bankhead and D. Sharp, 'Risk of ovarian cancer in women with symptoms in primary care: Population based case-control study', *BMJ*, vol. **339**, b2998, 2009.

[5] NICE, 'Ovarian cancer: The recognition and initial management CG122'. Apr. 2011, updated Oct. 2023. Accessed: 19 Nov. 2025. [Online]. Available: www.nice.org.uk/guidance/CG122.

[6] J. Zurawski, R. Knapp, N. Einhorn et al., 'An initial analysis of preoperative serum CA125 levels in patients with early stage ovarian carcinoma', *Gynecol Oncol*, vol. **30**, pp. 7–14, 1988.

[7] U. Menon, A. Ryan, J. Kalsi et al., 'Risk algorithm using serial biomarker measurements doubles the number of screen detected cancers compared with single threshold rule in the United Kingdom collaborative trial of ovarian cancer screening', *J Clin Oncol*, vol. **33**, pp. 2062–2071, 2015.

[8] S. Buys, E. Partridge, A. Black et al., 'Effect of screening on ovarian cancer mortality: The Prostate, Lung, Colorectal and Ovarian (PLCO)

cancer screening randomized controlled trial', *JAMA*, vol. **305**, no. 22, pp. 2295–2303, 2011.

[9] I. Jacobs, U. Menon, A. Ryan et al., 'Ovarian cancer screening and mortality in the UK Collaborative Trial of Ovarian Cancer Screening (UKCTOCS): A randomized controlled trial', *Lancet*, vol. **387**, no. 10022, pp. 945–956, 2016.

[10] Y. Woo, M. Kyrgiou, A. Bryant et al., 'Centralisation of services for gynaecological cancers: A Cochrane systematic review', *Gynecol Oncol*, vol. **126**, pp. 286–290, 2012.

[11] I. Jacobs, D. Oram, J. Fairbanks et al., 'A risk of malignancy index incorporating CA125, ultrasound and menopausal status for the accurate preoperative diagnosis of ovarian cancer', *Br J Obstet Gynaecol*, vol. **97**, pp. 922–929, 1990.

[12] J. Kaijser, A. Sayasneh, K. Van Hoorde et al., 'Presurgical diagnosis of adnexal tumours using mathematical models and scoring systems: A systematic review and meta analysis', *Hum Reprod Update*, vol. **20**, pp. 449–462, 2014.

[13] A. Rosenthal, L. Fraser, R. Manchanda et al., 'Results of annual screening in phase I of the United Kingdom familial ovarian cancer screening study highlight the need for strict adherence to screening schedule', *J Clin Oncol*, vol. **31**, no. 1, pp. 49–57, 2013.

[14] T. Rebbeck, H. Lynch, S. Neuhausen et al., 'Prophylactic oophorectomy in carriers of BRCA1 or BRCA2 mutations', *N Engl J Med*, vol. **346**, pp. 1616–1622, 2002.

[15] S. Domchek, T. Friebel, C. Singer et al., 'Association of risk reducing surgery in BRCA1 or BRCA2 mutation carriers with cancer risk and mortality', *JAMA*, vol. **304**, no. 9, pp. 967–975, 2010.

[16] N. Nik, R. Vang, S. Ie-Ming et al., 'Origin and pathogenesis of pelvic (ovarian, tubal and peritoneal) serous carcinoma', *Ann Rev Pathol*, vol. **9**, pp. 27–45, 2014.

[17] H. Kuhl and H. Schneider, 'Progesterone: Promoter or inhibitor of breast cancer', *Climacteric*, vol. **16**(suppl. 1), pp. 54–68, 2013.

[18] Scottish Intercollegiate Guidelines Network, 'Sign 135: Management of epithelial ovarian cancer'. Nov. 2013. Accessed: 19 Nov. 2025. [Online]. Available: www.sign.ac.uk.

[19] W. Foulkes, K. Metcalfe, P. Sun et al., 'Estrogen receptor status in BRCA1 and BRCA2 related breast cancer: The influence of age, grade and histological type', *Clin Cancer Res*, vol. **10**, no. 6, pp. 2029–2034, 2004.

[20] L. Havrilesky, P. Moorman, W. Lowery et al., 'Oral contraceptive pills as primary prevention for ovarian cancer: A systematic review and meta-analysis', *Obstet Gynecol*, vol. **122**, no. 1, pp. 139–147, 2013.

[21] P. Moorman, L. Havrilesky, J. Gierisch et al., 'Oral contraceptives and risk of ovarian cancer and breast cancer among high-risk women: A systematic review and meta-analysis', *J Clin Oncol*, vol. **31**, no. 33, pp. 4188–4198, 2013.

Chapter 27

The Management of Endometrial Hyperplasia and Carcinoma in Primary Care

Dileep Wijeratne and Inga Chen

Key Points

- The natural history of endometrial cancer is a progression through various stages of endometrial hyperplasia offering opportunities for treatments if the problem is identified at an early stage, before progression to cancer.
- Endometrial cancer is the commonest gynaecological malignancy in the UK and the incidence is increasing alongside the current obesity epidemic.
- The majority of cases of endometrial hyperplasia and cancer result from unopposed oestrogenic stimulation of endometrial growth. Risk factors include obesity, increasing age, anovulatory conditions such as polycystic ovarian syndrome (PCOS) and women with a uterus using oestrogen-only hormone replacement therapy (HRT).
- Postmenopausal bleeding (PMB) is the commonest presentation of endometrial malignancy. Women presenting with PMB require cervical examination to exclude a cervical cause, and referral using the urgent two-week suspected cancer pathway.
- In younger women presenting with menstrual dysfunction, a risk stratification is required to determine who can be managed in primary care and which women require early investigations.
- Measurement of endometrial thickness using ultrasound scanning, preferably by the transvaginal route, is usually the first-line investigation to exclude endometrial malignancy. In postmenopausal women endometrial thickening provides a reliable recommendation for further endometrial assessment.
- The management of endometrial hyperplasia without atypia is usually by medical means using intrauterine progestogen alongside management of any treatable cause, such as weight reduction. Oral progestogens are considered as second-line treatment.
- Monitoring of women with endometrial hyperplasia without atypia is important to ensure disease regression. This will be recommended or managed by secondary care.
- Hysterectomy is the first-line treatment for women with endometrial hyperplasia with atypia, provided they are considered fit for major surgery.
- The majority of women with endometrial cancer are diagnosed at stage 1 disease which, with early surgical treatment, has five-year survival rates of at least 92%.

Introduction

Endometrial cancer is the most common gynaecological malignancy in the UK with around 9,800 cases diagnosed every year [1]. The natural history of endometrial cancer is that of a progression through various stages of endometrial hyperplasia which, if left untreated, can progress to cancer. The incidence of endometrial hyperplasia is at least three times higher than that of endometrial cancer [2]. Early detection of endometrial hyperplasia therefore offers an opportunity for intervention and treatment before progression to endometrial cancer occurs.

The incidence of both endometrial cancer and endometrial hyperplasia has been steadily rising over the past 20 years, mainly due to increasing levels of obesity. Despite this, mortality from endometrial cancer has not increased. This is due, in large part, to the presence of clear guidelines, robust referral pathways and well-coordinated care for women presenting with symptoms such as postmenopausal bleeding. Accordingly, around 74% of cases of endometrial cancer are diagnosed at stage 1 disease, for which early treatment confers a five-year survival rate of around 92% [1].

In the coming years, an increasing number of younger women will present to primary care with symptoms of menstrual dysfunction in the context of risk factors for endometrial hyperplasia and cancer. Risk stratification of these women, followed by prompt referral for appropriate investigations and treatment, will be key in ensuring that deaths from endometrial cancer remain low. In addition, primary care will have an increasingly prominent role in supervising the treatment of endometrial hyperplasia (especially in cases of medical/conservative management). In acknowledgement of this changing landscape, this chapter discusses in detail:

1. Risk factors common to endometrial hyperplasia and cancer.
2. Classification of endometrial hyperplasia.
3. The risk of progression of each hyperplasia subtype to endometrial cancer.
4. Clinical presentation.
5. Investigations.
6. Management (conservative and surgical) and follow-up (with a focus on endometrial hyperplasia).

In addition, an illustrative case study is used to highlight some of the complexities in managing women with endometrial pathology.

Risk Factors for Endometrial Hyperplasia and Cancer

Both endometrial hyperplasia and endometrial cancer arise primarily in response to chronic oestrogenic stimulation of endometrial cell growth, unopposed by the suppressive effects of progesterone. Oestrogenic stimulation can be either intrinsic or extrinsic. Other factors such as genetic predisposition and immunosuppression can also play a role.

Obesity

- Androstenedione, produced by the theca interna cells of the ovary and the adrenal cortex, is converted to oestrogen (oestrone) by aromatase enzymes present in adipose tissue. Increased levels of peripheral adiposity are therefore associated with elevated levels of oestrone, thus increasing the overall potential for oestrogenic stimulation of the endometrium [3].

Table 27.1 Risk of atypical endometrial hyperplasia in relation to BMI [20]

BMI	Risk of atypical endometrial hyperplasia (odds ratio)
Normal BMI < 24.9	1.0
Overweight BMI 24.9–29.9	2.3
Obese BMI 30–39.9	3.7
Morbidly obese BMI 40 and above	13.0

- This is particularly relevant in situations where progesterone suppression is infrequent or absent, such as after the menopause or during episodes of amenorrhoea and anovulation seen in conditions such as polycystic ovarian syndrome.

Table 27.1 contains data from a case series of 446 women from the USA, illustrating the risk of developing atypical endometrial hyperplasia in relation to body mass index (BMI). In this series, morbid obesity conferred a 13-fold increase in the risk of developing atypical hyperplasia.

Other Forms of Endogenous Oestrogenic Stimulation

- Anovulatory menstrual cycles, whereby there is a significant reduction in the usual progestogenic suppression of the endometrium in the second half of the menstrual cycle, are more common at the extremes of reproductive life. Early menarche (at or before the age of 11) and late menopause (after the age of 55) are therefore relative risk factors for endometrial hyperplasia and cancer.
- Nulliparity confers a two- to threefold risk of developing endometrial cancer. There may be an association between the nulliparity and anovulatory menstrual cycles.

Exogenous Oestrogens

- *Oestrogen-only HRT* in women with an intact uterus (i.e. who have not undergone hysterectomy) has been shown to increase the risk of endometrial hyperplasia at all doses and is therefore not recommended [4].

- *Tamoxifen* is a selective oestrogen receptor modulator which has different effects depending on the site of action. In breast tissue, tamoxifen has an anti-oestrogenic effect, hence its use in the treatment of breast cancer. Tamoxifen has a pro-oestrogenic effect on the endometrium, increasing the risk of hyperplasia and carcinoma. This increase is not thought to be of significance in premenopausal women. The American College of Obstetricians and Gynaecologists suggests that postmenopausal women using tamoxifen should be 'closely monitored', but concludes, in keeping with the evidence, that there is no role currently for monitoring of asymptomatic women either by ultrasound or endometrial biopsy [5].

Oestrogen-Secreting Tumours

The prevalence of endometrial hyperplasia in women with *granulosa cell tumours* of the ovary has been estimated at up to 40% [6].

Genetic Risks

- *Lynch syndrome or HNPCC* (hereditary non-polyposis colorectal cancer, a DNA mismatch repair mutation) confers a lifetime risk of developing endometrial cancer of up to 50%. Although there is no clear evidence to guide practice, women with Lynch syndrome are frequently offered surveillance, usually after the age of 35, in the form of annual endometrial biopsy [6]. National Institute for Health and Care Excellence (NICE) guidelines now recommend that all women diagnosed with endometrial cancer are offered testing for Lynch syndrome, firstly by testing the malignant tissue for loss of mismatch repair (MMR) proteins and then germline testing if there are loss of these proteins detected [7].
- *Cowden syndrome* is a rare autosomal dominant disorder characterised by multiple harmatomatous growths and an increased risk of certain cancers. Women with Cowden syndrome have a lifetime risk of endometrial cancer of up to 19% [6].

Immunosuppression

Evidence from small case series involving renal graft recipients suggests that immunosuppressed individuals with abnormal uterine bleeding have up to a twofold increase in the incidence of endometrial hyperplasia at biopsy [8].

Diabetes Mellitus (Type 1 and Type 2)

Several studies have shown that diabetes is associated with an increased risk of developing endometrial cancer. This could be linked to obesity but there is some evidence that other factors like higher insulin levels may also contribute to this increase in risk [9].

Classification of Endometrial Hyperplasia

In 2014 the World Health Organization (WHO) proposed a simple revised classification which divides endometrial hyperplasia into two groups:

- hyperplasia without atypia
- atypical hyperplasia.

This new classification is based on the observation that from a clinical perspective, it is the presence or absence of nuclear atypia that is most significant with regards to risk of progression to endometrial cancer [10].

The Risk of Progression from Endometrial Hyperplasia to Endometrial Cancer

There is a paucity of high-quality data to help provide detailed and nuanced risk stratification with regards to the likelihood of endometrial hyperplasia progressing to cancer. However, the association between the presence of nuclear atypia and a significant risk of developing endometrial cancer is well established. The most useful general risk data comes from a retrospective case series of 170 patients. In the study, hysterectomy specimens were examined from women who had previously undergone endometrial sampling for abnormal menstrual bleeding. The time between endometrial sampling and hysterectomy ranged between 1 and 27 years (13 on average). The risk of progression to endometrial cancer based on the study's findings is shown in Table 27.2 alongside a brief description of the histological features of each hyperplasia subtype.

Practice point: importantly, women found to have atypical hyperplasia on histology are at significant risk of having a co-existent endometrial

Table 27.2 Risk of progression to endometrial cancer based on endometrial hyperplasia subtype [21]

Hyperplasia category	Histological features	Risk of progression to endometrial cancer
Simple hyperplasia (no atypia)	Mildly crowded glands. Mitoses may or may not be present	1%
Complex hyperplasia (no atypia)	Very crowded, disorganised glands (> 50% gland-to-stromal ratio). Mitoses present	3%
Simple hyperplasia with atypia (rare)	Nuclear enlargement with either evenly dispersed or clumped chromatin	8%

carcinoma. Studies suggest that this risk may be as high as 50% [11].

Clinical Presentation

The commonest way that women with either endometrial cancer or hyperplasia present is with abnormal uterine bleeding. In some cases, such as with postmenopausal bleeding, the indication for referral and assessment is clear and straightforward. In other cases, the decision of when to refer for investigations can be more complex. In younger women presenting with abnormal bleeding, for example the majority will be cases of benign menstrual dysfunction as only 5.4% of cases of endometrial cancer present in women aged 35–44 [12]. However, adopting a holistic approach to clinical assessment by taking into account the risk factors described above can help identify the small number of younger women who may be at risk of endometrial hyperplasia and cancer.

Once the progression to *endometrial cancer* has occurred (most commonly endometrial adenocarcinoma), the histological appearance becomes that of small, round, back-to-back glands without any intervening stroma. There will be varying degrees of nuclear atypia, depending on the level of differentiation of the malignant cells.

Occasionally, women may also present without abnormal bleeding. For example, postmenopausal women may be found incidentally to have an abnormally thickened endometrium on ultrasound/CT/MRI after investigations for other conditions. Endometrial cancer can also occasionally be detected when malignant cells are seen on cervical cytology in postmenopausal women (reported as glandular cells).

With regards to abnormal uterine bleeding, symptoms that should lead to a suspicion of endometrial hyperplasia and cancer depend on age and associated risk factors:

- *Postmenopausal women*: Any type of bleeding, including spotting, bleeding when wiping after passing urine and staining of underwear, should prompt investigation. On average, 10% of women who present with PMB will be diagnosed with endometrial cancer. A further 5–15% will be diagnosed with endometrial hyperplasia [13].
- *Perimenopausal women (age 45 to menopause)*: Any abnormal bleeding in this age group should prompt further investigation; 13.9% of cases of endometrial cancer occur in women aged 45–54 [12]. Abnormal bleeding includes:
  - *Heavy menstrual bleeding*: heavy and/or prolonged period loss, which is usually subjectively reported but may be supplemented by objective evidence such as microcytic anaemia.
  - *Polymenorrhea*: frequent periods with an interval between onset of bleeding episodes less than 21 days.
  - *Intermenstrual bleeding*.
  - *Oligomenorrhoea/amenorrhoea*: an extended interval between episodes of bleeding may of course be a normal feature of the perimenopause. However, in women who are anovulatory (e.g. with PCOS) or have other risk factors such as severe obesity, endometrial pathology should be considered.
  - *Younger than 45 years*: Abnormal uterine bleeding (as described above) that occurs in the context of significant risk factors or failed medical management should prompt further investigation.

Urgency of Referral

Women presenting with postmenopausal bleeding should be referred for investigation via urgent two-week suspected cancer pathways. Often, they will be sent to a one-stop service where they will receive a pelvic ultrasound (see below) with or without hysteroscopy and biopsy, combined with visual examination of the perineum and cervix. In perimenopausal women, the majority of referrals to hysteroscopy will be via routine pathways unless the referring clinician feels that the symptomatology or risk factor profile warrants more urgent assessment. In light of the relatively low incidence of endometrial cancer in premenopausal women under the age of 45, it is unusual for women of this age group to be referred via suspected cancer pathways with regards to suspected endometrial pathology. However, as with older women, if there is a strong enough clinical suspicion based on risk factors (e.g. women with menstrual dysfunction and Lynch syndrome), then urgent referral pathways can be used.

Investigations

Radiological Imaging

Ultrasound

Ultrasound of the pelvis (ideally transvaginal) is usually the first-line investigation for women with postmenopausal bleeding. This is because measurement of the endometrial thickness is useful for ruling out endometrial cancer.

The British Gynaecological Cancer Society recommends an outpatient endometrial biopsy when the double layer endometrial thickness (ET) is ≥ 4 mm on transvaginal ultrasound scan (TVUS). When the ET is less than 4 mm and there are no irregularities, for example the presence of fluid, then no further investigations are required unless the patient is complaining of recurrent PMB in which case a biopsy is necessary. Using a 4 mm cut-off value for TVUS has a negative predicted value of > 99%, meaning the probability of cancer is less than 1% in these patients with an ET < 4 mm [15].

Ultrasound is less useful for risk stratification in premenopausal women as there is a significant overlap between normal ET and that caused by endometrial pathology. The main use of ultrasound in premenopausal women is to rule out other structural anomalies such as fibroids or endometrial polyps which may be contributing to the menstrual dysfunction. However, guidance from the Royal College of Obstetricians and Gynaecologists (RCOG) supports the use of ET measurement in women with PCOS/anovulation and amenorrhoea. A combination of a thickened endometrium and/or cystic appearances would warrant referral for hysteroscopy and endometrial assessment.

CT and MRI

There is little evidence for the use of CT in the diagnosis of endometrial hyperplasia and cancer. When an incidentally thickened endometrium is detected on CT scans undertaken for other reasons, this is usually followed up with a pelvic ultrasound scan.

MRI is currently used in the staging of endometrial cancer to detect invasive disease. It may have the future potential to diagnose possible endometrial hyperplasia and to be used in women with atypical hyperplasia undergoing surveillance (see below) to detect malignant change. More evidence is needed, however, before these uses can be adopted as widespread practice [16].

Hysteroscopy and Endometrial Biopsy

In women suspected of having endometrial hyperplasia or cancer, confirmation of the diagnosis requires histological examination of a specimen of endometrial tissue. Commonly, endometrial biopsy samples are obtained using miniature sampling devices (such as the Pipelle) in the context of an outpatient hysteroscopy service.

Outpatient versus Inpatient Hysteroscopy

Outpatient hysteroscopy can be undertaken using miniaturised hysteroscopes often without the need for anaesthesia or instrumentation of the cervix. The diagnostic accuracy for detecting endometrial hyperplasia and carcinoma is high. Outpatient hysteroscopy is well tolerated, requiring reduced time off work, reduced loss of income and reduced travel costs for women, in addition to substantially less cost per woman to the NHS [14].

For certain women, inpatient hysteroscopy under general anaesthesia is the preferred option. Such cases include: when outpatient hysteroscopy has failed – either due to patient discomfort or technical difficulties such as uterine position or cervical stenosis; when outpatient sampling has been insufficient for diagnosis; when the woman herself declines an outpatient procedure (e.g. due to vaginismus or anxiety).

Management and Follow-Up of Endometrial Hyperplasia and Early Endometrial Cancer

Endometrial Hyperplasia (without Atypia)

The majority of cases of hyperplasia without atypia will regress back to normal endometrium during a period of observation. Data from cohort studies suggests spontaneous regression rates of around 74% at six months for (both simple and complex) hyperplasia without atypia. Observation alone, while addressing reversible risk factors such as HRT use and obesity, is therefore an acceptable treatment option [17].

Treatment with progestogens is associated with a higher rate of regression back to normal endometrium when compared with observation alone. Treatment is recommended either when women are symptomatic or if there is no regression after an initial period of observation (usually six months). Treatment may also be useful where risk factor modification may be difficult (such as in treating severe obesity) [16].

Risk Factor Modification

- *Obesity*: Tackling obesity is complex, but the usual principles of multidisciplinary management apply. There is evidence that the incidence of asymptomatic hyperplasia is reduced in severe obesity after bariatric surgery (surgery is not indicated for this reason alone).
- *HRT*: Women who present with abnormal bleeding and hyperplasia while on HRT should have a review of their need for ongoing HRT. Women who wish to continue and are taking sequential preparations should be switched to a continuous combined preparation. For women on continuous combined HRT preparations, a manipulation of the regimen to increase the proportion of progestogen may be enough to induce regression of the hyperplasia when atypia is not present. This is particularly important in postmenopausal women, as they will have no endogenous progesterone production. Women already taking an appropriate form of continuous combined HRT who develop hyperplasia should be advised to stop [16].
- *Tamoxifen*: Women who develop endometrial hyperplasia while taking tamoxifen will need a joint decision between oncology and gynaecology regarding ongoing management.

Progestogenic Suppression

Progestogens antagonise the stimulatory effects of oestrogens on the cells of the endometrium. The two modes of treatment which can reliably deliver high enough concentrations of progestogens to the endometrium are oral progestogens and the levonorgestrel-releasing intrauterine system (Mirena ®).

Intrauterine (LNG-IUD) versus Oral Progestogens

- The LNG-IUD is recommended as the first-line treatment as it achieves the highest concentration of progestogen at the endometrium, resulting in higher rates of regression [16].
- Evidence is available from randomised controlled trials (RCTs) comparing LNG-IUD with continuous oral progestogens for the treatment of simple hyperplasia. After six months, regression rates for LNG-IUD varied between 88 and 100%. For continuous oral progestogens, regression rates varied between 56 and 95% [16].
- One RCT reported follow-up results at two years. For the oral progestogen group, the regression rate was 64%; for the LNG-IUD group, the rate was 100%.
- For women with complex hyperplasia, a systematic review of uncontrolled observational studies found regression rates of 66% with oral progestogens and up to 92% with the LNG-IUD [18].
- The minimal systemic absorption of hormone via the LNG-IUD helps to produce a more favourable side effect profile, thus aiding compliance [16].
- In women of reproductive age, LNG-IUD also provides effective contraception.
- Some women will receive a diagnosis of endometrial hyperplasia after investigations for heavy menstrual bleeding for which LNG-IUD is also the recommended first-line treatment.

In light of the lower rates of disease regression and poorer compliance, oral progestogens are only recommended when the LNG-IUD is unacceptable to women or when its use is contraindicated (such as in women with suspected or confirmed pelvic infection or those undergoing investigations for cervical neoplasia).

Continuous oral progestogen regimens should be used, rather than cyclical schedules, which are known to be significantly less effective in inducing regression to normal endometrium.

The two continuous oral progestogen regimens with the strongest evidence base are:

- norethisterone 10–15 mg/day
- medroxyprogesterone 10–20 mg/day.

In women with endometrial hyperplasia without atypia, treatment with either the LNG-IUD or oral progestogens should continue for a minimum of six months [16].

Follow-Up for Women Undergoing Risk Factor Modification/Progestogenic Suppression

Endometrial surveillance in the form of a repeat endometrial biopsy should be undertaken at a minimum of six-monthly intervals. A shorter interval may be required in some women depending on the severity of risk factors (e.g. postmenopausal women undergoing HRT modifications may require repeat biopsies at three-monthly intervals) [16].

Generally, women can be discharged when they have had two consecutive six-monthly biopsies that show normal endometrium. However, women should be advised to report any symptom recurrence as this may represent the recurrent development of hyperplasia [16].

Women who have persistent, significant risk factors (such as obesity with a BMI of over 35) are at higher risk of relapse and should be advised to have yearly surveillance, even when regression has been achieved [16].

Women who have the LNG-IUD inserted should be advised to continue treatment for the duration of its five-year lifespan unless they wish it to be removed for fertility purposes. Endometrial biopsies can be easily taken with the IUD in situ.

Surgical Treatment of Endometrial Hyperplasia without Atypia

Hysterectomy is not offered as a first-line treatment in hyperplasia without atypia. The specific circumstances in which hysterectomy would be offered to women not wishing to preserve their fertility include:

- When progression to atypical hyperplasia occurs during follow-up.
- When the endometrium does not revert to normal after 12 months of treatment with progestogens.
- If there is a relapse of hyperplasia after completing progestogen treatment.
- If a woman has persistent, severe bleeding symptoms.
- If a woman declines to undergo endometrial surveillance or comply with medical treatment.

Endometrial ablation is not recommended in the treatment of endometrial hyperplasia because complete and permanent destruction of the endometrium cannot be guaranteed in every case. The adhesions that form after ablation may also render any further endometrial biopsies difficult or impossible [16].

Atypical Endometrial Hyperplasia

Hysterectomy

In women diagnosed with endometrial hyperplasia with atypia, the first-line treatment is total hysterectomy (removal of uterus and cervix) due to the high risk of co-existing malignancy or the high risk of progression to adenocarcinoma.

In postmenopausal women with atypical hyperplasia, the fallopian tubes and ovaries should also be removed at the time of hysterectomy as this will reduce the chance of ovarian malignancy in the future. For premenopausal women, the decision of whether to remove the ovaries will be individualised after discussion with a gynaecologist [19].

An RCT has compared total laparoscopic hysterectomy with open hysterectomy for women with atypical hyperplasia or grade I endometrial cancer. There were no differences in the rates of major complications between either approach and both allowed adequate visualisation of the abdominal cavity to assess for further disease. Laparoscopic hysterectomy, however, was associated with a shorter hospital stay, less pain and faster resumption of daily activities [19].

Women Unsuitable for Surgery/Wishing Fertility Preservation

In premenopausal women found to have atypical hyperplasia who wish to preserve their fertility or in women who are unsuitable for surgery, progestogenic suppression with careful surveillance is the mainstay of treatment. As in the case of non-atypical hyperplasia, the treatment of choice is the LNG-IUD. Importantly, there is a paucity of clear evidence to guide treatment and follow-up in these cases.

Prior to commencing treatment with progestogens, women with atypical hyperplasia should be reviewed in a gynaecology/oncology multidisciplinary team meeting. Further investigations will likely be recommended, including MRI to rule out invasive endometrial cancer and measurement of CA 125 levels to help exclude ovarian cancer. An individualised plan for follow-up will usually be formulated with review intervals for repeat endometrial biopsies being set at three to six months until two negative biopsies are obtained. Thereafter, long-term follow-up is usually recommended, either every 6–12 months or until hysterectomy can be performed. At each follow-up a detailed history of bleeding symptoms and pelvic examination should also be undertaken.

In women wishing to conceive, at least one normal endometrial biopsy should be obtained before pregnancy is attempted. In these cases, the chance of a live birth is around 25% and assisted conception has been shown to be associated with more live births (30%) compared to natural conception (15%) and may also prevent relapse. An early referral for specialist fertility advice may therefore also be indicated.

Once fertility is no longer required, hysterectomy is recommended, due to the high risk of relapse and progression to endometrial cancer [16].

Endometrial Cancer

The treatment of endometrial cancer depends upon the stage at presentation and is planned and undertaken by multidisciplinary gynaecology/oncology services. It is worth noting that 74% of cases of endometrial cancer are diagnosed at stage 1 disease, for which early treatment in the form of total hysterectomy and bilateral salpingo-oophorectomy confers a five-year survival rate of 92% [1].

Conclusion

Diagnosis and management of endometrial hyperplasia is important both in terms of treating menstrual dysfunction and preventing endometrial cancer. The diagnosis of endometrial pathology can, however, be challenging, especially in younger women where there is a significant overlap in symptomatology with benign menstrual dysfunction. In this chapter we have highlighted how a holistic approach to history-taking and examination can help to identify those women who warrant further assessment and treatment. We have also discussed the need for careful follow-up for women undergoing treatment or observation and highlighted some of the complex multidisciplinary challenges that can arise, especially in women of child-bearing age (see also case scenario below).

Case Scenario 27.1

Mrs B is a 39-year-old lady of South-East Asian (Bangladeshi) origin. She visits her GP requesting assistance due to an inability to conceive for approximately two years. She has one child, born by normal delivery five years ago. Prior to conception she had been prescribed a six-month course of clomiphene citrate for the purposes of ovulation induction. Until recently, her periods had been irregular with a cycle length varying between two and four months. In the past 12 months, however, her periods have become more frequent and heavy. She has occasionally had to take some time off work due to tiredness. Mrs B has a BMI of 33, an increase from her previously recorded value from five years ago, which was 28.

- *With regards to risk factors for endometrial pathology, what are the concerning features of this history?*

Previous oligomenorrhoea and requiring ovulation induction for conception are suggestive of a diagnosis of polycystic ovarian syndrome. Taking into account the WHO's reclassification of BMI categories based on ethnicity, a BMI of 33 falls into the 'severe obesity' category for a lady of South-East Asian origin. The history therefore combines a risk of excess oestrogenic stimulation secondary to obesity with episodes of absent progestogenic suppression secondary to anovulation. The new onset of heavier and more frequent menstruation may therefore represent the development of new endometrial pathology.

- *What would be the appropriate next steps in the investigation and management of this lady?*

An important first step in this case would be careful counselling that the focus of care should shift, for the time being at least, away from fertility concerns towards the exclusion of endometrial pathology. The most important investigation would be hysteroscopy and endometrial biopsy. As the incidence of endometrial cancer is low in premenopausal women under the age of 45, fast-track referral is not indicated. This lady could therefore be referred as routine to a direct access outpatient hysteroscopy service if available, or for review by a gynaecologist. Mrs B underwent outpatient hysteroscopy and endometrial biopsy. The biopsy results revealed endometrial hyperplasia with atypia.

- *What is the risk of progression to endometrial cancer and what are the options for management? Based upon the best available evidence, the risk of hyperplasia with atypia progressing to endometrial cancer is up to 29%. There is also a significant risk (up to 37%) of co-existing carcinoma that was not detected at biopsy.*

Mrs B's case is reviewed at a gynaecology oncology multidisciplinary team meeting and the recommendation made for hysterectomy. Mrs B is emphatic, however, that she wishes to maintain her fertility. In association with the gynaecology oncology team, a plan is made for progestogenic suppression using a Mirena® coil, with repeat endometrial biopsies planned at three-monthly intervals.

- *Which other referrals might be helpful in this situation?*

Mrs B's major risk factor for developing hyperplasia is her obesity. She accepts referral for dietary support from a nutritionist. She declines referral for a specialist fertility consultation.

Unfortunately, at three and six months, there is no evidence of regression in Mrs B's atypical hyperplasia. Furthermore, Mrs B's BMI increases over this time to 34 and she states that worry over her risk of developing cancer is a significant contributory factor to this. After further discussion with her gynaecologist, she decides to opt for a hysterectomy. The procedure is uncomplicated, and Mrs B makes a full recovery. Histopathological examination of the uterus confirms the diagnosis of endometrial hyperplasia with atypia.

References

[1] Cancer Research UK, 'Uterine cancer statistics'. Accessed 19 Nov. 2025. [Online]. Available: www.cancerresearchuk.org/health-professional/cancer-statistics/statistics-by-cancer-type/uterine-cancer.

[2] S. D. Reed, K. M. Newton, W. L. Clinton et al., 'Incidence of endometrial hyperplasia', *Am J Obstet Gynecol*, vol. **200**, no. 6, 678, 2009.

[3] E. R Simpson, 'Role of aromatase in sex steroid action', *J Mol Endocrinol*, vol. **25**, pp. 149–156, 2000.

[4] S. Furness, H. Roberts, J. Marjoribanks and A. Lethaby, 'Hormone therapy in postmenopausal women and risk of endometrial hyperplasia', *Cochrane Database Syst Rev*, vol. **8**, CD000402, 2012.

[5] American College of Obstetricians and Gynecologists, 'Committee opinion: Tamoxifen and uterine cancer'. 2014. Accessed 19 Nov. 2025. [Online]. Available: www.acog.org/clinical/clinical-guidance/committee-opinion/articles/2014/06/tamoxifen-and-uterine-cancer.

[6] L. M. and J. Berek, 'Endometrial cancer: Clinical features and diagnosis, prognosis and screening'. 2024. Accessed 19 Nov. 2025. [Online]. Available: www.uptodate.com/contents/endometrial-carcinoma-clinical-features-diagnosis-prognosis-and-screening.

[7] NICE, 'Testing strategies for Lynch syndrome in people with endometrial cancer'. Accessed 19 Nov. 2025. [Online]. Available: www.nice.org.uk/guidance/dg24.

[8] K. Bobrowska, P. Kaminski, A. Cyganek et al., 'High rate of endometrial hyperplasia among renal transplanted women', *Transplant Proc*, vol. **38**, pp. 177–179, 2006.

[9] R. Kaaks, A. Lukanova and M. Kurzer, 'The effect of diabetes on the risk of endometrial cancer: An updated systematic review and meta-analysis', *Cancer Epidemiol Biomarkers Prev*, vol. **11**, no. 10, pp. 1231–1241, 2002.

[10] R. J. Kurman, M. L. Carcangiu, C. S. Herrington and R. H. Young (eds.), *WHO Classification of Tumours of Female Reproductive Organs*, 4th ed. IARC, 2014.

[11] A. N. Fader and W. K. Huh, 'Endometrial hyperplasia'. StatPearls. Accessed 19 Nov. 2025. [Online]. Available: www.ncbi.nlm.nih.gov/books/NBK560693.

[12] SEER Cancer Stat Facts, 'Uterine cancer'. National Cancer Institute. Accessed 19 Nov. 2025. [Online]. Available: https://seer.cancer.gov/statfacts/html/corp.html.

[13] American College of Obstetricians and Gynecologists, 'ACOG practice bulletin: Management of endometrial cancer', *Obstet Gynecol*, vol. **106**, no. 2, 413, 2005.

[14] Royal College of Obstetricians and Gynaecologists, 'Best practice in outpatient hysteroscopy: Green-Top Guideline No. 59'. 2011, updated August 2024. Accessed 19 Nov. 2025. [Online]. Available: www.rcog.org.uk/globalassets/documents/guidelines/gtg59hysteroscopy.pdf.

[15] British Gynaecological Cancer Society. Accessed 19 Nov. 2025. [Online]. Available: www.bgcs.org.uk.

[16] Royal College of Obstetricians and Gynaecologists, 'Management of endometrial hyperplasia: Green-Top Guideline No. 67'. Feb. 2016.

[17] N. Terakawa, J. Kigawa, Y. Taketani et al. (Endometrial Hyperplasia Study Group), 'The behavior of endometrial hyperplasia: A prospective study', *J Obstet Gynaecol Res*, vol. **23**, pp. 223–230, 1997.

[18] I. D. Gallos, M. Shehmar, S. Thangaratinam et al., 'Oral progestogens vs levonorgestrel-releasing intrauterine system for endometrial hyperplasia: A systematic review and meta-analysis', *Am J Obstet Gynecol*, vol. **203**, no. 6, 547, 2010.

[19] M. J. Mourits, C. B. Bijen, H. J. Arts et al., 'Safety of laparoscopy versus laparotomy in early-stage endometrial cancer: A randomized control trial', *Lancet Oncol*, vol. **11**, pp. 763–771, 2010.

[20] M. Epplein, S. Reed, L. Voigt et al., 'Risk of complex and atypical endometrial hyperplasia in relation to anthropometric measures and reproductive history', *Am J Epidemiol*, vol. **168**, no. 6, pp. 563–570, 2008.

[21] R. J. Kurman, P. F. Kaminski and H. J. Norris, 'The behavior of endometrial hyperplasia: A long-term study of "untreated" hyperplasia in 170 patients', *Cancer*, vol. **56**, pp. 403–412, 1985.

The Management of Fibroids in Primary Care

Elizabeth Burt and Ertan Saridogan

Key Points

- Uterine fibroids are very common, but a significant proportion are asymptomatic.
- Symptoms are usually related to abnormal menstruation, pressure or fertility.
- The aetiology of fibroids is unclear, but is likely to be related to sex steroids, genetics and stem cell biology.
- Submucosal fibroids tend to cause more symptoms compared to intramural and subserosal fibroids.
- Consider referral to secondary/tertiary care when the uterus is palpable abdominally, its length is longer than 12 cm on ultrasound or at hysteroscopy, there are submucosal fibroids or there are pressure or fertility symptoms.
- The main diagnostic tools are history, abdominal and pelvic examination, and pelvic ultrasound examination. Occasionally there may be a role for MRI.
- Treatment should be tailored individually based on severity of symptoms, location/size of fibroids, fertility plans and acceptability of the options.
- Medical treatment options include levonorgestrel-releasing intrauterine device (LNG-IUD) 52 mg Mirena® or Levosert®, tranexamic acid, mefenamic acid, combined oral contraceptive pill, cyclical or long-acting progestogens and gonadotrophin-releasing hormone analogues and gonadotrophin-releasing hormone antagonists.
- Combined oral contraceptive pill, progestogens, LNG-IUD, tranexamic acid and mefenamic acid can be started in the primary care setting.
- Non-medical options include hysteroscopic or abdominal (open or laparoscopic) myomectomy, uterine artery embolisation and hysterectomy.

Case Scenario 28.1

Beatrice attends your practice. She is a 35-year-old nulliparous Afro-Caribbean lady. She has a long history of heavy periods, which are disrupting her daily life.

Introduction

Fibroids, also known as leiomyomas, are benign tumours of the uterine myometrium. They are extremely common, affecting up to 70–80% of women by the age of menopause [1]. Their high prevalence within the female population coupled with their related symptomatology renders them a source of significant morbidity, accounting for a significant proportion of primary care consultations. Fibroids may cause a wide spectrum of clinical presentations with varying severity, making both their diagnosis and management a challenge.

Epidemiology

Fibroids mainly affect women in their reproductive years. With fibroids being rare prior to menarche and known to shrink in size after the menopause, it is thought that oestrogen and progesterone are the driving hormones responsible for fibroid stimulation and maintenance.

Fibroids are common in all ethnicities; however, the prevalence is higher in Afro-Caribbean women, with 60% of these women having fibroids detected by the age of 35, increasing to 80% by the age of 49. In contrast, Caucasian women have an incidence of 40% at the age of 35, rising to 70% by the age of 49 [1]. This also highlights that the prevalence of fibroids increases progressively with age from puberty to menopause, with the peak age being the fifth decade. Afro-Caribbean women also have a distinctive natural history of fibroids, with fibroids occurring at an earlier age, being more numerous and clinically more apparent in comparison to their Caucasian counterparts.

Other risk factors increasing the susceptibility of uterine fibroids include environments with heightened and prolonged oestrogen and progesterone exposure. This would include early menarche, with later menarche appearing protective. In addition, increasing parity is also protective against fibroid development. Obesity, which is associated with a hyperoestrogenic state due to increased adipose production of oestrogen, is associated with an increased risk of fibroids, as is polycystic ovary syndrome [2–4].

Histology and Aetiology

Fibroids are benign monoclonal tumours of the smooth muscle. The typical histological appearance is of spheres of myometrial cells nesting within increased amounts of extracellular matrix [4]. Alternative histological appearances may be apparent when fibroids undergo degeneration, and this may occur when they outgrow their vascularity and undergo infarction and necrosis.

Fibroids range in size and can be solitary or occur in clusters. Most classically they occur within or around the uterine myometrium, but more rarely may be situated extra-uterine in the cervix, broad ligament or be peritoneal.

The aetiology of fibroids is still largely elusive but is likely to be multifactorial. The growth of fibroids has been linked to sex steroids, genetics and stem cell biology.

Classification

Fibroids are classified according to their location within the myometrium. This in turn may be correlated to their clinical significance and their associated symptomatology and is vital for the planning and recommendation of treatment strategies.

Submucosal

Submucosal fibroids (Figure 28.1a) are the least common of the fibroids, representing just 5%. Because of their position, these are most likely to cause the most bothersome clinical symptoms, such as abnormal uterine bleeding (AUB) and fertility difficulties. Less frequently they may prolapse into the cervical canal or vagina.

These can be further subdivided depending on the degree of their projection within the endometrial cavity. Type 0 submucosal fibroids are polyp-like and are completely within the uterine cavity. Type 1 fibroids have less than 50% of the fibroid within the myometrium, while type 2 have more than 50% within the myometrium. This classification is particularly helpful when planning endoscopic surgical treatment.

Intramural

Intramural fibroids are located within the myometrium, and although they are the most common type of fibroids, they are less likely to manifest symptoms unless very large (Figure 28.1b).

Subserosal

Subserosal fibroids are situated within the myometrium under the uterine serosa (Figure 28.1c). These are the least likely to cause symptoms. These tend to be related to pressure symptoms but are only problematic if large.

Pedunculated

Pedunculated fibroids are connected to the uterus by a stalk and may cause pressure symptoms or cause acute pain as a result of torsion (Figure 28.1d).

Presentation

Fibroids produce a heterogeneous array of symptoms. The majority of women are asymptomatic, with an incidental diagnosis being made during ultrasound or surgery for other indications. Fibroids, however, may cause extreme symptoms, with significant impact on quality of life. Symptoms attributable to fibroids may be related to their position within the endometrial cavity, their sheer size or from their effect on endometrial milieu and function. The symptoms can be grouped as menstrual disturbances, pressure symptoms and impact on fertility.

Symptoms associated with fibroids

- HMB
- Urinary frequency, nocturia
- Pelvic mass
- Pain
- Dyspareunia
- Constipation
- Sub-fertility

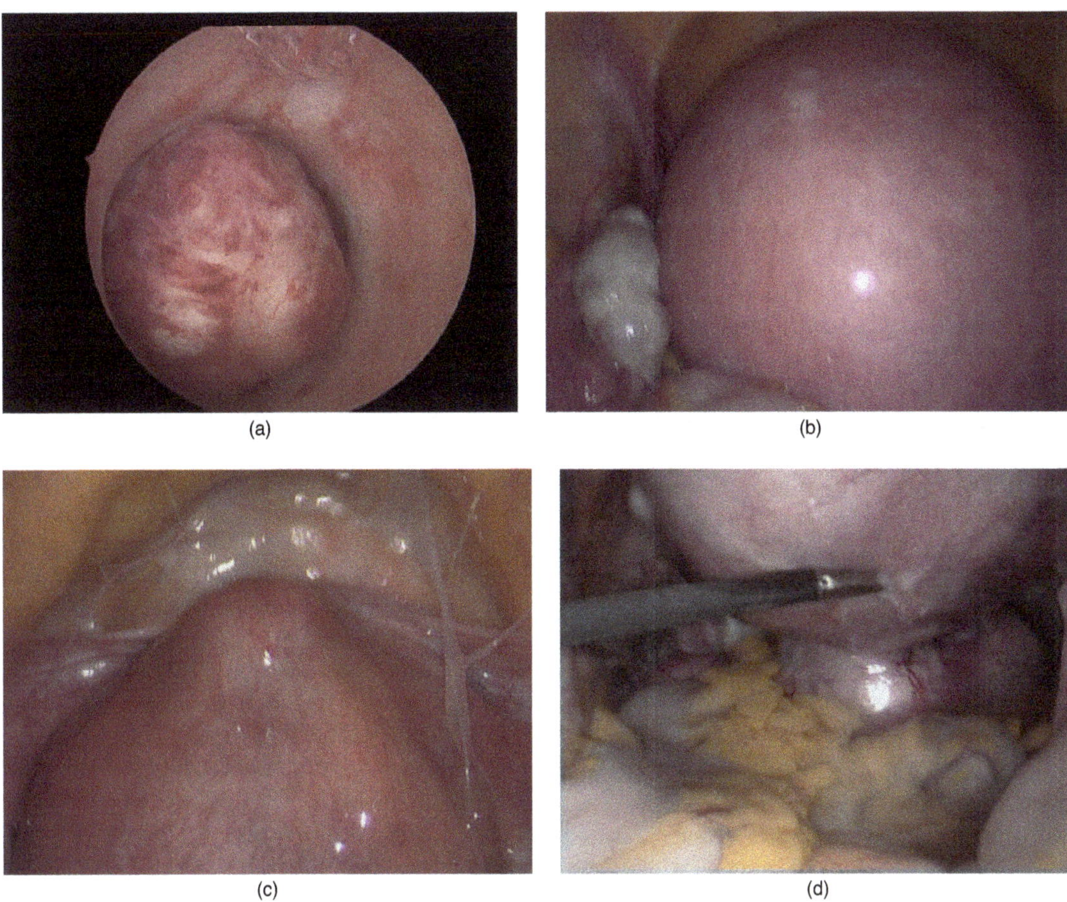

Figure 28.1 (a) Submucosal fibroid. (b) An enlarged uterus due to a large intramural fibroid. (c) Anterior wall subserosal fibroid. (d) Posterior wall pedunculated fibroid.

History

Specific questions in the history should cover:

- acute or chronic heavy menstrual bleeding (HMB)
- intermenstrual or post-coital bleeding
- dysmenorrhoea
- urinary symptoms (frequency, nocturia, incontinence)
- bowel symptoms (constipation, pressure on rectum)
- palpable or visible abdominal mass
- fertility desires
- smear history
- impact on quality of life.

Alarm symptoms in gynaecological presentation

- Acute menorrhagia > 45 years
- Intermenstrual bleeding
- Post-coital bleeding
- New rapid growing pelvic mass
- Features of cancer – unexplained weight loss
- Pelvic mass (not fibroid)

Examination

An abdominal examination may reveal a palpable or even visible mass, which is often described as having a knobbly consistency. A bimanual vaginal examination may be necessary to further assess the size of the uterus, which is commonly documented in relation to the size of a gravid uterus.

HMB and Dysmenorrhoea

This is the most common presentation, with HMB affecting 64% of women with fibroids [5]. These symptoms are most attributed to submucous fibroids, but may also be seen with larger intramural fibroids, or when the overall uterine size is very large.

Chronic heavy cyclical uterine bleeding may be a result of the disruption of the endometrium; alternatively, it has been postulated that fibroids have a direct effect on myometrial contractility and endometrial function, affecting both decidualisation and haemostasis.

Sequalae from HMB includes anaemia and, in addition, may cause psychological implications if it affects and restricts a woman's day-to-day life.

A history of HMB may be obtained, but it is important to recognise that post-coital bleeding and intermenstrual bleeding are not classical features of fibroids and caution should be exercised [6]. Furthermore, the duration of the HMB is an important factor. Acute menorrhagia starting over the age of 45 should prompt alarm bells and referral should be made for further endometrial assessment to rule out other conditions such as endometrial hyperplasia and malignancy.

To exclude significant anaemia a full blood count (FBC) should be considered, especially if any signs (pallor) or symptoms of anaemia (tiredness, shortness of breath, dizziness) are disclosed.

Pelvic Mass

Because of the size of the fibroid, women may present with the feeling of a pelvic or abdominal 'lump' that may have gradually increased in size over a number of years.

The growth of fibroids tends to be slow; the rare instance of leiomyosarcoma should be considered in a rapidly growing mass, although most fast-growing fibroids are benign.

Pain and Pressure Symptoms

Large subserosal fibroids may result in many pressure symptoms secondary to their compression of adjacent pelvic structures. This includes:

- lumbar and sacral nerve trunks resulting in chronic pelvic pain
- bladder and ureters causing urinary symptoms (frequency and nocturia) and less frequently hydronephrosis
- rectum leading to constipation
- cervix causing dyspareunia
- inferior vena cava and pelvic veins with subsequent vascular stasis leading to increased susceptibility to the development of deep vein thrombosis.

Acute abdominal pain may be related to pedunculated subserosal fibroids. These may undergo torsion with subsequent infarction.

Sub-fertility

Most women with fibroids are fertile, but the relative risk of conception, implantation and successful ongoing pregnancy is lower in the presence of large fibroids. Compounding the detrimental impact of fibroids on fertility further is their association with increased risk of miscarriage [7]. This is apparent in both spontaneous and assisted-conception pregnancies. It would seem intuitive that submucous fibroids which distort the cavity would be primarily responsible for this effect; however, it also appears that intramural fibroids reproduce this correlation, which may in part be related to their compression of the fallopian tubes, affecting gamete transfer or the effect on uterine contractility and blood flow. In contrast, subserosal fibroids are less likely to impact fertility outcomes, although with any type of large fibroids there may be significant distortion to the pelvic anatomy affecting the relationship between the fallopian tubes and ovaries, resulting in compromised ovum capture and gamete/embryo transport.

Sarcoma

Uterine sarcoma is a rare cancer and is frequently a histological diagnosis made post hysterectomy. More common in postmenopausal women, the majority are de novo lesions, and only 1:700 (0.14%) of presumed benign fibroids are indeed leiomyosarcomas [8]. As this is a rarity, diagnosis may pose a challenge and depends on excellent clinical acumen and a high index of suspicion in those women, especially postmenopausal, presenting with a pelvic mass, which has enlarged rapidly.

Obstetric

It is important to reiterate to women that the majority of those with fibroids experience an entirely normal pregnancy. However, in pregnancy, fibroids tend to grow rapidly and may be associated with acute pain, malpresentation and postpartum haemorrhage, with complications occurring in 10–40% of women [9]. It is thought that the size of the fibroids may be proportionally related to the chance of complications; however, often women with very large fibroids have no difficulties.

With an increase in endogenous oestrogen, pregnancy is associated with promotion of fibroid growth. This may lead to degeneration causing acute pain during pregnancy. Malpresentation, especially breech, which is more common in the presence of fibroids, is in turn associated with an exponential risk of caesarean section. Abnormal uterine contractility has been implicated in the association between fibroids and postpartum haemorrhage.

Case Scenario 28.2

Beatrice has a very clear history of chronic HMB with no other worrying symptoms. On examination, a bulky uterus can be palpated just above the pubic symphysis, approximately 14-week pregnancy size.

You organise a pelvic ultrasound and FBC.

Diagnosis

From a thorough history and examination, fibroids can be highly suspected and empirical medical treatment may be considered in primary care. An ultrasound should be arranged to confirm the diagnosis and plan further management and/or referral. Fibroid mapping is the detection and delineation of their classification, size and number.

Ultrasound

Ultrasound examination is the mainstay of diagnosis, with transvaginal ultrasound having a sensitivity of 100% and specificity of 94% for the detection of submucous fibroids; coupled with good patient acceptability, this is now the first-line investigation [10].

Fibroids classically appear as well-circumscribed hypoechoic lesions. Because of their histological makeup, they have a typical 'whorled' appearance and acoustic shadowing is seen.

Subserous fibroids distort the external uterine contour, while submucous fibroids protrude into the endometrial cavity. In order to aid the diagnosis of submucous fibroids and their differentiation from an endometrial polyp, either three-dimensional ultrasound or saline infusion sonohysterography may be employed.

Sarcomatous changes are neither well described nor specific, therefore making their diagnosis problematic. Uterine sarcomas tend to be large (> 8 cm), have less defined demarcation, may exhibit foci of haemorrhage or necrosis and have amplified vascularity [8].

MRI

MRI is often not a prerequisite for fibroid diagnosis, the exception being when it is indicated prior to complex surgery or if fibroids are suspected in more rare locations. MRI is also advantageous to assess the suitability for and predict success of uterine artery embolisation. For fibroid detection, MRI demonstrates a sensitivity of 88–93% and a specificity of 66–91% [11].

Case Scenario 28.3

Beatrice's transvaginal ultrasound demonstrated a 3 cm type 1 submucosal fibroid. The FBC was normal. Referral to secondary care is required due to the presence of a submucosal fibroid. In the interim, she would like to discuss possible treatment to alleviate her HMB.

Treatment Options

The majority of asymptomatic fibroids do not warrant treatment. See on which cases should be referred to secondary care. Optimal treatment and patient satisfaction are dependent on tailored therapeutic strategies. Factors to consider include:

- symptoms
- size and position of fibroids
- age
- patient wishes
- fertility desires.

Surgery remains the only definitive treatment for fibroids; however, because of the inherent risks of surgery, this is not acceptable to many women and thankfully many other options exist to circumvent the immediate need for surgery.

When to refer women with fibroids to secondary care

- Fibroids palpable abdominally
- Submucosal fibroids

- Alarm symptoms
- Medical management has failed
- Uterine length is greater than 12 cm on ultrasound or at hysteroscopy
- Pressure symptoms
- Fertility/obstetric problems

Expectant Management

The natural history of fibroids is not well established, with the growth of fibroids being both variable and unpredictable. For women who have non-troublesome small, non-intracavitary fibroids, a conservative approach should be advocated [12].

Counselling women with regards to the conceivable future risks associated with their fibroids can be a clinical challenge. It has been found that the largest fibroid may have a 35% volume increase per year, but equally up to one-fifth of fibroids may become smaller [13]. Fibroid growth may be correlated to their initial size at presentation and their position. Higher growth rate is associated with fibroids measuring less than 20 mm and greater than 50 mm and those that are intramural [13].

Women who are approaching menopausal age may wish to delay treatment as with menopause fibroids shrink, with associated symptoms diminishing.

Medical Management

Medical management can be further categorised into symptom relief and that used as an adjunct prior to surgery.

LNG-IUD: Mirena® or Levosert®

Marketed in the UK as Mirena® or Levosert®, the LNG-IUD is the preferred choice as first-line treatment for HMB in women who are not trying to get pregnant. It provides local release of progestogens, which, in turn, suppresses endometrial growth. LNG-IUD may reduce the bleeding by 90%, and up to 20% of women may be amenorrhoeic after 12 months. In addition to being highly efficacious for HMB, it delivers reliable long-term contraception, and it is licensed for up to five years' use for HMB. If HMB remains under control, Mirena® can be used for up to eight years as its licence has been extended to eight years for contraceptive purposes.

LNG-IUD has specific beneficial effects on fibroid-related bleeding and a positive effect is witnessed on fibroid size reduction [14]. The National Institute for Health and Care Excellence (NICE) recommend LNG-IUD only in the presence of fibroids less than 3 cm, but in clinical practice it is often used in the presence of bigger fibroids.

The main disadvantage of LNG-IUD cited by many women is the irregular bleeding, which may be troublesome for the first six months, and other progesterone-related side effects might be described. In the presence of submucous fibroids, fitting may be difficult and, together with a large uterine cavity, expulsion may be more common. Therefore, LNG-IUD is less effective in women with large/multiple and submucosal fibroids.

Combined Oral Contraceptive Pill (COCP)

The COCP has been an established form of contraception for the last 50 years and, more recently, additional benefits have also come to light, making the COCP an attractive choice of treatment for a multitude of gynaecological conditions. Specifically, for use in HMB, the COCP reduces the production of gonadotrophins, inhibits folliculogenesis and, in turn, prevents endometrial proliferation. Once thought to be linked to fibroid growth, this fear has now been allayed and on the contrary, the COCP may be associated with a 17% reduction in growth [5]. Correspondingly the COCP delivers an overall 50% reduction in menstrual blood loss, including that attributable to fibroids [15].

Cyclical and Long-Acting Progestogens

For those with HMB and who have fibroids less than 3 cm in diameter, which do not distort the cavity, cyclical or long-acting progestogens may be trialled as per NICE guidelines for HMB [16].

Cyclical progesterone such as norethisterone or medroxyprogesterone acetate may be used. It has been found that long courses of treatment from day 5–26 of the menstrual cycle are superior to treatment only given in the luteal phase and can reduce blood loss by 80%. In general, cyclical progestogens are less effective in reducing menstrual blood loss than LNG-IUD, tranexamic acid and COCP. Cyclical progestogen does not provide contraception and may be useful in women who have contraindications to the COCP. Furthermore, women using cyclical progestogens are less likely to experience troublesome intermenstrual bleeding compared to LNG-IUD, but use can be limited due to progestogenic side effects [16].

Long-acting progesterone such as intramuscular or subcutaneous depot medroxyprogesterone acetate (Depo Provera) can be given every 12 weeks and provide both contraceptive cover and induce amenorrhoea in up to 50% of users. As it prevents folliculogenesis, there is also a reduction in oestradiol concentration, which can impact bone density if used longer term (more than two years), but this effect is reversible with restoration when it is stopped.

Tranexamic Acid and NSAIDs

For women wishing to avoid hormonal/contraceptive preparations, the combination of mefenamic acid and tranexamic acid is often prescribed. Mefenamic acid is a non-steroidal anti-inflammatory drug (NSAID), which inhibits prostaglandin synthesis, and tranexamic acid is a plasminogen activator inhibitor, which acts as an antifibrinolytic agent.

Often a trial of three months is suggested, and mefenamic and tranexamic acid have been shown to reduce menstrual blood flow by 25% and 50%, respectively. Used solely at the time of menstruation, both are generally well tolerated. They may be used individually, in combination or in parallel to other treatment, such as LNG-IUD.

Preoperative Treatment

To facilitate surgical management, concurrent medical treatment may be clinically warranted in the preoperative planning period. The intended benefits are reduction in bleeding, optimisation of haemoglobin, to permit a less invasive surgical route and to overall lessen surgical morbidity risk.

Gonadotrophin-Releasing Hormone Agonist (GnRHa)

GnRHa are synthetic molecules which block the GnRH receptor at the level of the pituitary, thereby modifying the release of follicle-stimulating hormone (FSH) and luteinising hormone (LH). Initially causing an elevated level of release, there is subsequent downregulation and hypogonadotrophism. This simulates a temporary menopausal state. Deprived of the stimulatory effect of oestradiol and progesterone, amenorrhoea occurs and fibroid regression is observed, which can be in the order of 50% volume reduction.

The side effect profile of GnRHa is comparable to an artificial menopause with hot flushes, vaginal dryness, mood swings and bone density loss. This, therefore, restricts its continuing usage and currently can only be used for six months. An alternative to prevent these side effects is to use concomitant add-back therapy; however, this combination is less efficacious in the context of fibroid volume reduction and does not fully mitigate the side effects. The side effects, except osteoporosis with more than six months' usage, are transitory complaints and fully reversible on cessation of the medication; equally fibroids tend to regrow post-treatment within approximately three months.

Gonadotrophin-Releasing Hormone Antagonists

Relugolix is a gonadotrophin-releasing hormone antagonist which suppresses pituitary production of LH and FSH, therefore reducing endogenous oestrogen and progesterone levels. Unlike GnRHa, they do not cause the initial elevation of gonadotrophins and can be taken orally. Relugolix is currently marketed under the brand name of Ryeqo®. It is combined with add-back oestradiol and the progesterone norethisterone; this prevents hypoestrogenic side effects, as well as maintaining bone density. Because of its inhibitory effect on folliculogenesis and ovulation, it also has a contraceptive effect. Its use is associated with an 80% reduction in menstrual bleeding, and a reduction in pain and overall uterine volume [17].

Summary of Medical Options

See Table 28.1.

Case Scenario 28.4

After full discussion, Beatrice was not keen on hormonal preparations and decided to try the combination of tranexamic acid and mefenamic acid. This has reduced her bleeding to a more manageable level. She is subsequently seen in secondary care and counselled regarding further treatment options.

Table 28.1 Medical management of fibroids

Pharmacological agent	Mechanism of action	Reduction in menorrhagia	Reduction in fibroid growth	Side effects
LNG –IUD Mirena®, Levosert®	Prevents endometrial proliferation	90%	Reduction in uterine volume	• Irregular bleeding • Expulsion • Progesterone effects • Ovarian cysts
Tranexamic acid	Antifibrinolytic	50%	-	• Gastrointestinal effects
Mefenamic acid	Inhibits prostaglandin synthesis	25%	-	• Gastrointestinal effects
COCP	Inhibits folliculogenesis, ovulation and induces endometrial atrophy	50%	17%	• Thromboembolic events • Breakthrough bleeding • Progesterone effects
Cyclical and long-acting progestogens	Endometrial suppression and inhibits folliculogenesis	80%	-	• Progestogenic effects • Reduction in bone mineral density (long-acting progestogens)
GnRHa	Downregulation at pituitary levels reducing gonadotrophin release	Amenorrhoeic during treatment	50%	• Menopausal symptoms • Bone demineralisation
Gonadotrophin-releasing hormone antagonist with add-back HRT	Inhibits pituitary release of gonadotrophins	80%	Reduction in uterine volume	• Menopausal symptoms • Headache • Arthralgia • Cough • Nausea • Anaemia • Fatigue

Uterine Artery Embolisation (UAE)

UAE is a minimally invasive, surgery-sparing technique. This is a percutaneous procedure performed by interventional radiologists. A catheter is inserted into the femoral artery and, using fluoroscopic guidance, the uterine arteries are injected with an embolic agent. This in turn induces avascular necrosis within the fibroids.

Patient satisfaction post procedure is high, with an associated 40–70% reduction in fibroid volume and 80–90% of patients having significant symptom relief after one year [18]. Results are comparable to both hysterectomy and myomectomy, but in favour of UAE it is associated with shorter hospital stay and is overall more cost-effective [19–21].

Although UAE is considered both safe and efficacious, women should be fully aware of the fact that fibroid shrinkage is not permanent and up to one-third of women may require further treatment [22].

Although complications of UAE are rare, they may include premature ovarian failure (1%), which is more common in those over the age of 45, postembolisation syndrome and the need for urgent hysterectomy.

Desire for pregnancy was once considered a relative contraindication as UAE was thought to affect endometrial blood flow, which in turn may affect implantation and placentation; nevertheless, successful pregnancies have been reported after UAE. Although data is minimal, the consensus is that UAE is associated with an increased rate of miscarriage compared to untreated fibroids and myomectomy (35% vs. 17% vs. 23%). Caesarean section delivery and postpartum haemorrhage are also higher post-UAE. Reassuringly, other pregnancy outcomes, namely intrauterine growth restriction, malpresentation and preterm delivery, are not amplified after UAE [23]. Because of the potential impact on fertility and pregnancy outcomes, many clinicians do not offer UAE as a first-line treatment for fibroids in women planning to become pregnant in the future.

Transcervical Ultrasound-Guided Radiofrequency Ablation Uterine Fibroids (Sonata®)

Sonata®, approved by NICE in 2021, is a new treatment for fibroids. It is a minimally invasive procedure that uses intrauterine ultrasound and targeted radiofrequency to treat fibroids of varying sizes and locations. It can be carried out under local or general anaesthesia. Treatment can lead to a > 50% reduction in menstrual bleeding, a reduction in total uterine volume and a reduction in symptom severity. The procedure has good patient acceptability, and women can expect to return to normal daily activity within one to two days [24]. Procedure risks are minimal but may include pain, fibroids sloughing, infection and vaginal discharge.

Surgical Management

Surgical intervention may be indicated in a variety of circumstances:

- failure of medical treatment
- large fibroids
- pressure symptoms
- intracavitary fibroids
- patient wishes.

Hysterectomy is obviously contraindicated in those wishing to conceive and therefore other uterus-preserving surgical options exist.

Myomectomy

Myomectomy, which is the surgical removal of fibroids with preservation of the normal myometrium, can be further classified depending on the surgical route employed. Preoperative treatment with GnRHa may be recommended.

Transcervical Resection of Fibroids (TCRF)

Submucous fibroids, which are predominately intracavitary (i.e. type 0, type 1 and some type 2), are amenable to resection via the vaginal route with hysteroscopy. Subject to the size of the fibroids, this may be carried out either as an outpatient or under general anaesthesia. This is a relatively short procedure and well tolerated with a reduction in bleeding in 90% of patients [11]. Potential complications include haemorrhage, infection, uterine perforation, irrigation fluid overload and intrauterine adhesions.

Pertinent to fertility, the elimination of submucosal fibroids appears to enhance conception and reduce miscarriage rates [7].

Open/Laparoscopy Myomectomy

Abdominal myomectomy can be either open (laparotomy) or via laparoscopy. With the advent of morcellation, even large fibroids can be treated laparoscopically with the associated benefits of minimal access surgery. Care should be taken with morcellation; if there is any suspicion of malignancy, morcellation may cause dissemination.

Hysterectomy

This is the only option that conveys symptom relief with no possibility of fibroid recurrence. Hysterectomy may be completed through the abdominal, vaginal or laparoscopic route; the decision will depend on the preoperative size and location of the fibroids and experience of the surgeon.

Hysterectomy is only an option for women who have completed their family with no desire for further fertility and may not be suitable for women who have significant surgical risks.

Case Scenario 28.5

After further consultation in secondary care, given Beatrice's principal complaint of HMB in the presence of an intracavitary fibroid, a TCRF was advised. This was performed as a day case with excellent postoperative recovery.

References

[1] D. Baird, D. Dunson, M. Hill, D. Cousins and J. M. Schectman, 'High cumulative incidence of uterine leiomyoma in black and white women:

Ultrasound evidence', *Am J Obstet Gynecol*, vol. **188**, no. 1, pp. 100–107, 2003.

[2] D. Valez Edwards, D. Baird and K. Hartmann, 'Association of age at menarche with increasing number of fibroids in a cohort of women who underwent standardized ultrasound assessment', *Am J Epidemiol*, vol. **178**, no. 3, pp. 426–433, 2013.

[3] D. Baird and D. Dunson, 'Why is parity protective for uterine fibroids?', *Epidemiology*, vol. **14**, no. 2, pp. 247–250, 2003.

[4] N. Chabbert-Buffet, N. Esber and P. Bouchard, 'Fibroid growth and medical options for treatment', *Fertil Steril*, vol. **102**, no. 3, pp. 630–639, 2014.

[5] R. Moroni, C. Vieira, R. Ferriani, F. Candido-dos-Reis and L. Brito, 'Pharmacological treatment of uterine fibroids', *Ann Med Health Sci Res*, vol. **4** (suppl. 3), pp. S185–S192, 2014.

[6] NICE, 'Heavy menstrual bleeding: Assessment and management'. NICE clinical guideline 44. Accessed: 19 Nov. 2025. [Online]. Available: www.guidance.nice.org.uk/cg44.

[7] E. Pritts, W. Parker and D. Olive, 'Fibroids and infertility: An updated systematic review of the evidence', *Fertil Steril*, vol. **91**, no. 4, pp. 1215–1223, 2009.

[8] H. Brölmann, V. Tanos, G. Grimbizis et al., 'Options on fibroid morcellation: A literature review', *Gynecol Surg*, vol. **12**, no. 1, pp. 3–15, 2015.

[9] X. Guo and J. Segars, 'The impact and management of fibroids for fertility: An evidence-based approach', *Obstet Gynecol Clin North Am*, vol. **39**, no. 4, pp. 521–533, 2012.

[10] BMJ Best Practice, 'Uterine fibroids'. Accessed: 19 Nov. 2025. [Online]. Available: http://bestpractice.bmj.com/best-practice/monograph/567.html.

[11] A. Khan, M. Shehmar and J. Gupta, 'Uterine fibroids: Current perspectives', *Int J Women's Health*, vol. **29**, no. 6, pp. 95–114, 2014.

[12] NICE, 'Fibroids: Clinical knowledge summaries'. 2013. Accessed: 19 Nov. 2025. [Online]. Available: cks.nice.org.uk/fibroids.

[13] D. Mavrelos, J. Ben-Nagi, T. Holland et al. 'The natural history of fibroids', *Ultrasound Obstet Gynecol*, vol. **35**, no. 2, pp. 238–242, 2010.

[14] U. Sangkomkamhang, P. Lumbiganon and M. Laopaiboon, 'Progestogens or progestogen-releasing intrauterine systems for uterine fibroids', *Cochrane Database Syst Rev*, vol. **2**, CD008994, 2013.

[15] S. Gupta, 'Non-contraceptive benefits of the combined oral contraceptive pill', *TOG*, vol. **15**, no. 2, pp. 138–139, 2013.

[16] M. Bofill Rodriguez, A. Lethaby, C. Low and I. T. Cameron, 'Cyclical progestogens for heavy menstrual bleeding', *Cochrane Database Syst Rev*, vol. **8**, no. 8, CD001016, 2019.

[17] A. Al-Hendy, A. Lukes, A. Poindexter et al., 'Treatment of uterine fibroid symptoms with relugolix combination therapy', *N Engl J Med*, vol. **384**, no. 7, pp. 630–642, 2021

[18] Royal College of Obstetricians and Gynaecologists, 'Clinical recommendations of the use of uterine artery embolization (UAE) in the management of fibroids'. 2013. Accessed: 19 Nov. 2025. [Online]. Available: www.rcog.org.uk/globalassets/documents/guidelines/23-12-2013rcogrcruae.pdf.

[19] I. Pinto, P. Chimeno, A. Romo et al., 'Uterine fibroids: Uterine artery embolization versus abdominal hysterectomy for treatment – A prospective, randomized, and controlled clinical trial', *Radiology*, vol. **226**, no. 2, pp. 425–431, 2003.

[20] M. Mara, J. Maskova, Z. Fucikova et al., 'Midterm clinical and first reproductive results of a randomized controlled trial comparing uterine fibroid embolization and myomectomy', *Cardiovasc Intervent Radiol*, vol. **31**, no. 1, pp. 73–85, 2008.

[21] I. Manyonda, M. Bratby, J. Horst et al., 'Uterine artery embolization versus myomectomy: Impact on quality of life – Results of the FUME (Fibroids of the Uterus: Myomectomy versus Embolization) Trial', *Cardiovasc Intervent Radiol*, vol. **35**, no. 3, pp. 530–536, 2012.

[22] J. Moss, K. Cooper, A. Khaund et al., 'Randomised comparison of uterine artery embolisation (UAE) with surgical treatment in patients with symptomatic uterine fibroids (REST trial): 5-year results', *BJOG*, vol. **118**, no. 8, pp. 936–944, 2011.

[23] H. Homer and E. Saridogan, 'Uterine artery embolization for fibroids is associated with an increased risk of miscarriage', *Fertil Steril*, vol. **94**, no. 1, pp. 324–330, 2010.

[24] S. Chudnoff, R. Guido, K. Roy, D. Levine, L. Mihalov and J. G. Garza-Leal, 'Ultrasound-guided transcervical ablation of uterine leiomyomas', *Obstet Gynecol*, vol. **133**, no. 1, pp. 13–22, 2019.

Chapter 29

Osteoporosis and Fracture Prevention in Primary Care

Danny Murphy

Key Points

- Osteoporosis increases the risk of fracture. Osteoporotic fractures cause increased mortality and morbidity, as well as reduced mobility, independence and quality of life.
- We should formally assess fracture risk in all high-risk patients using FRAX or QFracture. Specifically, this includes all women aged 65 and older, all men aged 75 and over and those who are younger but have an increased fracture risk – for those aged under 50, there needs to be a major risk factor such as current or frequent steroid use, untreated premature menopause or a previous fragility fracture.
- The evidence base for bone-sparing drug treatments is summarised in Scottish Intercollegiate Guidelines Network (SIGN) and National Osteoporosis Guidelines Group UK (NOGG) guidelines.
- Fracture risk changes as we age; bone health and treatments for osteoporosis should be reviewed at three- to five-year intervals.
- Women treated with steroids or aromatase inhibitors are at risk of rapid bone loss; treatment may be appropriate at a higher bone mineral density than for other cohorts.

Introduction

Osteoporosis increases the risk of fracture. Osteoporotic fractures cause increased mortality and morbidity, and reduce mobility, independence and quality of life. In the UK each year there are around 300,000 fragility fractures which present to hospital, including 70,000 hip fractures [1]. People who have sustained one fragility fracture are at increased risk of additional fractures. One in three women, and one in five men, will sustain at least one osteoporotic fracture in their lifetime [2].

Osteoporosis is defined as 'a disease characterised by low bone mass and structural deterioration of bone tissue with increase in susceptibility to fragility fracture' [2]. Fragility fractures are fractures which result from mechanical forces that would not normally cause a fracture, for example those caused by a fall from standing height or less, or by normal activities such as lifting a shopping bag or turning over in bed [1]. Fragility fractures occur most commonly in the spine (vertebrae), hip (femoral neck or proximal femur) or distal radius; they can also occur in the humerus, pelvis and other long bones. We wouldn't consider fractures in the skull, face or long bones of the hand or foot to be fragility fractures.

Osteoporosis is diagnosed using a dual-energy x-ray absorptiometry (DXA) scan to measure bone mineral density (BMD) at the femoral neck and lumbar spine. A T-score of ≤ -2.5 standard deviations defines osteoporosis; a T-score of -1 to -2.5 represents osteopenia or bone thinning, and a T-score of > -1 is normal [3].

Getting Started on Fracture Prevention

The steps in diagnosing and managing osteoporosis and preventing fractures are as follows:

- identify who is at risk
- assess their fracture risk
- consider reversible causes of low bone density
- reduce the risk of fracture
- ensure that treatment and bone health are reviewed.

Identify Who Is at Risk

We should formally assess fracture risk in all high-risk patients using FRAX or QFracture [4,5]. Box 29.1 gives a list of those who are considered high risk.

Box 29.1 Patients Who Are High Risk for Osteoporosis and Issues to Take into Consideration [1]

- All women aged ≥ 65.
- All men aged ≥ 75.
- Postmenopausal women and men older than 50 who have had a fragility fracture.
- Women and men aged over 50 with any of the following risk factors for fracture:
  - current use of oral corticosteroids, or frequent recent use
  - history of falls
  - family history of hip fracture
  - body mass index (BMI) < 18.5 kg/m^2
  - smoking
  - alcohol intake > 14 units/week
  - secondary medical causes of osteoporosis:
    - hypogonadism, including menopause < 40, use of aromatase inhibitors or GnRH antagonists
    - endocrine conditions – diabetes, Cushing's, hyperthyroidism, hyperparathyroidism and hyperprolactinaemia
    - conditions associated with malabsorption – IBD, coeliac disease, chronic pancreatitis
    - rheumatoid arthritis (RA) and inflammatory arthritis
    - haematological malignancy
    - COPD
    - chronic liver failure
    - CKD Group 3 or worse (eGFR < 60 ml/min)
    - immobility.
- Men or women starting a treatment that might significantly affect bone density (e.g. hormone deprivation therapy to treat cancer).

Consideration should be given as to whether any of the secondary causes listed in Box 29.1 can be treated to reduce risk.

We should not routinely assess fracture risk in people younger than 50 unless they have a major risk factor for fracture such as current or frequent steroid use, untreated premature menopause (younger than 45) or a previous fragility fracture, as they are unlikely to be at high risk of fracture. Risk assessment tools may underestimate fracture risk in certain circumstances, for example if a person has a history of multiple falls and/or fractures, has had previous vertebral fracture(s) or has a high alcohol intake or high-dose steroid use [1].

How Should I Assess Fracture Risk?

Online fracture risk assessment tools FRAX or QFracture [4,5] should be used both to assess the need for a DXA scan and to help guide decisions about treatment before and after DXA scanning. The FRAX tool calculates a 10-year risk of fracture based on individual risk factors and allows the direct application of a person's 10-year fracture risk to NOGG intervention thresholds [6]. Most patients should have a FRAX calculated, and their fracture risk plotted against age (using the 'view NOGG guidance' button on the FRAX website) before a DXA scan is requested – this gives a graphic which puts the patient in a green, amber or red zone (Figure 29.1).

- Patients in the green zone are at low risk of fragility fracture and do not require a DXA scan.
- Patients in the amber zone should be given bone health advice and referred for a DXA scan to measure BMD.
- Patients in the red zone can be offered osteoporosis treatment to reduce their risk of fracture without having a DXA scan.

When using QFracture, SIGN and the National Institute for Health and Care Excellence (NICE) propose requesting a DXA scan if the 10-year fracture risk is close to 10%. If the DXA confirms osteoporosis, then drug treatment should be considered.

Local DXA scanning units provide guidance on who should be scanned based on these guidelines. Giving as much information as possible on the referral form will help to inform the clinical report and treatment recommendations.

SIGN [7] does not recommend starting therapy based on clinical risk factors alone without BMD assessment, but the NICE CKS page suggests considering this for those who have had a past vertebral fracture [3], and NOGG [6] recommend that this is done when certain patients are starting oral glucocorticoids. This includes the following groups:

- anyone with a prior fragility fracture
- women aged ≥ 70
- postmenopausal women and men aged ≥ 50 who are starting a dose ≥ 7.5 mg of prednisolone (or equivalent) for over three months
- postmenopausal women and men aged ≥ 50 who have a FRAX probability of major osteoporotic fracture or hip fracture which exceeds the intervention threshold.

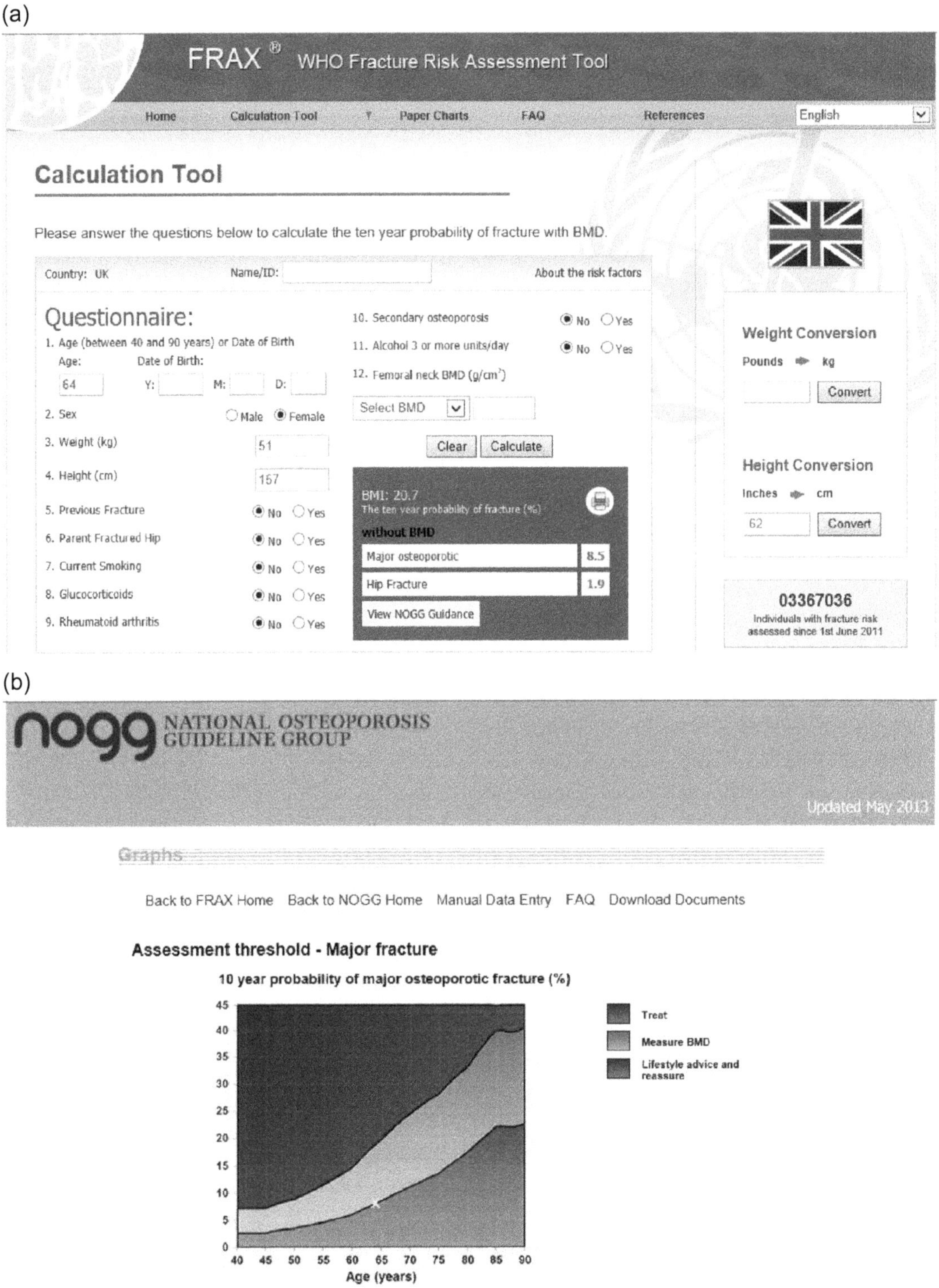

(a)

FRAX® WHO Fracture Risk Assessment Tool

Home | Calculation Tool | Paper Charts | FAQ | References | English

Calculation Tool

Please answer the questions below to calculate the ten year probability of fracture with BMD.

Country: UK Name/ID: About the risk factors

Questionnaire:

1. Age (between 40 and 90 years) or Date of Birth
   Age: 64 Date of Birth: Y: M: D:
2. Sex ○ Male ◉ Female
3. Weight (kg) 51
4. Height (cm) 157
5. Previous Fracture ◉ No ○ Yes
6. Parent Fractured Hip ◉ No ○ Yes
7. Current Smoking ◉ No ○ Yes
8. Glucocorticoids ◉ No ○ Yes
9. Rheumatoid arthritis ◉ No ○ Yes
10. Secondary osteoporosis ◉ No ○ Yes
11. Alcohol 3 or more units/day ◉ No ○ Yes
12. Femoral neck BMD (g/cm^2)
    Select BMD

Clear | Calculate

BMI: 20.7
The ten year probability of fracture (%)
without BMD

Major osteoporotic	8.5
Hip Fracture	1.9

View NOGG Guidance

Weight Conversion
Pounds ➡ kg
Convert

Height Conversion
Inches ➡ cm
62 Convert

03367036
Individuals with fracture risk assessed since 1st June 2011

(b)

nogg NATIONAL OSTEOPOROSIS GUIDELINE GROUP

Updated May 2013

Graphs

Back to FRAX Home | Back to NOGG Home | Manual Data Entry | FAQ | Download Documents

Assessment threshold - Major fracture

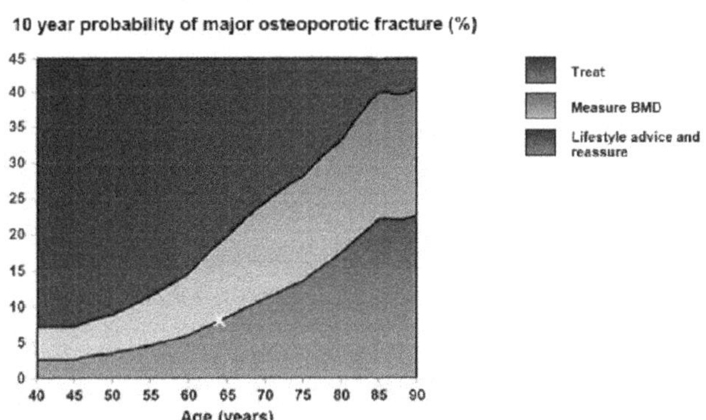

Figure 29.1 (a) FRAX calculator. (b) NOGG guidance graph.

Box 29.2 Lifestyle Advice for Good Bone Health

- Exercise regularly.
- Eat a balanced diet, including adequate calcium and vitamin D.
- Stop smoking.
- Drink alcohol only within recommended limits.

Management Principles

Management of People at Low Risk of Fracture

People at low risk of fracture by FRAX/QFracture score do not need a DXA scan or drug treatment. They should be offered lifestyle advice and consideration of diet and calcium and vitamin D supplementation which might be bought over the counter. SIGN and NICE advise that adults should consume 700–1000 mg/day of calcium; patients who want to calculate their intake can do so using an online calculator, using supplementation if their diet is not adequate in this respect [9].

Relevant lifestyle advice is shown in Box 29.2; this cohort should be offered a repeat bone health assessment in five years, or earlier if clinical circumstances change. Patients who want more information can be signposted to the website of the Royal Osteoporosis Society [8].

Management of People at Moderate Risk of Fracture and Osteopenia

Patients in the FRAX/NOGG amber zone, or who have a QFracture risk of close to but below 10%, should be given bone health advice and referred for a DXA scan to measure BMD. Their risk can then be recalculated using FRAX with the addition of the DXA scan result.

Management of People at High or Very High Risk of Fracture

UK national guidelines are not consistent on the management of this cohort. Table 29.1 outlines the view of NICE and NOGG, whereas Figure 29.2 shows a more complex algorithm from the SIGN guideline.

For those at a high risk of fracture, clinical risk factors alone may predict risk to a degree that is not improved by adding a DXA scan [10].

Table 29.1 UK guidelines for the management of those at high risk of fracture

	High risk
NICE [2,9]	• Treat all those with osteoporosis (T-score ≤ −2.5) on DXA [2]. • Treat adults at a 'high risk of fragility fracture' – 'high risk' in this context is undefined [9]. • Consider drug treatment without a DXA if there has been a previous vertebral fracture [2].
NOGG [6]	• Offer drug treatment to people at high and very high risk of fracture. • If a DXA scan is not practical (e.g. due to frailty), use the online NOGG intervention thresholds, based on FRAX, to guide treatment decisions. • Consider drug treatment in those with a prior fragility fracture, particularly in older people.

Considering this fact, and combining these three guidelines, a pragmatic approach is therefore as follows:

- Consider empirical treatment for those at very high risk, without DXA scanning – for example, those who have had a vertebral fracture.
- Where a DXA has been done, combine bone densitometry with a risk factor calculation such as FRAX or QFracture and treat those at high risk of fracture.
- Where a DXA has not been done and there is no clinical event to justify empirical treatment, request a DXA and reassess fracture risk using FRAX and including the BMD measurement.
- Offer lifestyle advice.
- Prescribe a bisphosphonate and calcium/vitamin D supplement if dietary intake is less than 700 mg/day. Vitamin D monotherapy can be considered if a person's calcium intake is greater than 700 mg/day.
- Consider treating without a BMD, based on NOGG/FRAX intervention thresholds, if a DXA scan is impractical, for example due to frailty.

Vitamin D supplementation at a population level, and at a daily dose of 10 μg/400 IU, is recommended for everyone in England during the winter months (October to March) [11] and all year round for those who have dark skin, cover up most of their skin when outdoors, live in care homes or do not go outside very often [11].

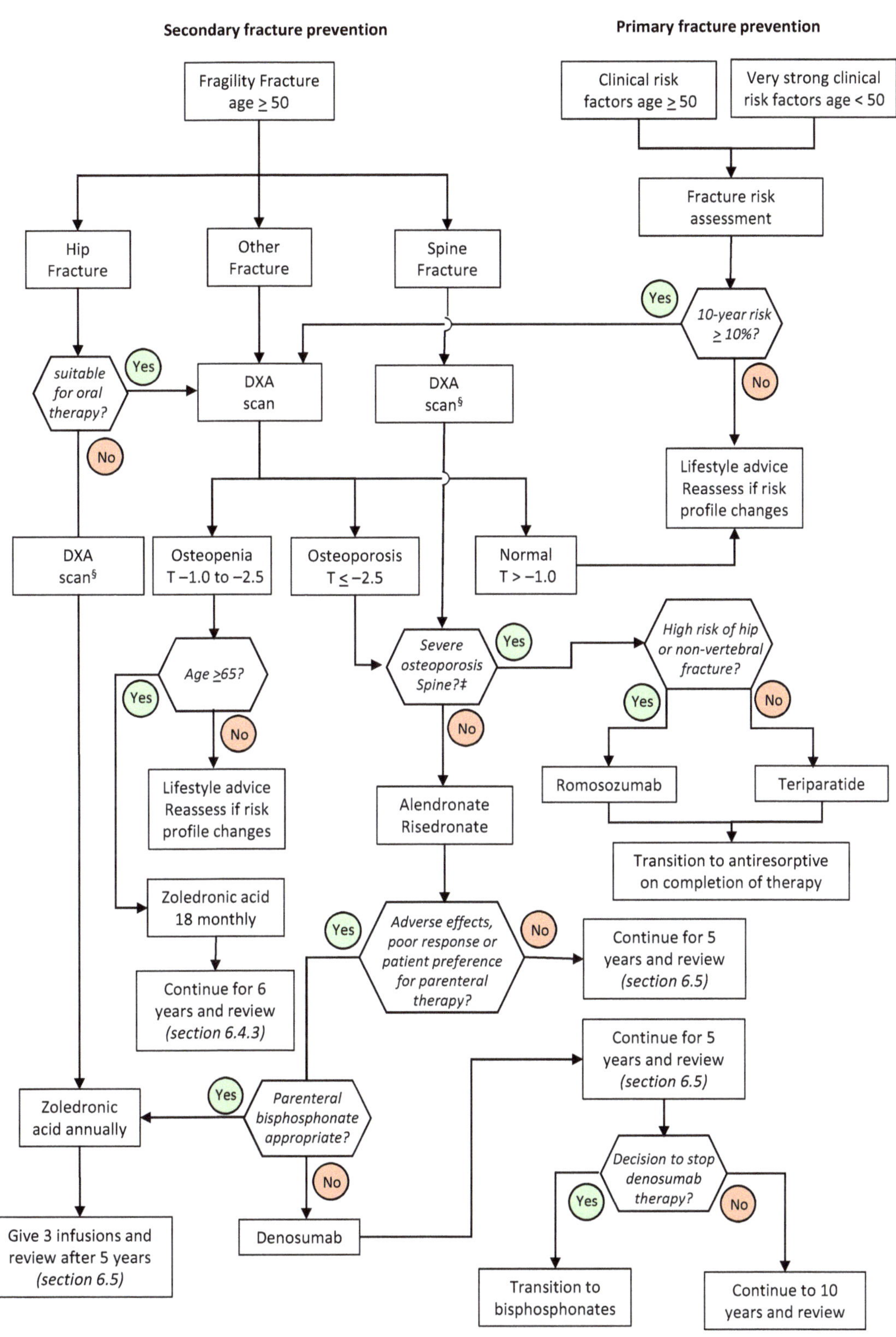

Figure 29.2 SIGN algorithm for the management of those at high or very high risk of fracture [7].

Table 29.2 Treatment options for osteoporosis and those who have had a fragility fracture.

Clinical situation	SIGN [7]	NICE [2]
T ≤ −2.5 but without severe osteoporosis in the spine	• Alendronate. • Risedronate. • If not tolerated, poor response or patient prefers parenteral therapy, consider denosumab or annual zoledronic acid.	• Does not differentiate depending on spinal osteoporosis. • Recommends alendronate or risedronate for all those with T ≤ −2.5. • Consider this also for those taking an equivalent corticosteroid dose of prednisolone 7.5 mg daily for 3 months or longer.
T ≤ −2.5 with severe osteoporosis in the spine	• Romosozumab if there is a high risk of hip or non-vertebral fracture. • Teriparatide if there isn't a high risk of hip or non-vertebral fracture. • Transition to an anti-resorptive agent after the course above is finished.	• If not tolerated or contraindicated, consider specialist referral for consideration of zoledronic acid, strontium ranelate, raloxifene, denosumab or teriparatide.
T −2.5 to −1.0 (osteopenia)	• Zoledronic acid 18 monthly if aged ≥ 65. • Lifestyle advice if aged < 65, with a reassessment if the risk profile changes.	• Modify risk factors where possible, treat any underlying conditions and repeat the DXA at an appropriate interval using clinical judgement (usually within 2 years).

Details of Drug Therapy for Osteoporosis

Management again varies depending on which guideline is being used – this is outlined in Table 29.2.

When to Refer

This will be an individual decision, based on clinical judgement, which guideline is being followed, local pathways and access to parenteral therapy locally. Referral might be considered in the following groups of people:

- Patient with osteoporosis who also have cystic fibrosis or chronic kidney disease with an eGFR <30 ml/min/1.73m2 [7].
- Anyone who has been treated in primary care but is intolerant of both alendronate and risedronate [2,7].
- People who prefer parenteral therapy [2].
- People older than 50 with a history of a vertebral fracture and a T-score of < −1.5 at any site, or a spinal T-score of < −4.0 [12].
- More than two vertebral fractures of any age independent of BMD.
- High-dose glucocorticoid therapy (> 7.5 mg of prednisolone or equivalent for more than three months) [6].
- People with multiple clinical risk factors for fracture [6].
- People who sustain a fragility fracture on bisphosphonate treatment, after checking adherence and for secondary causes of osteoporosis. NOGG defines poor adherence as less than 80% of the treatment being taken correctly [2,6].
- People where oral bisphosphonates are contraindicated or caution should be advised – reasons might include the following [13,14,15,16]:
  - Alendronate:
    - Inability to sit or stand upright for at least 30 minutes after taking the medication.
    - Abnormalities of the oesophagus or other factors which delay oesophageal emptying such as stricture or achalasia, or any symptomatic oesophageal disease.
    - Upper gastrointestinal bleeding.
    - Dysphagia.
    - Gastritis.
    - Within one year of a peptic ulcer.
    - Past surgery to the upper gastrointestinal tract.
  - Risedronate:
    - Pregnancy and lactation.
    - Severe renal impairment with a creatinine clearance < 30 ml/min.
    - Upper gastrointestinal disorders.

- Both alendronate and risedronate:
  - Hypersensitivity to the active substance or any excipients.
  - Hypocalcaemia.
  - Elderly patients with a current or recent history of upper gastrointestinal disease or bleeding.
  - Atypical femoral fractures.

Pharmacological Therapy: Anti-resorptive Agents

This class of drug includes bisphosphonates, oestrogens and monoclonal antibodies such as denosumab. They depress osteoclasts and reduce bone resorption.

Bisphosphonates

Once-weekly alendronate and risedronate are first-line therapy for prevention and treatment of osteoporotic fractures. Bisphosphonates reduce the risk of fragility fracture by at least 50% [17,18,19].

Bisphosphonates are poorly absorbed orally and need to be taken exactly as directed to optimise bone-sparing effects and minimise upper gastrointestinal intolerance. They should be taken first thing in the morning, on an empty stomach, with a full glass of tap water, and no other food, drink or medication taken for at least 30 minutes (alendronate and risedronate) and at least 60 minutes with ibandronate [13,14,20]. Patients should stay upright to minimise oesophageal damage. Alendronate effervescent tablets, dissolved in water to produce a buffered alendronate solution for once-weekly treatment, can be used in those who develop gastrointestinal side effects with tablet formulations, or those at risk of oesophageal ulceration.

When starting treatment, patients should receive education regarding osteoporosis and how to take their medication and be encouraged to report upper gastrointestinal symptoms. If these occur, bisphosphonate therapy should be stopped. An enquiry into adherence should be made at every review [21]. Continuation of alendronate with a proton pump inhibitor is not recommended because of an increased fracture risk with this combination [22]. Once symptoms have settled, a further trial of the same or a different oral bisphosphonate is appropriate, but if the patient remains intolerant, they should be referred for initiation of intravenous or subcutaneous therapy.

In December 2014, the Medicines and Healthcare Products Regulatory Agency (MHRA) issued guidance on use and safety of bisphosphonates [23]. The guidance discussed the following:

- Oesophageal reactions – minimise by avoiding use if there is stricture or achalasia. Ensure that patients follow dosing instructions. Consider carefully before using with Barrett's oesophagus.
- Osteonecrosis of the jaw – an area of exposed or dead bone in the jaw for > eight weeks in a patient who has had bisphosphonate. More common in those receiving intravenous bisphosphonates for cancer than with oral bisphosphonates for osteoporosis. If poor dental health or for intravenous bisphosphonates, then dental examination recommended prior to treatment. Patients should maintain good oral hygiene, have regular dental review and report dental problems.
- Atrial fibrillation – small increased risk if treated with zoledronate or pamidronate; recent review suggests not with alendronate.
- Atypical femoral fractures – stress-type fractures of the femoral shaft after minimal or no trauma, often bilateral. Patients may have thigh pain for several weeks before the completed fracture occurs (they should be warned to report this and be referred for x-ray). Associated with long-term anti-resorptive therapy – all patients should be reviewed after five years' bisphosphonate use. Optimal duration of therapy to reduce risk of conventional fractures while minimising atypical fractures is unknown, as is the prevalence, therefore difficult to advise people (also occur with strontium ranelate or denosumab).
- Adverse effects on renal function – intravenous zoledronate. Patients should be well hydrated prior to therapy and renal function monitored. Zoledronate not recommended if eGFR < 35 mmol/L. (Alendronate is not recommended if eGFR < 35 or risedronate if < 30.)

Zoledronate is a potent bisphosphonate given annually by intravenous infusion. It reduces vertebral, non-vertebral and hip fractures and

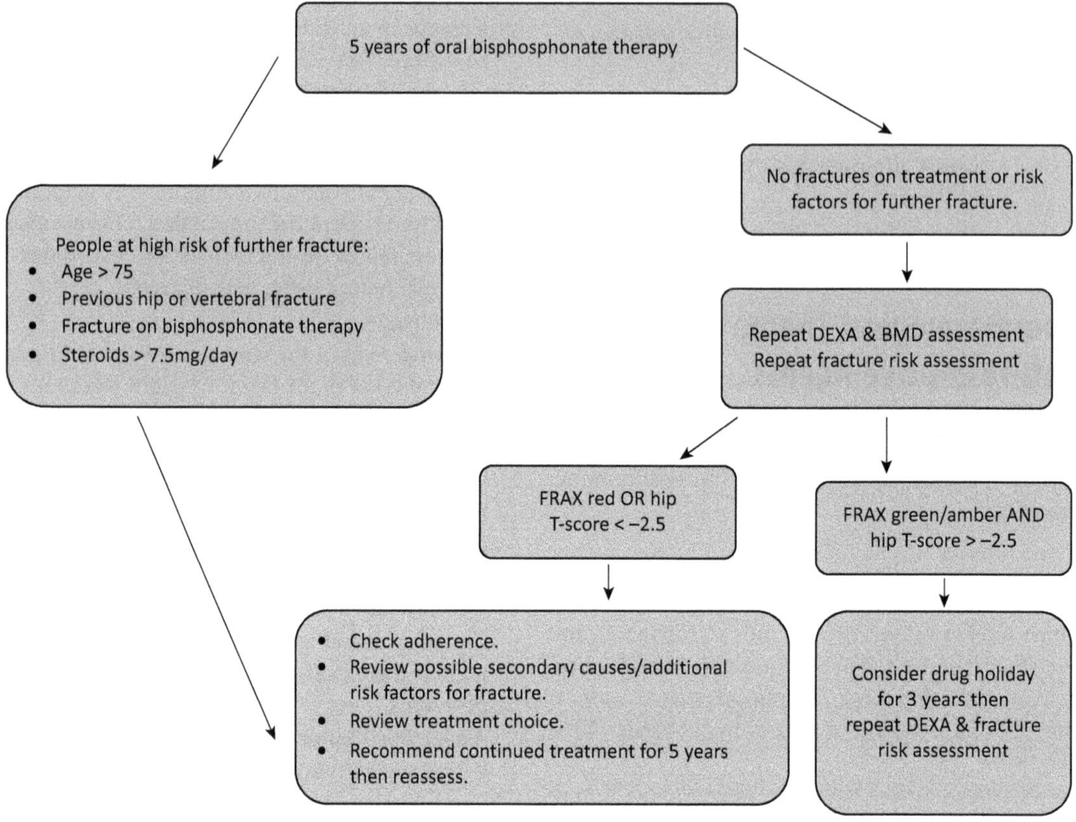

Figure 29.3 Issues to consider when deciding whether a patient should have a 'bisphosphonate holiday' [6,7].

reduces mortality in post-hip-fracture patients. Up to one-third of people develop a flu-like reaction within three days after the first infusion; this is much less common after subsequent infusions [24,25].

Bisphosphonate Treatment Duration and 'Holidays': Who, When and for How Long?

There is a concern that long-term use of bisphosphonates can increase the risk of rare complications such as avascular necrosis of the jaw and atypical femoral fractures. For this reason, in most cases bisphosphonates should be prescribed for an initial period of five years, and fracture risk then reassessed.

Bisphosphonates have a long duration of action. Patients at medium or low risk of further fracture can therefore consider a temporary break in therapy – this is often termed a 'bisphosphonate holiday'.

Figure 29.3 is a suggested algorithm to use when considering a bisphosphonate holiday, written using information from the SIGN and NOGG guidelines.

If a bisphosphonate treatment holiday is offered, fracture risk should be reassessed earlier than three years if there is a new fragility fracture, or if new risk factors develop (such as the initiation of oral steroid therapy).

For those in whom the decision at five years is to continue for another five years, there is little evidence to support treatment decisions after 10 years of bisphosphonate therapy. Most patients, at this point, may benefit from a two-year treatment holiday to reduce the risk of atypical fracture; some high-risk patients, particularly those who have fractured on treatment, may require ongoing treatment.

Prescribing decisions in these circumstances should be taken on an individual shared-decision basis, with uncertainties about risk versus benefit discussed with the patient. Specialist advice and support may be appropriate.

Denosumab

Denosumab is a fully human monoclonal antibody to the RANK ligand which is involved in differentiation and maturation of osteoclasts. Denosumab reduces hip, vertebral and non-vertebral fractures and effects are sustained while on treatment; 60 mg is given twice yearly by subcutaneous injection. Usually initiation occurs in specialist care with ongoing treatment in primary care under a resourced shared care agreement. Denosumab is contraindicated in patients with hypocalcaemia.

NICE TA 204 [26] recommends denosumab for secondary prevention in postmenopausal women at increased risk of osteoporotic fragility fractures who are unable to comply with the special instructions for taking oral alendronate and risedronate or etidronate, or who are intolerant of these or have a contraindication to them. It can also be used for primary prevention in those who are unable to use oral bisphosphonates and meet the NICE criteria in terms of age, risk factors and T scores. SIGN recommend its use in postmenopausal women with osteoporosis who cannot use or tolerate bisphosphonates, and as shown in Figure 29.2.

It is important to be aware that on stopping denosumab treatment, BMD can rapidly decline to levels below those at treatment initiation. This significantly increases fracture risk, particularly of vertebral fracture. It is important that people on denosumab treatment maintain adherence. Denosumab should not be stopped without a plan in place to mitigate this risk, and specialist advice should be sought in this circumstance.

Hormone Replacement Therapy (HRT) [7]

Oestrogen-containing HRT can reduce the risk of fracture; some preparations are licensed for the prevention of osteoporosis in postmenopausal women. HRT may be considered for the prevention of osteoporosis in younger postmenopausal women. A shared decision-making approach should be taken, balancing the risks and benefits of HRT against those of bisphosphonate treatment.

Calcitriol and raloxifene are used less than they used to be; they are less effective than bisphosphonates in reducing the risk of non-vertebral and hip fractures. Strontium ranelate is also used less than it used to be due to increased risks of venous thromboembolism, myocardial infarction and cerebrovascular disease.

Pharmacological Therapy: Anabolic Drugs

Anabolic drugs increase bone density rather than reducing bone turnover. Anabolic agents should be considered in those at very high risk of fracture.

Teriparatide (Recombinant Parathyroid Hormone)

Daily subcutaneous injections of 20 mcg teriparatide for up to 18 months increase bone formation more than resorption, particularly at spinal sites, resulting in significant reductions in vertebral and non-vertebral fractures.

UK national guidance for the use of teriparatide varies. Teriparatide should be considered in the following circumstances:

- Postmenopausal women with severe osteoporosis or very high fracture risk, to prevent fractures or in those with a history of at least two moderate or one severe low trauma vertebral fractures [6,7].
- People at very high risk of fracture [6].
- People older than 50 with a history of a vertebral fracture and a T-score of < −1.5 at any site, or a spinal T-score of < −4.0 [12].
- Postmenopausal women or men aged 50 or older who are intolerant of bisphosphonate therapy, particularly with a history of vertebral fractures [6].

Teriparatide is contraindicated in people with hypercalcaemia, severe renal impairment, malignancy, pregnancy and lactation. Teriparatide should not be prescribed without specialist guidance.

Romosozumab

Romosozumab is a monoclonal antibody given monthly by subcutaneous injection; it works by inhibiting sclerostin in bone. It is given as a 12-month treatment course, usually followed by an anti-resorptive agent. It works by both inhibiting bone reabsorption and stimulating new bone formation. It is approved for use in the UK in postmenopausal women with a previous fragility fracture who are at high risk of future fracture [27].

Romosozumab increases the risk of hypocalcaemia in patients with an eGFR of < 30 ml/min/

1.73 m^2. It is contraindicated in patients with ischaemic heart and cerebrovascular disease; there is conflicting evidence about any increased risk of cardiovascular disease in people who do not have established cardiovascular disease. Romosozumab should not be initiated without specialist involvement.

Fracture Prevention and Special Groups

Patients Taking Aromatase Inhibitors

Aromatase inhibitors induce bone loss in women, increasing the risk of fracture.

All women who are either commencing aromatase inhibitor therapy or have treatment-induced menopause should have their fracture risk assessed; aromatase inhibitor therapy should be considered to be a secondary cause of osteoporosis. DXA should be requested when indicated.

Women at high risk of fracture should be started on drug treatment to reduce the risk of fracture. Women whose risk lies close to the intervention threshold should have a further bone health assessment in one to two years.

Women who are treated with a bisphosphonate as part of their cancer treatment should have a bone health review at cessation of bisphosphonate treatment [6].

Patients Taking Corticosteroids

People currently taking or frequently using steroids are at increased risk of osteoporosis and fracture.

Risk assessment using FRAX or QFracture should be undertaken in the following groups [1]:

- People younger than 40 with current or recent use of high-dose corticosteroids (7.5 mg prednisolone or equivalent) for three months or more [1].
- People older than 40 with current use of oral corticosteroids, or frequent recent use. Frequent use is not defined in guidelines but many consider that 3 or more courses in 12 months is a reasonable pragmatic threshold.
- Treatment decisions in people taking corticosteroids:
- Assess the need for treatment following fracture risk assessment and BMD measurement if indicated.
- Bone turnover reduces and fracture risk increases very quickly on starting corticosteroids; if BMD assessment is suggested when assessing fracture risk, consider starting bisphosphonate therapy while awaiting BMD assessment in people at high risk of fracture. This includes [6]:
  - Anyone with a previous fragility fracture.
  - Women older than 70.
  - Postmenopausal women on high-dose steroids (≥ 7.5 mg/day of prednisolone or equivalent over three months (NB: this is equivalent to ≥ 30 mg/day of prednisone for four weeks over three months).
  - Postmenopausal women with a FRAX fracture probability exceeding the treatment threshold.
- In those where treatment is recommended, continue treatment with bisphosphonates and/or calcium and vitamin D until treatment with oral corticosteroids has stopped.
- Consider requesting specialist advice for patients younger than 50 who are assessed to be at high risk of fracture.
- Reassess fracture risk using FRAX after stopping steroid treatment to determine the need for further treatment.

Premenopausal Women

Most premenopausal women with osteoporotic fractures will need initial specialist assessment. Caution is advised in prescribing bisphosphonates in women of childbearing age; while there is no clear evidence that bisphosphonates are harmful in pregnancy and lactation, it is generally advised that bisphosphonates should not be used for at least three months before conception and while lactating [28].

References

[1] NICE, 'CG 146. Osteoporosis: Assessing the risk of fragility fracture'. 2017. Accessed: 3 Jun. 2024. [Online]. Available: www.nice.org.uk/guidance/cg146.

[2] NICE CKS, 'Osteoporosis – Prevention of fragility fractures'. 2023. Accessed: 3 Jun. 2024. [Online]. Available: https://cks.nice.org.uk/topics/osteo

porosis-prevention-of-fragility-fractures/background-information/prevalence.

[3] NHS, 'Osteoporosis'. 2022. Accessed: 3 Jun. 2024. [Online]. Available: www.nhs.uk/conditions/osteoporosis.

[4] University of Sheffield, 'FRAX Fracture risk assessment tool'. Accessed: 3 Jun. 2024. [Online]. Available: https://frax.shef.ac.uk/FRAX.

[5] ClinRisk, 'QFracture'. Accessed: 3 Jun. 2024. [Online]. Available: https://qfracture.org/index.php.

[6] NOGG, 'Clinical guideline for the prevention and treatment of osteoporosis'. 2021. Accessed: 3 Jun. 2024. [Online]. Available: www.nogg.org.uk/full-guideline.

[7] SIGN, '142. Management of osteoporosis and the prevention of fragility fractures'. 2020. Accessed: 3 Jun. 2024. [Online]. Available: www.sign.ac.uk/media/1741/sign142.pdf.

[8] Royal Osteoporosis Society. Accessed: 3 Jun. 2024. [Online]. Available: https://theros.org.uk.

[9] Bone Health and Osteoporosis Foundation, 'Steps to estimate your calcium intake'. Accessed: 3 Jun. 2024. [Online]. Available: www.bonehealthandosteoporosis.org/patients/treatment/calciumvitamin-d/steps-to-estimate-your-calcium-intake.

[10] J. A. Kanis, A. Oden, O. Johnell et al., 'The use of clinical risk factors enhances the performance of BMD in the prediction of hip and osteoporotic fractures in men and women', *Osteoporos Int*, vol. **18**, no. 8, pp. 1033–1046, 2007.

[11] Public Health England, 'Statement from PHE and NICE on vitamin D supplementation during winter'. Accessed: 3 Jun. 2024. [Online]. Available: https://www.gov.uk/government/publications/vitamin-d-supplementation-during-winter-phe-and-nice-statement.

[12] NICE, 'TA161. Raloxifene and teriparatide for the secondary prevention of osteoporotic fragility fractures in postmenopausal women'. Feb. 2018. Accessed: 3 Jun. 2024. [Online]. Available: www.nice.org.uk/guidance/ta161.

[13] SPC, 'Alendronic acid 70mg'. Apr. 2022. Accessed: 3 Jun. 2024. [Online]. Available: www.medicines.org.uk/emc/product/5206/smpc#gref.

[14] SPC, 'Risedronate sodium 35mg'. Dec. 2020. Accessed: 3 Jun. 2024. [Online]. Available: www.medicines.org.uk/emc/product/4767/smpc#gref.

[15] BNF, 'Alendronic acid'. Feb. 2024. Accessed: 3 Jun. 2024. [Online]. Available: https://bnf.nice.org.uk/drugs/alendronic-acid.

[16] BNF, 'Risedronate sodium'. Feb. 2024. Accessed: 3 Jun. 2024. [Online]. Available: https://bnf.nice.org.uk/drugs/risedronate-sodium.

[17] C. Ayers, D. Kansagara, B. Lazur et al., 'Effectiveness and safety of treatments to prevent fractures in people with low bone mass or primary osteoporosis: A living systematic review and network meta-analysis for the American College of Physicians', *Ann Intern Med*, vol. **176**, no. 2, pp. 182–195, 2023.

[18] K. N. Tu, J. D. Lie and C. K. V. Wan, 'Osteoporosis: A review of treatment options'. *P&T*, vol. **43**, no. 2, pp. 92–104, 2018.

[19] SPC, 'Risedronate sodium 35mg'. Dec. 2020. Accessed: 3 Jun. 2024. [Online]. Available: www.medicines.org.uk/emc/product/4767/smpc#gref.

[20] SPC, 'Ibandronic acid 150mg'. Accessed: 3 Jun. 2024. [Online]. Available: www.medicines.org.uk/emc/product/4135/smpc#gref.

[21] NICE, 'QS149. Osteoporosis'. Accessed: 3 Jun. 2024. [Online]. Available: www.nice.org.uk/guidance/qs149.

[22] Specialist Pharmacy Service, 'Using bisphosphonates with proton pump inhibitors'. Apr. 2023. Accessed: 3 Jun. 2024. [Online]. Available: www.sps.nhs.uk/articles/using-bisphosphonates-with-proton-pump-inhibitors-ppis.

[23] MHRA, 'Bisphosphonates: Use and safety'. Dec. 2014. Accessed: 3 Jun. 2024. [Online]. Available: www.gov.uk/government/publications/bisphosphonates-use-and-safety/bisphosphonates-use-and-safety.

[24] LiverTox, 'Clinical and research information on drug-induced liver injury'. National Institute of Diabetes and Digestive and Kidney Diseases, 2012.

[25] E. L. Greear, P. Patel and A. Bankole, 'Zoledronate'. StatPearls Publishing, 2024.

[26] NICE, 'TA204. Denosumab for the prevention of osteoporotic fractures in postmenopausal women'. Oct. 2010. Accessed: 3 Jun. 2024. [Online]. Available: www.nice.org.uk/guidance/TA204.

[27] NICE, 'TA791. Romosozumab for treating severe osteoporosis'. May 2022. Accessed: 3 Jun. 2024. [Online]. Available: www.nice.org.uk/guidance/TA791.

[28] Best Use of Medicines in Pregnancy, 'Bisphosphonates'. 2017. Accessed: 3 Jun. 2024. [Online]. Available: https://www.medicinesinpregnancy.org/leaflets-a-z/alendronic-acid/.

Chapter

30 Management of the Patient with Benign and Malignant Breast Conditions in Primary Care

Jo Marsden

Key Points

- Most people significantly overestimate their risk of being diagnosed with and dying from breast cancer.
- Most breast symptoms are due to a benign cause.
- Most people diagnosed with breast cancer have no known risk factors other than age and sex.
- Most people with lifestyle risk factors never get breast cancer.
- High-risk familial breast cancer accounts for < 2% of annual UK breast cancer diagnoses.
- Most benign breast conditions are not associated with an increased risk of breast cancer.
- The benefits from mammographic screening are considered to outweigh the risks.
- Eighty per cent of people treated for breast cancer survive for at least 10 years.
- Uptake of healthy lifestyle behaviours after breast cancer improves all-cause and breast cancer mortality.

Case Scenario 30.1

Deborah, aged 52, has been diagnosed with a screen-detected right breast cancer. She is anxious that current hormone replacement therapy (HRT) use may have 'caused' her cancer, especially as her mother was diagnosed with it in her 70s, and that it was 'missed' by tests, done for a right-sided breast lump six years ago. Deborah asks about treatment. What can you advise her?

Introduction

Breast cancer is the commonest female malignancy in the UK [1] and encompasses invasive breast cancer and non-invasive ductal carcinoma in situ (DCIS). Between 2017 and 2019 an annual average of 56,900 and 8,500 new cases of invasive and non-invasive cancer were diagnosed respectively, with about one-third presenting via the NHS Breast Screening Programme (NHSBSP) [1,2]. The UK lifetime risk of diagnosis in women is one in seven [1,2] (Figure 30.1).

A full-time GP is likely to diagnose approximately one or two people with breast cancer annually but will see many more with breast symptoms and possibly unnecessary concern about risk of malignancy and mortality. Across all ages, UK deaths from breast cancer have fallen by around 40% since the 1970s; survival continues to improve. Currently around three-quarters of women in England who have breast cancer survive for 10 years or more, with 10-year survival rising to 87% for those aged 55–64. Improvements in survival mean that breast cancer is the most prevalent UK malignancy (total number of people living with the condition at a specific time). To place this in context with all-cause mortality, breast cancer is not in the five commonest causes of death for women in England and Wales in 2024 – these range from dementia (15% of deaths) to malignancy of the respiratory tract at (4.2%), with deaths from breast cancer making up 3.5% [3].

When Should Symptomatic People Be Referred to a Breast Clinic for Assessment?

GPs have an important role in determining whether breast symptoms warrant referral; guidance is available to support this, as shown in Table 30.1. These criteria apply to both women and men [4].

In the absence of other symptoms, breast pain (mastalgia) is usually benign and, in the absence of a lump, highly unlikely to be associated with cancer. It is common in premenopausal women, often (but not always) cyclical, variable in character and usually self-limiting. Simple analgesia and topical anti-inflammatories may help. There is limited evidence that dietary intervention or evening primrose oil have any more than a placebo effect [5]. Non-cyclical mastalgia is often musculoskeletal; costochondritis (Tietze's syndrome) is a particular variant. Referral is recommended when initial treatment fails, or unexplained symptoms persist; the establishment of a 'primary care breast pain clinic' has helped in some areas to reassure this cohort of women and reduce suspected cancer referrals. No cancers were found in one cohort of 177 women with breast pain only [6]. The Association of Breast Surgery is currently reviewing safety, patient experience and resource implications for breast pain referral pathways [7].

Table 30.1 Suspected cancer referral criteria – breast cancer

Refer people using a suspected cancer pathway referral if they are:

- Aged ≥ 30 with an unexplained breast lump with or without pain.
- Aged ≥ 50 with any of the following symptoms in one nipple only:
  - discharge
  - retraction
  - other changes of concern.

Consider a suspected cancer pathway referral in people:

- With skin changes that suggest breast cancer.
- Aged ≥ 30 with an unexplained lump in the axilla.

Consider non-urgent referral in people aged under 30:

- With an unexplained breast lump with or without pain.

Any referring health professional should understand the procedures which are likely to be offered. The diagnosis of breast symptoms involves triple assessment [8]:

- Clinical examination.
- Imaging; in general, mammography is first line for those aged ≥ 40 (or younger women with a suspicious ultrasound) and ultrasound is first line for women aged < 40.
- Tissue biopsy; image-guided tissue sampling when a solid, discrete lump is confirmed on imaging (i.e. fine needle aspiration cytology, core biopsy). Free-hand core biopsy and nipple discharge cytology may sometimes be appropriate.

When triple assessment is negative for cancer, people are advised to seek advice from their GP if

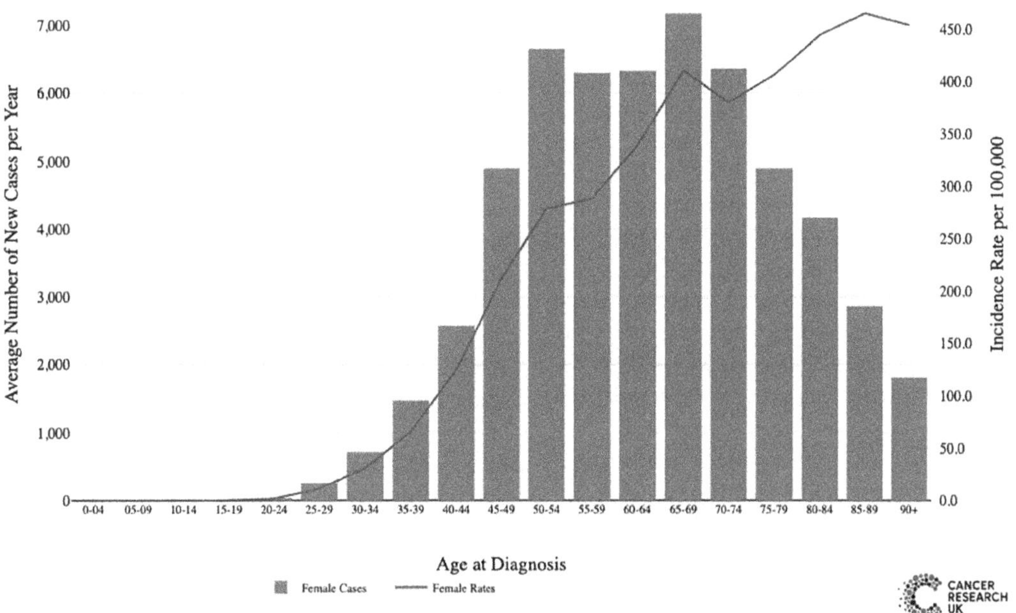

Figure 30.1 Breast cancer: average number of new cases per year and age-specific incidence rates per 100,000 population, females, UK, 2016–2018. Prepared by Cancer Research UK – original data sources are available from www.cancerresearchuk.org/cancer-info/cancerstats (accessed January 2024). Reproduced with permission.

they remain concerned or if there is a change in symptoms or signs (they can be re-referred). If Deborah's previous breast lump was evaluated by triple assessment, it is highly unlikely that her cancer was 'missed'. Delayed diagnosis of breast cancer after a false- negative triple assessment is approximately 0.2% [9].

Breast Screening

Women aged 50–70 are eligible for participation in the NHSBSP and are invited by their local screening centre for a mammogram every three years. Those over 70 can request screening but will not be automatically invited. Trans men and those of the female sex who identify as non-binary are eligible to participate if they have not had a bilateral mastectomy, as are trans women and those of the male sex who identify as non-binary who have received female sex hormones. Someone of the female sex who has changed the gender marker on their notes to male will not automatically be invited for screening but can request it [10]. The UK AgeX Trial is evaluating the risks and benefits of an additional screen for those aged 47–49 and 71–73, with the first outcome report scheduled for December 2026. The aim of screening mammography is to diagnose breast cancer at an earlier stage, before it becomes symptomatic, so reducing the complexity of treatment and increasing survival [10,11,12,13].

There has been extensive debate about the benefits and harms of screening. In 2012, an independent UK review concluded that the NHSBSP probably prevents around 1,300 breast cancer deaths each year, but that around 19% of cancers diagnosed by screening are over-diagnosed; that is, they would never have come to clinical attention during the woman's lifetime. As it is not possible to reliably identify these 'over-diagnosed' cancers, some women will receive unnecessary treatment with the risk of side effects (99% will have surgery, 80% radiotherapy, 70% adjuvant endocrine therapy and 26% chemotherapy). For every breast cancer death prevented by the NHSBSP, three women will be over-diagnosed and have unnecessary treatment [12].

Other possible harms of screening include the following:

- false-positive results (i.e. anxiety due to recall for further investigation)
- false-negative results (i.e. failure to diagnose a pre-existing cancer)
- radiation exposure. For every 10,000 women who have three-yearly mammograms between the age of 47 and 73, the radiation exposure will be associated with an excess diagnosis of three to six breast cancers [13].

Overall, the benefits from NHSBSP participation are considered to outweigh the risks and survey data suggests that being informed of the risks and benefits does not put women off attending [14,15].

Risk Factors for Breast Cancer

Little is known about the exact cause of most breast cancers; the aetiology is complex and involves interplay between genetic, reproductive, lifestyle and environmental factors. An individual's risk of diagnosis is affected by non-modifiable and modifiable factors (Table 30.2).

Non-modifiable Risk Factors

These establish individual baseline risk and are listed in Table 30.2. Most people are at population or average baseline risk, (i.e. relative risk of 1.0), which is determined by increasing age and being female (80% of breast cancers are diagnosed in women over 50). Only a minority have a baseline risk greater than that of the population due to the influence of other non-modifiable risk factors, which are now discussed.

Familial Breast Cancer

DNA repair gene mutations are necessary for the malignant transformation of normal breast epithelial cells. In most people these mutations are acquired during their lifetime, leading to 'sporadic' breast cancer. Only 5–10% of breast cancers are due to inheritance of mutations in specific genes [16,17].

When concern is expressed about familial risk, a family history should be taken to determine whether referral to a breast clinic, specialist family history clinic or regional genetics centre is warranted (Box 30.1). This is not indicated if breast cancer has been diagnosed in only one first-degree or second-degree relative over 40 and there are no other concerning features in the family history (see Box 30.1), where the unaffected relative is managed as if they are at population risk in primary care [18].

- People at moderate increased risk are eligible for annual mammographic surveillance

Table 30.2 Breast cancer risk factors categorised by type and associated conferred relative risk

High risk (relative risk > 4.0)		**Relative risk**
Female sex	*Non-modifiable*	100
Increasing age (< 65 vs. ≥ 65 years)	*Non-modifiable*	5.8
Inherited high-risk susceptibility gene (e.g. BRCA1)	*Non-modifiable*	18
Inherited high-risk susceptibility gene (e.g. BRCA2)	*Non-modifiable*	15
High-risk benign breast condition atypical ductal hyperplasia (ADH)	*Non-modifiable*	~ 4
High-risk benign breast condition lobular carcinoma in situ (LCIS)	*Non-modifiable*	~ 9
Percentage mammographic breast density (> 75% vs. < 0.5%)	*Non-modifiable*	4.6
Moderate risk (relative risk 2.1–4.0)		
First-degree relative with premenopausal breast cancer	*Non-modifiable*	3.3
Low risk (relative risk 1.1–2.0)		
First-degree relative with postmenopausal breast cancer	*Non-modifiable*	1.8
Young age at menarche (< 12 years vs. > 15 years)	*Non-modifiable*	1.3
Older age at menopause (> 55 years vs. < 45 years)	*Non-modifiable*	1.2–1.5
Proliferative benign breast disease without epithelial atypia	*Non-modifiable*	< 2
Ionising background radiation (cosmic, gamma, internal, per Sv)	*Non-modifiable*	1.02
Age at first full-term pregnancy (nulliparous or first child over 30 vs. < 20)	*Modifiable*	1.7–1.9
Nulliparity (vs. any parity)	*Modifiable*	1.3
No breastfeeding (vs. breastfeeding)	*Modifiable*	1.1
Postmenopausal body mass index (80th percentile ≥ 55 years vs. 20th percentile)	*Modifiable*	1.2
Alcohol (2 drinks per day vs. no drinks)	*Modifiable*	1.2
Hormonal oral combined contraceptives	*Modifiable*	1.2
Combined HRT (current use at least 5 years vs. none)	*Modifiable*	1.3
Physical activity (sedentary vs. active)	*Modifiable*	1.8
Current smoking (vs. never)	*Modifiable*	1.1

Population risk is 1.0. Reproduced with permission by The International Menopause Society (IMS).

between the ages of 40 and 49 (sometimes extended to 59), thereafter surveillance as part of the NHSBSP. Anti-oestrogenic chemoprevention may be discussed.

- People confirmed or very likely to be at high risk due to an inherited high-risk-susceptibility gene may be recommended surveillance (mammography +/− MRI), prophylactic surgery (mastectomy, oophorectomy) or offered anti-oestrogenic chemoprevention as appropriate.
- Genetic testing is undertaken in those who may be at high risk, on the recommendation of a specialist genetic service.

Deborah has no other cancers in her family other than her mother's breast cancer at the age of 70 and is not of Jewish ancestry. She can be reassured about her family history and that if she has any daughters, her diagnosis at the age of 52 does not increase their individual risk unless there is other information from their father's family history which changes this.

Benign Breast Conditions

A range of non-malignant conditions arise from the breast stroma (fat and supportive connective tissue) and epithelium (duct-alveolar lobule). They can be categorised as follows.

- Non-fibrocystic benign conditions. These are not associated with an increased breast cancer risk. Examples include infection and inflammatory changes.
- Fibrocystic changes. Incidence begins to rise during the second decade of life, peaks in the fourth and fifth decades and declines thereafter. Endogenous sex hormones and HRT are implicated in the aetiology, although oral contraceptives appear to reduce the incidence of

some types (e.g. fibroadenoma). Risk is also increased in women with familial breast cancer [19]. Histological categorisation according to the estimated risk of a subsequent breast cancer diagnosis does not correlate with symptoms

Box 30.1 Family History Indicating an Increased Risk of a Cancer-Causing Gene

Criteria in the family history which mean that advice should be sought from secondary care, even if the index patient does not otherwise fulfil the criteria for referral:

- bilateral breast cancer
- male breast cancer
- ovarian cancer
- Jewish ancestry
- sarcoma in a relative younger than age 45 years
- glioma or childhood adrenal cortical carcinomas
- complicated patterns of multiple cancers at a young age
- paternal history of breast cancer (two or more relatives on the father's side of the family).

(Table 30.3). The only category associated with a significant risk is atypical ductal hyperplasia (ADH/ALH), which is considered a marker of increased risk and an non-obligate precursor [20].

- Lobular carcinoma in situ (LCIS). Despite its name, this is not malignant. It is another marker for increased risk and also a non-obligate breast cancer precursor (Table 30.2a) [20]. Collectively, ADH, ALH and LCIS are considered 'high-risk' benign breast conditions.

Asymptomatic Women with Higher Breast Density and No Other Risk Factors

Higher mammographic density may reduce screening sensitivity and cancer detection and is associated with an increased risk of breast cancer. A UK randomised trial is currently evaluating whether adding extra imaging (e.g. automated whole breast ultrasound, contrast enhanced spectral mammography or abbreviated MRI) to the standard of care offered by the NHSBSP (i.e. three-yearly surveillance mammograms) improves small cancer detection rates in the screening population [23]. A UK randomised

Table 30.3 Benign breast change and subsequent risk of invasive breast cancer

Pathology and baseline relative risk for breast cancer			Symptoms	Management
Normal tissue, no benign change		1.0	-	-
Fibrocystic change				
Non-proliferative change	• Fibroadenoma • Duct ectasia • Solitary cysts	1.0	Lump (+/– pain), nipple discharge or inversion or incidental finding.	Reassure and discharge once the diagnosis is confirmed.
Proliferative disease without atypia	• Multiple cysts • Ductal papilloma • Radial scar • Sclerosing adenosis • Epithelial hyperplasia	1.1 – 1.9	Lump (+/– pain), nipple discharge or inversion or incidental finding.	Reassure and discharge once the diagnosis is confirmed.
Proliferative disease with atypia	• Atypical ductal hyperplasia (ADH) and atypical lobular hyperplasia (ALH)	~ 4	None, usually an incidental biopsy finding.	Surveillance mammography. The optimal frequency and duration are unknown. Currently most units undertake annual mammography for 5 years [9].
LCIS	-	~ 10	None, usually an incidental biopsy finding.	As for proliferative disease with atypia, above.

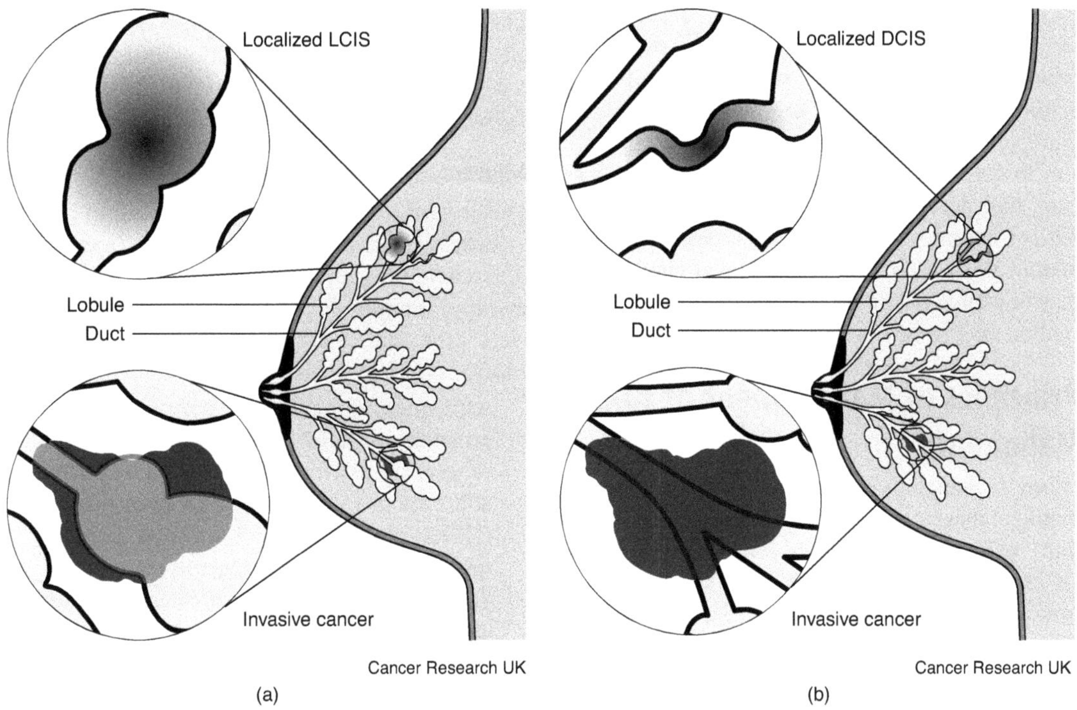

Figure 30.2 In situ carcinoma (LCIS (a), DCIS (b)) is restricted to the breast ducts and lobules in contrast with invasive breast cancer, where malignant cells invade through the duct wall into the surrounding breast tissue. Source: www.cancerresearchuk.org/about-cancer/type/breast-cancer/about/types/lcis-lobular-carcinoma-in-situ and www.cancerresearchuk.org/about-cancer/type/breast-cancer/about/types/dcis-ductal-carcinoma-in-situ (accessed January 2024). Reproduced with permission.

trial has shown that added imaging with abbreviated MRI and contrast enhanced spectral mammography may lead to earlier detection of cancer when screening women with dense breasts but the risks (e.g. overdiagnosis) and benefits (e.g. reduced breast cancer mortality) are unresolved [21].

Modifiable Risk Factors

These include lifestyle and some reproductive factors; individual impact is determined by baseline risk, increasing as this rises. All, including HRT, are associated with a low estimated risk which means most women exposed will not be diagnosed with breast cancer because of this (Table 30.2). Their effect is largely mediated via exposure to female sex hormones, changes to sex hormone metabolism or the presence of a greater proportion of less differentiated breast epithelial cells, which are more susceptible to malignant transformation when exposed to carcinogens (e.g. nulliparity, late age at first full-term pregnancy, not breastfeeding). In people with familial breast cancer or a benign breast condition, more robust evidence is required to clarify how modifiable factors influence risk [22,23,24]. In the absence of such, it is pragmatic to assume that risk estimates are similar to those at population risk.

Deborah should be reassured that her HRT use was unlikely to have resulted in her diagnosis. Evidence suggests that exogenous sex hormone exposure promotes the development of cancer from pre-existing occult lesions and that the natural history of the disease is not changed [25]. When counselling women about breast cancer, advice should be individualised, accounting for personal, non-modifiable risk; the risk associated with HRT should be placed in context with other modifiable factors.

Breast Cancer Prevention

Primary prevention is aimed at reducing exposure to risk factors. For those at population risk, it is estimated up to 25% of breast cancer diagnoses could be avoided by adopting healthy lifestyle choices (e.g. increasing physical activity, minimising alcohol intake and maintaining a normal body mass index (BMI)) [26,27]. However, we can't identify which individuals will benefit from this; such measures have no impact on hormone-insensitive cancers. Except for promoting breastfeeding, reproductive factors are not easily modifiable as they stem from prolonged, endogenous hormonal exposure. Screening and breast self-examination (BSE) are examples of secondary prevention measures, which aim to detect disease at an early stage to facilitate cure. BSE does not reduce breast cancer mortality but is recommended to raise awareness and earlier presentation [28]. In addition, those at familial risk, may be offered risk reducing surgery and chemoprevention after review in secondary/tertiary care.

Principles of Management of Breast Malignancy

When malignancy is confirmed by triple assessment, management is coordinated by the breast unit multidisciplinary team. Treatment for both DCIS and invasive breast cancer is determined by tumour characteristics and national guidelines [29].

Ductal Carcinoma in Situ (DCIS)

Malignant cells are confined to the breast ducts and cannot metastasise to ipsilateral axillary nodes or other parts of the body (Figure 30.2b).

Treatment

This is aimed at local control by removing the affected breast tissue and minimising the risk of local recurrence, of which 50% may be further DCIS and 50% may be invasive cancer. The mainstay of treatment is surgery, which may be combined with radiotherapy. If the DCIS is oestrogen receptor positive (ER+ve), tamoxifen or an aromatase inhibitor may be considered. Recurrence/progression risk is greatest with high-grade DCIS. There is current uncertainty as to whether low- or intermediate-grade DCIS progresses if left untreated; a UK randomised trial comparing local treatment with mammographic surveillance is underway [30].

Invasive Breast Cancer

This is a systemic condition from the outset, as malignant epithelial cells can invade surrounding breast tissue and metastasise (Figure 30.2). While most presentations do not have detectable systemic disease and are considered to be 'early' breast cancer, management assumes that there are undetectable, occult systemic micro-metastases. The aim of treatment for early breast cancer is twofold.

Local Control Treatment

This is used to prevent local progression and complications such as skin ulceration and reduce the risk of recurrence in the breast and ipsilateral axillary glands (i.e. surgery, radiotherapy).

Adjuvant, Systemic Therapy

This is used to prevent the development of distant metastases by eradicating occult micro-metastases (i.e. chemotherapy, anti-oestrogenic endocrine therapy, immunotherapy, targeted drugs such as Herceptin and bisphosphonates). Selection of adjuvant therapy is based on the following.

- Assessment of the receptor status (i.e. oestrogen, progesterone, HER2 receptors). Most breast cancers are oestrogen receptor (ER) positive (~ 80%), about 15% are HER2 receptor positive (HER2) positive and 15% are triple receptor negative [31]. Anti-oestrogenic, endocrine therapy (e.g. tamoxifen, aromatase inhibitors, luteinising hormone-releasing hormone agonists) is prescribed for ER-positive cancer. The type and duration of anti-oestrogenic therapy is determined by menopausal status, side effects and recurrence risk. Treatment may continue for up to 10 years. Herceptin is used in cancers that are HER2+ve.
- Assessment of individual risk of systemic recurrence using prognostic factors is used to inform decisions about the use of chemotherapy. Tumour profiling tests can be offered to guide decisions about chemotherapy where the estimated risk of distant recurrence is indeterminate (e.g. Oncotype DX, Endopredict and Prosigna).

Overall, 5- and 10-year survival rates for breast cancer are 87% and 78%, respectively [1], although this is affected by stage at diagnosis. Five-year survival for stage 1 cancer is close to 100%, but this falls to around 25% for advanced, stage 4 disease [32]. Although the latter is incurable and can only be palliated, many women maintain a good quality of life with supportive treatments.

Breast Cancer Follow-Up

The aim of follow-up for early stage breast cancer is:

- to detect recurrence of a previous breast cancer or a new primary breast cancer

- to manage physical and psychological health problems induced by breast cancer diagnosis and treatment and enhance quality of life.

Follow-Up Appointments

There is a move away from long-term, routine, outpatient-based appointments, instead tailoring care to individual need at the completion of 'active' or primary treatment (i.e. surgery, chemotherapy, Herceptin and radiotherapy). Regular follow-up does not reduce mortality and clinical time released can improve access for those with complex post-treatment problems [33]. Personalised care and support planning aims to identify and address physical, psychological and social needs at the earliest opportunity. End of treatment summaries should be provided to the person and their primary care physician [34]. These offer information about the following:

- signs of symptoms of potential recurrence (Table 30.4)
- post-treatment imaging schedules (see below)
- named breast clinical nurse specialist contact details in case of concerns about recurrence or side effects
- support for improving long-term health (see below).

Some trusts offer clinical nurse specialist telephone follow-up in addition to this.

Imaging after a Diagnosis of DCIS or Invasive Breast Cancer

- This depends on age and management:
  - Under 50; annual mammograms until the age of 50, then refer to the NHSBP.
  - Over 50; breast conserving surgery; DCIS/triple receptor negative breast cancer annual mammogram for 5 years, other invasive breast cancer annual mammograms for 5 years 1,2,3,5) then NHSBSP
  - Over 50 post mastectomy; 50 to 60 biennial mammogram, > 60 refer to NHSBSP. [8,29]
- Imaging investigations for systemic recurrence are not undertaken in the absence of symptoms.
- DEXA scans are recommended in those with invasive breast cancer, not receiving bisphosphonates and commencing aromatase inhibitors or ovarian ablation/suppression therapy, or who have a treatment-induced menopause.

Lifestyle Behaviours

Healthy lifestyle interventions have been shown to reduce recurrence [35]. The National Institute for Health and Care Excellence (NICE) recommends achieving and maintaining a healthy weight, limiting alcohol intake to below five units per week and regular physical activity. [29].

Conclusion

Health professionals in primary care have a key role in aligning expectations surrounding the diagnosis and management of benign and malignant breast conditions. This can be achieved by supporting people's information needs, clear communication of risk, providing reassurance as needed and, for those with breast malignancy, directing appropriate contact with specialist breast services during treatment through to survivorship, while promoting preventative long-term health improvement behaviours.

Table 30.4 Signs and symptoms of breast cancer recurrence

Symptoms and signs around a scar, or in the breast or chest area that could indicate local recurrence	Symptoms and signs that do not improve over a few weeks and for which there is no obvious cause that could indicate systemic recurrence
• A change in shape and size of the breast • A new breast lump or thickening • Skin puckering, dimpling, redness or rash • Swelling in the arm • Pain • Nipple discharge • Change in nipple shape or inversion • Axillary or supraclavicular lymphadenopathy	• Pain in the back or hips • Unexplained weight loss and loss of appetite • Nausea • Abdominal discomfort or swelling • Unexplained tiredness • A persistent dry cough and shortness of breath • Severe headaches, especially if worse in the mornings • Scans and blood tests are only done at the advent of systemic symptoms. Investigations in asymptomatic patients do not reduce breast cancer mortality and impair quality of life

References

[1] Cancer Research UK, 'Breast cancer statistics'. Accessed: 20 Feb. 2024. [Online]. Available: www.cancerresearchuk.org/health-professional/cancer-statistics/statistics-by-cancer-type/breast-cancer#heading-Zero.

[2] Cancer Research UK Early Diagnosis Data Hub, 'Proportion of cases by route to diagnosis'. May 2022. Accessed: 20 Feb. 2024. [Online]. Available: https://crukcancerintelligence.shinyapps.io/EarlyDiagnosis/_w_8877a5e7177e415ea064fc6ea06f094f/?Tab=hometab.

[3] Office of National Statistics. Nomis. Mortality statistics - underlying cause, sex and age (2013 to 2024). https://www.nomisweb.co.uk/datasets/mortsa.

[4] NICE, 'NG12. Suspected cancer: Recognition and referral'. Jan 2026. Accessed: 20 Feb. 2024. [Online]. Available: www.nice.org.uk/guidance/ng12.

[5] NICE CKS, 'Breast pain – Cyclical'. Aug. 2021. Accessed: 20 Feb. 2024. [Online]. Available: https://cks.nice.org.uk/topics/breast-pain-cyclical.

[6] M. Jahan, T. Bartholomeuz, N. Milburn et al., 'Transforming the 2-week wait (2WW) pathway: Management of breast pain in primary care', *BMJ Open Qual*, vol. **11**, no. 1, e001634, 2022.

[7] Association of Breast Surgery, 'Breast pain pathways'. Accessed: 20 Feb. 2024. [Online]. Available: https://associationofbreastsurgery.org.uk/professionals/clinical/aspire-breast-pain-pathway-rapid-evaluation/breast-pain-pathways.

[8] Royal College of Radiologists, 'Guidance on screening and symptomatic breast imaging'. 5th ed. 2019. Accessed: 20 Feb. 2024. [Online]. Available: https://www.rcr.ac.uk/media/043jyjqj/guidance-on-screening-and-symptomatic-breast-imaging-2025.pdf.

[9] NHS England, 'Clinical guidelines for the management of breast cancer: West Midlands expert advisory group for breast cancer'. Dec. 2016. Accessed: 20 Feb. 2024. [Online]. Available: www.england.nhs.uk/mids-east/wp-content/uploads/sites/7/2018/02/guidelines-for-the-management-of-breast-cancer-v1.pdf.

[10] NHS breast cancer screening: information for trans and non-binary people. https://www.gov.uk/government/publications/nhs-population-screening-information-for-transgender-people/nhs-population-screening-information-for-trans-people.

[11] Oxford Population Health CEU, 'AgeX trial'. Accessed: 20 Feb. 2024. [Online]. Available: www.ceu.ox.ac.uk/research/agex-trial.

[12] Independent UK Panel on Breast Cancer Screening, 'The benefits and harms of breast cancer screening: An independent review', *Lancet*, vol. **17**, no. 380(9855), pp. 1778–1786, 2012.

[13] H. Barton, D. Shatti, C. A. Jones et al., 'Review of radiological screening programmes for breast, lung and pancreatic malignancy', *Quant Imaging Med Surg*, vol. **8**, no. 5, pp. 525–534, 2018.

[14] D. Ritchie, G. Van Hal and S. Van den Broucke, 'Factors affecting intention to screen after being informed of benefits and harms of breast cancer screening: A study in 5 European countries in 2021', *Arch Public Health*, vol. **80**, no. 1, 143, 2022.

[15] National Institute for Health and Care Research, 'Benefits of the NHS breast screening programme outweigh small risk of overdiagnosis'. Jul. 2022. Accessed: 20 Feb. 2024. [Online]. Available: www.nihr.ac.uk/news/benefits-of-the-nhs-breast-screening-programme-outweigh-small-risk-of-overdiagnosis/31011.

[16] NICE CKS, 'Breast cancer – Managing FH'. Mar 2024. Accessed: 20 Feb. 2024. [Online]. Available: https://cks.nice.org.uk/topics/breast-cancer-managing-fh.

[17] CRUK, 'Family history of breast cancer and inherited genes'. Accessed: 20 Feb. 2024. [Online]. Available: www.cancerresearchuk.org/about-cancer/breast-cancer/risks-causes/family-history-and-inherited-genes.

[18] NICE, 'CG164. Familial breast cancer: Classification, care and managing breast cancer and related risks in people with a family history of breast cancer'. Nov 2023. Accessed: 20 Feb. 2024. [Online]. Available: www.nice.org.uk/guidance/cg164.

[19] A. Johansson, A. E. Christakou, A. Iftimi et al., 'Characterization of benign breast diseases and association with age, hormonal factors, and family history of breast cancer among women in Sweden', *JAMA Netw Open*, vol. **4**, e2114716, 2021.

[20] M. Morrow, S. J. Schnitt and L. Norton, 'Current management of lesions associated with an increased risk of breast cancer', *Nat Rev Clin Oncol*, vol. **12**, pp. 227–238, 2015.

[21] University of Cambridge, Department of Radiology, 'BRAID trial'. Accessed: 20 Feb. 2024. [Online]. Available: https://www.cam.ac.uk/research/news/enhanced-breast-cancer-screening-in-the-uk-could-detect-an-extra-3500-cancers-per-year-trial-shows.

[22] S. Y. Cohen, C. R. Stoll, A. Anandarajah et al., 'Modifiable risk factors in women at high risk of

breast cancer: A systematic review', *Breast Cancer Res*, vol. **25**, 45, 2023.

[23] B. Park, J. L. Hopper, A. K. Win et al. (KOHBRA Study Group), 'Reproductive factors as risk modifiers of breast cancer in BRCA mutation carriers and high-risk non-carriers', *Oncotarget*, vol. **8**, pp. 102110–102118, 2017.

[24] R. Arthur, Y. Wang, K. Ye et al., 'Association between lifestyle, menstrual/reproductive history, and histological factors and risk of breast cancer in women biopsied for benign breast disease', *Breast Cancer Res Treat*, vol. **165**, pp. 623–631, 2017.

[25] R. T. Chlebowski, G. L. Anderson, A. K. Aragaki et al., 'Association of menopausal hormone therapy with breast cancer incidence and mortality during long-term follow-up of the women's health initiative randomized clinical trials', *JAMA*, vol. **324**, pp. 369–380, 2020.

[26] K. F. Brown, H. Rumgay, C. Dunlop et al., 'The fraction of cancer attributable to modifiable risk factors in England, Wales, Scotland, Northern Ireland, and the United Kingdom in 2015', *Br J Cancer*, vol. **118**, pp. 1130–1141, 2018.

[27] Y. B. Zhang, X. F. Pan, J. Chen et al., 'Combined lifestyle factors, incident cancer, and cancer mortality: A systematic review and meta-analysis of prospective cohort studies', *Br J Cancer*, vol. **122**, pp. 1085–1093, 2020.

[28] T. T. Ngan, N. T. Q. Nguyen, H. Van Minh et al., 'Effectiveness of clinical breast examination as a "stand-alone" screening modality: An overview of systematic reviews', *BMC Cancer*, vol. **20**, no. 1, 1070, 2020.

[29] NICE, 'NG101. Early and locally advanced breast cancer: Diagnosis and management'. Jan. 2024. Accessed: 20 Feb. 2024. [Online]. Available: www.nice.org.uk/guidance/ng101/chapter/Recommendations#diagnostic-assessment-and-adjuvant-therapy-planning.

[30] Association of Breast Surgery, 'LORIS trial'. Accessed: 20 Feb. 2024. [Online]. Available: https://associationofbreastsurgery.org.uk/professionals/research/trials/closed/loris.

[31] CRUK, 'Tests on your breast cancer cells'. Accessed: 20 Feb. 2024. [Online]. Available: www.cancerresearchuk.org/about-cancer/breast-cancer/getting-diagnosed/tests-breast-cancer-cells.

[32] CRUK, 'Survival for breast cancer'. Accessed: 20 Feb. 2024. [Online]. Available: www.cancerresearchuk.org/about-cancer/breast-cancer/survival.

[33] NHS England, 'Personalised care and improving quality of life outcomes'. Accessed: 20 Feb. 2024. [Online]. Available: www.england.nhs.uk/cancer/living.

[34] NHS England, 'Patient initiated follow-up'. Accessed: 20 Feb. 2024. [Online]. Available: www.england.nhs.uk/outpatient-transformation-programme/patient-initiated-follow-up-giving-patients-greater-control-over-their-hospital-follow-up-care.

[35] Y. B. Zhang, X. F. Pan, J. Chen et al., 'Combined lifestyle factors, incident cancer, and cancer mortality: A systematic review and meta-analysis of prospective cohort studies', *Br J Cancer*, vol. **122**, pp. 1085–1093, 2020.

Index

For EU product safety concerns, contact us at Calle de José Abascal, 56–1°, 28003 Madrid, Spain or eugpsr@cambridge.org.

www.ingramcontent.com/pod-product-compliance
Ingram Content Group UK Ltd.
Pitfield, Milton Keynes, MK11 3LW, UK
UKHW050132230726
473566UK00012B/555

* 9 7 8 1 0 0 9 4 9 2 7 4 4 *